GLOBAL BEHAVIORAL RISK FACTOR SURVEILLANCE

GLOBAL BEHAVIORAL RISK FACTOR SURVEILLANCE

Edited by

David V. McQueen

National Center for Chronic Disease Prevention & Health Promotion
Atlanta, Georgia

and

Pekka Puska

World Health Organization
Geneva, Switzerland

Kluwer Academic/Plenum Publishers
New York, Boston, Dordrecht, London, Moscow

Library of Congress Cataloging-in-Publication Data

Global behavioral risk factor surveillance/edited by David McQueen and Pekka Puska.
   p.   cm.
   Includes bibliographical references and index.
   ISBN 0-306-47777-7
     1. World health.   2. Health behavior—Cross-cultural studies.   3. Health risk
assessment—Cross-cultural studies.   4. Public health—Cross-cultural studies.   I. McQueen,
David V.   II. Puska, Pekka.

   RA441.G557 2003
   362.1—dc21

2003050651

ISBN 0-306-47777-7

©2003 Kluwer Academic/Plenum Publishers, New York
233 Spring Street, New York, New York 10013

http://www.kluweronline.com/

10 9 .8 7 6 5 4 3 2 1

A C.I.P. record for this book is available from the Library of Congress

FOREWORD

Surveillance is a fundamental component of modern public health, and in the past three decades behavioural risk factor surveillance has become a critical tool for the scientific development of chronic disease prevention and health promotion. We should be encouraged by the global development of risk factor surveillance that is highlighted in this book, while at the same time recognise the enormous challenge ahead of us if we are to have a truly global system.

The chapters herein give a comprehensive look at the state of risk factor surveillance. It is based on work arising from four global meetings on surveillance—Atlanta 1999, Savannah 2000, Atlanta 2000, and Tuusula—attended by a broad range of people ranging from experts in doing surveillance to those using the fruits of surveillance, and from the most to the least economically developed countries. Despite decades of compelling evidence that these risks cause premature disease disparities in health, never before has there been such a concerted effort to come to grips with monitoring health-related behaviours in many settings. We can be encouraged by the involvement of many diverse individuals and organisations concerned about assessing the health of the globe.

The book shows the relevance of surveillance to three seminal events that have changed the landscape for public health in recent years. The first was the rise of chronic disease and health promotion into the mainstream of public health; the great epidemiologic transition that occurred throughout the 20th century was clearly recognised. The second was the recognition of the burden of chronic disease globally. The third was the rise of the need for evidence to illustrate the dimensions of the transition and the role of risk factors in this transition.

These three events alone are powerful reasons for the development of a global effort of behavioural risk factor surveillance. It is risk factor surveillance that tracks the change in behaviours related to the epidemiologic transition; it is risk factor surveillance that assesses the impact of the morbidity of illness; and it is risk factor surveillance that provides the evidence of changes over time, changes that we hope are in response to population-based public health and health promotion interventions that will precede the improvements in health outcomes.

Three essential points are made in this book about surveillance: time is a variable, a systems approach is important, and enduring partnerships in the execution of the effort of collecting and using data make a system invaluable. Although surveillance is in practice a very complex undertaking, understanding the basics that underpin all of this work is essential. Public health practitioners and researchers, faced with the critical demand to get on with the pressing public health tasks at hand, often do not reflect on why activities are carried out the way they are. Surveillance is no exception to this, but over the past few years and as a result of the meetings that generated so much of the content of this book, there has been more reflection on what constitutes the primary reason to carry out socio-behavioural monitoring of the population.

A critical message throughout the many presentations in the book is that risk factor surveillance is much more than just a technical exercise. Much effort is devoted to the technical issues of sampling, questionnaire design, appropriate analysis, and proper dissemination of results, but many of the real challenges in behavioural risk factor surveillance—particularly for the less economically developed regions—have to do with capacity building, sustainability, and overall maintenance of a stable, reliable, and valid monitoring system. And, of course, diminishing the risk of disease is what public health is supposed to be about. It is about time we kept score.

It is hoped that through this publication, with chapters presenting a wide spectrum of opinion and approaches, we can move forward to a concerted global effort to better understand the changes over time in risk factors for chronic disease. Only with this kind of information can public health intelligently address the global burden of disease.

Jim Marks, Director
National Center for Chronic Disease Prevention and Health Promotion
Centers for Disease Control and Prevention
Atlanta, Georgia

ACKNOWLEDGEMENTS

This book is a joint undertaking of many authors from around the world. It would not have been possible without the efforts of a number of key people who assisted at critical points in the development of the book. First and foremost we thank all the authors who responded to multiple requests for revision and assistance. We recognise that for many authors English was not their first language and that this resulted in considerably more effort on their part to meet our culture-bound requirements.

The editorial staff at the Centers for Disease Control and Prevention (CDC) was, as usual, competent and helped ensure all the pieces came together. Linda Elsner, who managed the texts in the middle and later stages of preparation and was absolutely invaluable in moving this effort along, provided primary assistance. Mary Hall, on the global health staff, provided important input and assistance at critical points in the project. Finally, many CDC staff provided support and assistance before, during, and after the surveillance meetings that provided much of the background material for the chapters.

CONTENTS

Alfred Rütten, Randall Rzewnicki, Heiko Ziemainz, Wil T. M. Ooijendijk, Frederico
Schena, Timo Stahl, Yves Vanden Auweele, and John Welshman

David H. Wilson

10. DID THEY USE IT? BEYOND THE COLLECTION
OF SURVEILLANCE INFORMATION

Judith M. Ottoson and David H. Wilson

11. HARMONISING LOCAL HEALTH SURVEY DATA.
THE EURALIM EXPERIENCE

Alfredo Morabia, Mary E. Northridge, Sigrid Beer-Borst, and Serge Hercberg
for the EURALIM Study Group

    4.   METHODS.. 213
        4.1. The Cardiovascular Disease Behavioral Risk Index (CaDRI).......... 213
        4.2. The Delphi Technique 214
        4.3. Data Analysis.. 215
    5.   RESULTS... 215
    6.   DISCUSSION... 219
    7.   REFERENCES 219

**16. PERSPECTIVES ON BUILDING INFRA-STRUCTURE,
     COMPARING DATA, AND USING SURVEILLANCE
     DATA IN DEVELOPING COUNTRIES** 221

David V. McQueen, Mary Hall, and Kelli Byers Hooper

    1.   INTRODUCTION 221
    2.   BACKGROUND 221
    3.   ISSUES.. 222
        3.1. Capacity... 222
        3.2. Comparability 223
        3.3. Data Use 224
    4.   THEMES 225
        4.1. Time as a Variable 226
        4.2. Sampling Methods 226
        4.3. Data Collection 226
        4.4. Data Analysis... 226
        4.5. How Data Are Used.. 226
        4.6. Limitations... 226
    5.   CONCLUSION 226

**17. NON-COMMUNICABLE DISEASE SURVEILLANCE
     IN LATIN AMERICA AND THE CARIBBEAN.
     ADVANCES SUPPORTED BY THE PAN AMERICAN
     HEALTH ORGANIZATION** 227

Stephen J. Corber, Sylvia C. Robles, Pedro Orduñez, and Paz Rodríguez

    1.   THE PAN AMERICAN HEALTH ORGANIZATION 227
    2.   SURVEILLANCE OF NON-COMMUNICABLE DISEASES.............. 228
        2.1. Questionnaire Development 229
        2.2. Survey Evaluation... 229
    3.   CONCLUSION 232
    4.   REFERENCES 232

CHAPTER 1

INTRODUCTION

David V. McQueen and Pekka Puska[*]

This book has had a relatively long gestation. This is attributable to a number of factors, not the least of which is the effort of the editors to manage manuscripts from multiple, geographically dispersed authors. English is not the first language of many authors, adding to the editorial effort to make sure that the writers' intent was faithfully conveyed. More important, as the book developed, so did the field of monitoring behavioural risk factors for chronic disease.

Initially this book was conceived as a classic scientific publication of conference proceedings following the first global conference on risk factor surveillance, which was held in Atlanta, Georgia, in the fall of 1999. Many excellent presentations were offered at that conference, and they alone could have formed the basis for a worthy publication. However, conference proceedings can be limiting and often result in publications of mixed quality and of little interest to those who did not participate. The surprise of the conference was the scope and size of the global interest in risk factor surveillance. An initial expectation of participation by perhaps 50 or 60 experts from around the world blossomed into a meeting nearly five times that size. Clearly the idea tapped a vein of interest heretofore unexplored.

Several key phenomena occurred at the Atlanta meeting. First, it was clear that there already was a global cohort of experts pursuing risk factor surveillance; second, the level of competency represented in the papers was very high; third, interest was keen in forming an informal network of experts; fourth, desire was strong to share approaches and findings among experts; and fifth, there was an expressed feeling of need for global leadership in risk factor surveillance. These five phenomena are reflected in many of the papers presented in this volume.

There was also a sense that many challenges lie ahead, and many important unresolved issues still need to be addressed for global risk factor surveillance to move forward. Underlying this expression of need was a sense of urgency driven by the changing burden of disease, the global epidemiologic transition to chronic diseases, and the necessity to document through surveillance the changes in the global picture. As a result, before the conference had ended many attendees argued for a series of smaller meetings to address very specific issues related to developed and less developed economies in countries. Others grasped the need for a regular series of larger scientific conferences

[*] David V. McQueen, Centers for Disease Control and Prevention, Atlanta, Georgia 30341-3717, USA; Pekka Puska, World Health Organization, CH-1211 Geneva, Switzerland.

where experts could gather and present the scientific evidence of their efforts. Thus was born a tradition of having a global conference every 2 years. The second global conference was held in Finland in 2001, and the third global conference will be convened in Australia in 2003.

As a result of all this dynamic activity generated from the Atlanta conference, this book "morphed" into something more than a routine proceedings report. It came to be more a reflection of the state of the art and the condition of risk factor surveillance around the globe, focusing more on the issues and challenges of that task than on the straightforward reporting of results of behavioural risk factor surveillance. Two smaller but critical meetings followed the initial Atlanta meeting. The first, in Savannah, Georgia, addressed issues that concerned those countries with advanced data collection efforts and developed surveillance activities—namely, issues of analysis, interpretation, and use of data. The second, also in Atlanta, was concerned with efforts in the less developed economies and struggled with the problems of building capacity, sustainability, and use of data. Finally, at the second global conference in Finland, many of these emerging challenges became topics of general discussion. No doubt the Australian conference will follow up on these challenges further.

This volume, therefore, reflects all of this activity to a degree. It recognizes that the quest for a global approach to risk factor surveillance is well under way, but hardly complete. It deals with many of the hard issues that face countries beginning to develop surveillance activities and presents some models and approaches that may ultimately yield a concerted, integrated global effort.

CHAPTER 2

WHY IS GLOBAL SURVEILLANCE NECESSARY?

Towards Global Surveillance of Non-Communicable Disease Risk Factors: Developments and Challenges

Pekka Puska[*]

1. INTRODUCTION

The "Global Issues and Perspectives in Monitoring Behaviors in Populations: Surveillance of Risk Factors in Health and Illness" conference, held in Atlanta in September 1999 and organised jointly by the U.S. Centers for Disease Control and Prevention (CDC) and the Finnish National Public Health Institute (KTL), was undoubtedly a landmark for developing international collaboration on the long road towards global non-communicable disease (NCD) risk factor surveillance. Practical background to the meeting included numerous contacts between KTL and CDC over the years with regard to chronic disease prevention and health promotion. During these contacts, the issue of surveillance and monitoring became increasingly important and obvious. Both institutes had accumulated a great deal of experience with behavioural surveillance systems over the years, and each had collaborated with a number of countries. Furthermore, both institutes realised the growing international interest in this topic because of the changing global burden of disease: NCD prevention and health promotion were becoming key topics in international public health, and monitoring target risk factors is a major component of the work. The aim of the Atlanta meeting was to start an international discussion to explore the feasibility of working globally to address NCD risk factor surveillance.

The role of CDC in organising the Atlanta meeting was crucial. CDC's substantial professional contribution helped to ensure the success of the meeting. We are grateful to Drs. J. Koplan, J. Marks, and D. McQueen and many others for their strong support. KTL, a national public health institute with close to 1,000 employees, also provided an important contribution to the organisation of the meeting. The institute has a history spanning over 90 years, and the development of the institute is very similar to that of CDC. In earlier years, KTL was an infectious disease control centre. With the changing public

[*] World Health Organization, CH-1211 Geneva, Switzerland.

health situation, the Finnish government realised the need for a more comprehensive institute. Increasing emphasis was placed on chronic diseases, environmental health, and health promotion. Thus KTL, like CDC, increasingly emphasised the big public health problems of chronic diseases, while maintaining infectious disease control as an important area of work.

In 1980, KTL implemented a strong chronic disease prevention and health promotion national monitoring system. This monitoring system has provided the foundation for national health activity. Information from the monitoring system has been a powerful tool for (1) health policy development, planning, evaluation, and decision making; (2) disease prevention and health promotion intervention planning, evaluation, and decision making; and (3) epidemiological and behavioural research. The information attracts media attention and directs the public health agenda.

In addition to CDC and KTL, the World Health Organization (WHO) gave valuable support to the Atlanta conference. At WHO headquarters in Geneva, a new department on NCD surveillance has recently been established within the Noncommunicable Diseases and Mental Health Cluster. Because of the growing global interest in the topic of NCD risk factor surveillance, many other agencies also supported the Atlanta meeting.

2. MAJOR ISSUES

Recent studies have shown how the global burden of disease is rapidly changing, such that NCDs are now the major health problem not only in the developed world, but also in the developing world (WHO, 1997). Cardiovascular diseases are responsible for one of every three deaths in the world, and many of these deaths are occurring in the "working age" population. Thus, surveillance and prevention of NCDs are major challenges for contemporary global health. Many industrialised countries have developed policies to address NCD prevention, but ministries of health from the developing world are increasingly turning to WHO for advice on the control of emerging heart disease, cancer, and injury epidemics.

At the Atlanta meeting, a number of major issues related to behavioural surveillance of NCD risk factors were discussed, including (1) general theoretical backgrounds behind surveillance and monitoring, (2) target groups for conducting surveillance and monitoring—populations, age groups, disadvantaged groups, high-risk groups, and so on, (3) types of indicators on which data should be collected, (4) how data should be collected, and (5) reporting and use of information beyond the mere collection of data.

Another central topic of the meeting was the added value of international cooperation for conducting surveillance of NCD risk factors. International collaboration should aim at some common indicators, standardised measurements, and practices. This step would allow comparisons of risk factor patterns, trends, and experiences.

The Atlanta meeting noted that we do not start from zero. Internationally, a great deal of progress has already been made on some of the key indicators, such as tobacco use. This progress has resulted in a number of good documents and very solid recommendations, including the WHO published recommendations on how to monitor smoking (WHO, 1998). Thus, good work has been done and much more work is currently under way. Recent information technology developments also provide great possibilities for international cooperation. The potential is huge.

One challenge faced at the Atlanta meeting is how to address all the complex issues related to global surveillance. A single surveillance system is not feasible and cannot solve all the problems. There are separate surveillance needs for diseases, health status, functional capacity, biological risk factors, nutrition, behavioural lifestyles, health services, and health promotion processes. Furthermore, the needs vary in the different parts of the world, in different countries, and in different communities. And, from a practical point of view, there are two main survey methods: the more expensive and labourious health examination surveys, and the cheaper health interviews or questionnaires. The balance that should be maintained between these two approaches remains unclear.

Important questions were raised at the meeting, such as "What should be the priorities of an international cooperation to address NCD risk factor surveillance?" and "What should be the surveillance priorities of countries?" While it is unrealistic to build the kind of comprehensive health monitoring system that is in place in the United States or Finland, the Atlanta meeting emphasised behavioural risk factor surveillance because risk-related behaviours are the direct targets of interventions and their measurement can take place through interviews that often are more feasible than expensive health examinations. Other important questions raised at the meeting included "What kinds of international networks are needed to collaborate on surveillance of NCD risk factors?", "How do we exchange results and experiences?", and "How do we address all the complex and relevant issues, particularly in the developing world?" To answer these questions, reference has often been made to useful experiences in infectious disease control. Chronic disease prevention and health promotion should learn from infectious disease experiences, but there is a major difference in surveillance. Infectious disease surveillance primarily targets diseases and their outbreaks, because this focus provides valuable information on the outbreak source. However, for cancer and heart disease, measuring disease rates does not help us take action because the length of time associated with disease development is too long. NCD prevention efforts target risk factors, usually behaviours, and consequently they should be the key items for surveillance. By demonstrating behavioural risk factor prevalence changes in the population, such as smoking rates, there is little doubt that cancer rates and heart disease rates will eventually improve.

3. INTERNATIONAL STRUCTURES

International cooperation has been very important for infectious disease control and surveillance. Strong international networks have been developed for rapid exchange of surveillance information by national public health institutes, which are usually the focal point institutions in the countries. When epidemics occur somewhere in the world, information reaches the responsible agencies in other countries rapidly. WHO has played an important role, together with the national public health institutes, and the international collaboration has often used the slogan that "infectious disease epidemics know no political borders." To date, nothing like this has taken place in the NCD field, even though NCDs are the major global public health problem today. And the situation in both the infectious and NCD disease fields is not really that different. While the causal agents for NCDs are lifestyles rather than bacteria or viruses, lifestyles also are not restricted by political borders. Commonly referred to as globalisation, lifestyles are communicated and transferred rapidly across countries in today's world. Therefore, why is it that the public health institutes are not taking on the challenge to start surveillance of determinants of these modern epidemics in the same way? Surveillance and monitoring systems are key areas of work for national health institutes. Even if many other agencies are involved, including non-governmental organisations and universities, the national public health institutes are the official instruments for health policy in their countries, and thus have particular responsibility.

Regarding international collaboration, an important question concerns leadership and networking. Recent developments have been very encouraging for strengthening WHO's response to the global burden of NCDs. Within the new Noncommunicable Diseases and Mental Health Cluster at WHO headquarters in Geneva, strong emphasis has been placed on developing approaches, methods, and international networking in the field of NCD surveillance and monitoring. The approaches developed are described in this book. The importance of risk factor surveillance can also be evidenced by the fact that *World Health Report 2002* will focus on risk factors.

With respect to population-based NCD prevention and health promotion, WHO finds that behavioural risk factor surveillance is an essential element for national programme planning. The key challenge is with regard to international collaboration. WHO's leadership is based on the fact that it is "the agency of countries," has good expertise, and has traditionally played a key role in global health monitoring efforts. One message from the Atlanta meeting is that as we look forward to the important role that WHO can play in this area, we also cannot leave the entire responsibility to WHO. It is very much the task of countries and their national institutes to be active in the development of NCD-related surveillance, especially that of behavioural risks factors.

4. RECENT PROGRESS

From the Atlanta meeting, it was quite obvious that a number of NCD-related behavioural risk factor monitoring activities are already going on in different parts of the world: (1) a number of countries have collaborated with CDC concerning their surveillance needs, (2) KTL has collaborated with the Baltic countries and some areas of Russia, using the Finbalt Health Monitor (Prättälä et al., 1999), (3) the European Union is proceeding with its health monitoring concepts, (4) WHO has collaborated with CDC on the behavioural risk factor surveillance component of the Mega Country Health Promotion Network, and (5) the WHO Pan American Health Organization also has made progress within the new CARMEN programme. These activities cover a variety of historical backgrounds, needs, and cultural settings, and are all quite different. Thus, it is not feasible to aim at one uniform global surveillance system. However, it is important to increase the international collaboration and communication to conduct more systematic NCD risk factor surveillance. Theoretical concepts and frameworks should be discussed, and standardisation can and should take place regarding the measurement of individual risk factors, like smoking or physical inactivity. We ultimately should aim for some level of "harmonisation" to increase international comparisons. Although direct comparisons of prevalence rates have many difficulties, such attempts are useful. Even more useful are comparisons of trends and experiences.

Following the Atlanta meeting, a great deal of progress has taken place. Several global, regional, and national meetings have been organised and more surveillance activities have been implemented. WHO also has strengthened its surveillance activity and contributions. The "Non-Communicable Disease Surveillance in the Americas— Second International Conference on Monitoring Health Behaviors: Towards Global Surveillance," which was held October 2001 in Tuusula, Finland, and co-sponsored by KTL, CDC, and WHO, reviewed the progress and challenges and paved the way towards global surveillance of behavioural risk factors—the cornerstone for global NCD prevention and health promotion.

5. REFERENCES

Prättälä, R., Helasoja, V., and the Finbalt Group, 1999, *Finbalt Health Monitor: Feasibility of a Collaborative System for Monitoring Health Behaviour in Finland and the Baltic Countries*, National Public Health Institute, Helsinki (Publication B21/1999).

World Health Organization, 1997, *World Health Report 1997: Conquering Suffering, Enriching Humanity*, WHO, Geneva.

World Health Organization, 1998, *Guidelines for Controlling and Monitoring the Tobacco Epidemic*, WHO, Geneva.

CHAPTER 3

THE WHO STEPWISE APPROACH TO SURVEILLANCE (STEPS) OF NON-COMMUNICABLE DISEASE RISK FACTORS

Ruth Bonita, Regina Winkelmann, Kathy A. Douglas, and Maximilian de Courten[*]

1. INTRODUCTION

Non-communicable diseases (NCDs) are responsible for a high proportion of death and disability in all countries. In developing countries the burden of disease caused by NCDs is increasing rapidly. If the current rapid increase in NCDs is left uncontrolled there will be significant social, economic, and health consequences for these populations which, in turn, will threaten to overwhelm already stretched health services. The most cost-effective approach to containing this emerging epidemic is primary prevention based on comprehensive, population-based programmes. Fortunately, the major risk factors—tobacco and alcohol use, physical inactivity, high blood pressure, and high cholesterol—of the most common NCDs are amenable to prevention. Although most of this evidence comes from developed countries, it appears that the causal relationships are broadly similar in developing countries.

The key information required for planning primary preventive programmes and for predicting the future caseload of NCDs is the population distribution of the major common risk factors. Data on these risk factors are available in many developed countries, but are missing for most of the developing world. This deficit seriously hinders efforts to combat this epidemic.

NCD surveillance programmes which could inform policy making require careful planning. Compared with communicable diseases, NCDs evolve over decades. Setting surveillance systems in place is the first step in a long-term process and, as such, requires long-term commitment. The increasing recognition of the emerging burden of NCDs in developing countries will stimulate this process.

[*] Ruth Bonita, Regina Winkelmann, and Kathy A. Douglas, Noncommunicable Diseases and Mental Health, World Health Organization, CH-1211 Geneva, Switzerland; Maximilian de Courten, World Health Organization, Suva, Fiji Islands.

2. THE EMERGING EPIDEMIC OF CHRONIC DISEASES

No matter what their stage of economic development or demographic and epidemiological transition, countries face an increasing burden of NCDs. In 1999, NCDs were estimated to be responsible for almost 60% of deaths in the world and 43% of the global burden of disease (World Health Organization [WHO], 2000a). On the basis of current trends, these diseases are predicted to account for 73% of global deaths and 60% of the global disease burden by the year 2020 (Murray and Lopez, 1996).

NCDs have for several decades been of major importance in developed countries and are now becoming recognised as a major public health threat in the developing world as well. For example, during the next 30 years, the burden of disease from NCDs for developing and newly industrialised countries is expected to rise by more than 60% (Murray and Lopez, 1996). In comparison, the increase in developed countries is expected to be less than 10%. The example of cardiovascular disease (CVD), which contributes a substantive part of both mortality and disease burdens, highlights the problem. In 1999, CVD (mainly heart disease and stroke) was responsible for approximately half of all NCD deaths and one fourth of the worldwide NCD burden. Low- and middle-income countries suffer the major impact of the CVD epidemic, with two thirds of global CVD deaths and three fourths of global CVD disability occurring in these countries (WHO, 2000c). Furthermore, CVD is more likely to affect people at younger ages in low- and middle-income countries: 47% of CVD deaths in developing countries are among people below the age of 70 years, but only 23% in established market economies are among people of this age (Murray and Lopez, 1996).

The underlying causes of this NCD epidemic are demographic changes and increases in population risk factor levels resulting from social and economic changes. Evidence is strong that smoking, high blood pressure, and high cholesterol explain approximately two thirds to three fourths of heart attacks and strokes (Vartiainen et al., 1995). It has also been shown that major changes in the rates of CVD can be explained to a great extent by changes in population risk factor levels (WHO, 2000a). A vast body of knowledge exists about the risk factors of NCDs, as does experience in preventing them. Although most of these data come from developed countries, the causal relationships appear broadly similar in developing countries. In a number of countries, developed and developing, a comprehensive, long-term approach could reduce risk factors in the population and in turn disease, disability, and death (WHO, 2000a).

Because these are chronic diseases, NCD prevalence tends to be disproportionately high compared with NCD incidence. The economic burden associated with NCDs is also increased by expensive modern medical and surgical treatment that is both labour-intensive and technologically sophisticated. Hence, the need to devote resources to preventing NCDs in the first place is urgent and governments need to set in place plans to control the emerging NCD epidemic. Prevention and control programmes require quantified goals and targets established within a given time frame. Assessment of progress towards these goals requires surveillance.

3. SURVEILLANCE

3.1. Definitions

In the context of NCDs, surveillance is the ongoing (continuous or periodic) collection and analysis of population-based data to measure the magnitude of the problem (risk factors or disease) and trends over time. It also implies timely dissemination to users (Last, 2001). A major goal of surveillance is to use the data collected for the formulation of policies and programmes to promote health and prevent disease (Berkelman et al., 1997; McQueen, 1999). In this sense, surveillance is also an essential tool for measuring the impact of preventive efforts. Surveillance offers a systematic approach to data collection that not only increases efficiency with regard to staffing and training, but also allows for consistent and comparable trend data to be collected routinely and for important health issues to be incorporated into the system as they emerge. Surveillance is based on a public health agenda, as opposed to a research agenda, to help ensure that the data collected are timely and directly responsive to the health needs of a nation's population.

"Risk factors" refer to any attribute, characteristic, or exposure of an individual which increases the likelihood of that person developing an NCD. Behavioural risk factors are actions that put individuals at health risk. Examples include the consumption of tobacco products and alcohol, physical inactivity, poor eating habits that contribute to obesity, behaviours that result in unintentional and intentional injuries (e.g., not using seat belts or carrying a weapon), and sexual behaviours that result in unintended pregnancies and sexually transmitted infections, including human immuno-deficiency virus (HIV) infection. Although health risk behaviour is often seen as a personal choice, social, economic, and political environments have a critical role in determining risk behaviour at the individual level.

A risk factor surveillance system that includes behavioural risk factors provides the evidence base for tracking changes in population health over time (Berkelman et al., 1997). Because behaviours can be modified, prevalence and trend data on key risk factors can be used to support the development of targeted NCD policies and programmes for improving health outcomes in the population. In addition, because multiple risk factors are integrated, interactions among the various factors can be examined. Inclusion of key physiological measures, such as height, weight, and blood pressure, also provide important measures of the population's changing health status.

3.2. The Role of WHO in Responding to the NCD Epidemic

In 2000, the WHO 53rd World Health Assembly passed the resolution *On the Prevention and Control of Noncommunicable Diseases* (WHO, 2000a) with the goal of supporting Member States in their efforts to reduce the toll of morbidity, disability, and premature mortality related to NCDs. This global strategy has three main objectives:

- map the emerging epidemics of NCDs and analyse their social, economic, behavioural, and political determinants to provide guidance for policy, legislation, and finance,

- reduce the level of exposure of individuals and populations to the common risk factors for NCDs, and
- strengthen health care for people with NCDs.

Risk factor surveillance contributes to this resolution by providing data on critical and modifiable risk factors associated with the leading causes of NCD mortality and morbidity. Further, such surveillance provides an effective source of evidence to help guide the development and implementation of targeted disease prevention and health promotion policies and programmes and to measure their impact.

The overall goal of the WHO global NCD surveillance strategy is to enable countries to build and strengthen capacity to conduct risk factor surveillance within the framework of an integrated, systematic approach aiming at sustainability of each country's NCD data collection. In this process, countries can use the data collected for decision making and also contribute to the collection of standardised information for global comparisons.

The WHO global NCD surveillance strategy includes the following components:

- identification of the key risk factors to be addressed together with recommended WHO standardised definitions,
- a co-ordinated approach for conducting risk factor surveillance that upholds scientific principles and is sufficiently flexible to meet local and regional needs,
- identification of additional behavioural risk factor indicators to be addressed according to each country's need,
- technical materials and tools to support the implementation of surveillance tools,
- effective communication strategies for providing data to policy and intervention programme planners, decision-makers, potential funding sources, and the general public, and
- use of state-of-the-art technology to share information both between and within countries.

3.3. Risk Factor Surveillance or Disease Surveillance?

The objective of the first phase of WHO's global NCD surveillance strategy is to focus on the risk factors that predict the major NCDs. The key to controlling the global epidemic of NCDs is primary prevention, and the aim is to avert the epidemics wherever possible and to reverse them where they have begun. Intervening with risk factors is the basis for NCD prevention, and surveillance is therefore targeted to risk factors. In a world of finite resources, priority should go to ensuring collection of at least the minimum data necessary for informing these programmes and monitoring their impact.

In primary prevention, surveillance of risk factors for disease has a higher priority than disease surveillance; information on diseases is not essential to planning and evaluating primary preventive activities. In this sense, the risk factors of today are the diseases of tomorrow. Of course, information on disease occurrence is important in assisting health services planning, determining public health priorities, and monitoring the long-term effectiveness of disease prevention campaigns. Therefore, where resources are available, data on diseases (e.g., heart disease, stroke, cancer, hypertension, and diabetes) should be included in the surveillance process.

Table 1. Risk factors common to major non-communicable diseases

Risk factor	Cardiovascular disease[a]	Diabetes	Cancer	Respiratory conditions[b]
		Disease		
Tobacco use	[	[	[	[
Alcohol use	[		[	
Nutrition	[	[	[	[
Physical inactivity	[	[	[	
Obesity	[	[	[	[
High blood pressure	[	[		
High blood lipids	[	[	[	
High blood glucose	[	[	[	

[a] Including heart disease, stroke, and hypertension.
[b] Including chronic obstructive pulmonary disease and asthma.

3.4. Choice of Risk Factors for Global NCD Surveillance

Emphasis in surveillance should be given to those risk factors amenable to intervention. Intervention strategies can often be delivered cost-effectively by community-wide activities (including information and education campaigns) and legislative reform or structural changes that encourage health-preserving behaviour.

The major risk factors for one NCD are also likely to affect the risk for one or more of the other NCDs (Table 1). Furthermore, relatively small numbers of risk factors account for a large fraction of the risk for NCD in a population (Stamler et al., 1999). All of these risk factors, except for high blood pressure and blood lipids, can be measured by self-completed questionnaires. In this model, hypertension and diabetes can be seen as both risk factors and NCDs. High blood pressure, which is positively related to stroke, heart attack, and cardiac and renal failure, and which influences morbidity and mortality from diabetes, is relatively easily measured. High blood lipids, which are positively related to heart disease and inversely related to stroke, require at least a fingerprick (if not venipuncture) blood sample. The method for assessing the presence of diabetes can be straightforward when fasting blood glucose is used. Assessment for high blood glucose, which is also positively related to diabetes, is important because the increase in diabetes prevalence has been rapid in many countries (King et al., 1998).

3.5. Choice of Core Measures

The choice of which risk factors to measure depends on whether modification of the risk factor is possible through primary prevention and on the frequency and severity of the NCDs to which each factor contributes. It is also determined by the ease of collecting the information in a standardised manner, the potential burden on participants, and the availability of resources. Taking these considerations into account, WHO derived the core measures for inclusion in their NCD surveillance strategy from the key risk factors listed in Table 1.

4. WHO STEPWISE APPROACH TO SURVEILLANCE (STEPS)

4.1. A Framework for NCD Risk Factor Surveillance

The WHO stepwise approach to surveillance (STEPS) is the WHO-recommended NCD surveillance tool. The framework is based on the concept that surveillance systems require standardised data collection as well as sufficient flexibility to be appropriate in a variety of countries' situations and settings, from the least to the most well resourced. This approach, therefore, allows for the development of an increasingly complex and comprehensive surveillance system depending on local needs (Figure 1).

The stepwise approach advocates that for sustainable surveillance, small amounts of good quality data are more valuable than large amounts of poor quality data or none at all. In STEPS, the recommended surveillance measures are categorised according to the degree of complexity in obtaining the data, such as questionnaires alone (Step 1), physical measures collected in the field (Step 2), or laboratory measurements requiring external expertise (Step 3).

Step 1 contains the core set of self-reported measures that all countries should assess. These risk factors include, apart from socio-economic data, tobacco and alcohol use data, information on nutritional indicators, and data on physical inactivity. Standard WHO definitions for measuring the prevalence of tobacco use (WHO, 1998) and alcohol consumption (WHO, 2000b) and internationally devised measures of physical activity (University of Pittsburgh, 2001) are recommended. The premise is that all countries can use the information not only for within-country trends, but also for between-country comparisons. The questionnaires must therefore be relatively simple and may not necessarily give a complete picture of each behaviour, but the questions have been selected as suitable measures to reflect trends. In effect, the minimum data form the basis for a global database.

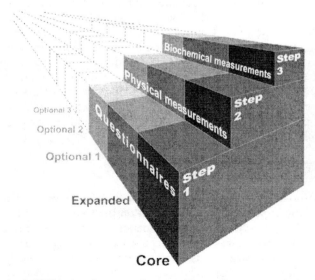

Figure 1. WHO's stepwise approach to surveillance of non-communicable disease risk factors.

Step 2 adds to the interview-based questionnaires by including simple physical measurements such as blood pressure, height, weight, and waist circumference. Because physical measures are involved, Step 2 requires a basic field survey. Steps 1 and 2 are desirable and appropriate for most developing countries, but even collection of data at Step 1 alone is useful when access to a field survey is not possible. Step 3 incorporates all of the above plus biochemical measures, the collection of which is even more elaborate, such as obtaining and analysing blood samples.

The overarching framework of the WHO global NCD surveillance initiative focuses on a limited number of risk factors, but synergies with existing and planned surveillance needs are possible. For example, WHO's mega-country surveillance initiative (WHO, 2001a) would increase the comprehensiveness of Step 1—the bottom row of the stepwise model (Figure 2).

Similarly, the incorporation of risk factors from other NCD areas, such as mental health and injuries, would further increase the model's breadth. To ensure consistency and comparability of basic global self-reported information, the core dimension of the framework contains the same minimum set of questions in Step 1. Above all, STEPS encourages obtaining core data on the established risk factors that determine the major disease burden. STEPS is also sufficiently flexible so that each country can incorporate optional modules related to local or regional interests. WHO's surveillance system can provide more in-depth information by including these optional modules. In countries where well-formulated health promotion activities have been instituted, such as campaigns to promote seat belt use, trend data on the use of seat belts would be appropriate. In some settings, the teams responsible for the surveillance process may also wish to add more sophisticated laboratory measures to the stepwise protocols recommended here.

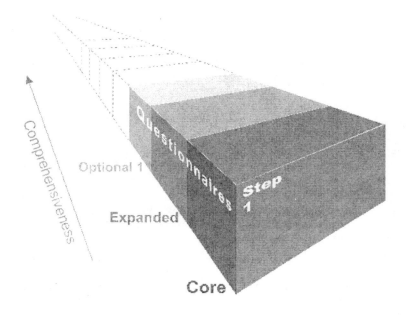

Figure 2. Behavioural risk factor surveillance (STEPS).

4.2. Inclusion of Additional NCD Risk Factors for Local Needs

WHO's recommendations for global NCD surveillance are limited to a core set of NCD risk factors. A number of other measures have been excluded from the minimum set of the framework because they do not meet the criteria outlined in Section 3.5. This is especially true for indicators for which it is difficult to ensure the cross-country consistency necessary to make meaningful comparisons. For example, measurement of general levels of psychological and social well-being are difficult to assess for cross-cultural comparisons. They will be useful only if governments are committed to improving physical, social, and occupational environments as well as encouraging individuals to adopt more health-promoting lifestyles. It is hoped that governments will respond to the 2001 World Health Report on mental health (WHO, 2001b) to institute such programmes. Methods to assess the effectiveness of mental health measures at a population level are likely to be specific to individual countries. Similarly, measures of perceived general quality of life are excluded from the core data because, from a surveillance perspective, the scope for a primary preventive response is not yet clear.

Use of psycho-active drugs is an important public health issue in some countries, and a case could be made for including use of psycho-active drugs in surveys of NCD risk factors. Indeed, surveys of the general population will be used to establish estimates for the prevalence of substance use. Because of differences in cultural contexts and because of the generally low prevalence of use, such measures are not considered core in global surveillance.

4.3. Choice of Summary Measures

The optimum statistical indicator for a given risk factor depends on how the risk factor is measured. With smoking, for example, the population fits into one of three, mutually exclusive categories—current daily smoker, ex-daily smoker, and non-smoker. The key indicator for such a categorical variable is the prevalence—that is, the proportion of the population in a given category at a given time. Judging whether prevalence changes or differences are statistically significant must take into account the level of statistical uncertainty surrounding each measurement, which is related to the size of the sample on which it is based. Large samples yield more precise estimates and will allow smaller differences or trends to be detected.

Indeed, a key feature of surveillance is the ability to measure changes over time. This ability requires careful planning in any baseline survey to ensure sufficient power to detect statistically significant changes between age groups, men and women, and population and geographic sub-groups.

In the assessment of the health of the whole population, measures of central tendency and dispersion provide important information: average blood pressure is as important to know as the prevalence of blood pressure above or below certain threshold values. Average systolic blood pressure and average diastolic blood pressure are simple, robust measures that can be directly comparable, no matter when and where they are measured.

The proportion of the population exceeding any given level of a continuous variable is directly related to the average level and the spread in the distribution of that population. Furthermore, for all of the continuous variables included in STEPS except alcohol use and serum cholesterol levels, the risk of the corresponding NCD increases in a continuous and graded fashion across the whole distribution of measurements (Eastern Stroke and Coronary Heart Disease Collaborative Research Group, 1998).

5. FROM SURVEYS TO SURVEILLANCE

For surveys in the STEPS framework to be used most effectively for public health, such as in setting priorities, developing programmes, and evaluating interventions, data must be collected, analysed, and used regularly and systematically. Although the interval between the episodes of data collection may vary depending on the different measurements involved and on the infra-structure currently available to countries, a move toward a more integrated surveillance perspective is needed. This perspective promotes population-based data collection, as opposed to a specific focus on one particular high-risk group. It also assumes ongoing collection of NCD risk factors that are directly relevant and important to public health, and a systematic approach in which an infra-structure for conducting surveillance can be developed, maintained, and expanded over time.

In some countries, surveillance of NCD risk factors has already been undertaken. We can learn from the experiences of these countries, and they can contribute to the collection of global NCD risk factor data. For countries that are just beginning, an appropriate first step towards initiating surveillance of NCD risk factors would be to conduct an initial "baseline" survey, following the WHO stepwise approach. This initial survey will provide very important information for determining the priorities for interventions and for raising public and political awareness concerning the likely extent of health problems. Nonetheless, it must be emphasised that the baseline survey is only the first step in what must become an ongoing surveillance activity.

The challenges in conducting surveillance of risk factors for NCDs are not to be under-estimated. For the results to have maximum utility, a lot of thought and preparation are required before even the first data are collected. Addressing the issues that must be considered in the planning stage (see Appendix) can be very helpful in clarifying what must be done before planning an initial, well-designed survey and beginning development of a surveillance infra-structure. Although presented as a sequence, these questions are actually inter-connected, with the answers to some directly influencing the answers to one or more of the other questions. Clearly, surveillance of NCD risk factors should not begin until all persons involved in its planning are comfortable that they have perspicuous and appropriate answers to each of the questions.

6. CONCLUSION

All countries face an increasing burden of NCDs, regardless of their stage of economic development or demographic and epidemiological transition. Surveillance of NCD risk factors provides information of central importance for planning and evaluating disease prevention and health promotion programmes and policies. Which risk factors to measure is each country's choice that will depend on the frequency and severity of the NCDs to which each factor contributes, the ease of collecting the information, the burden on participants, and the availability of resources.

The stepwise approach developed by WHO (STEPS) recommends that countries begin to collect consistent information on critical risk factors. At a minimum, these risk factors should include, together with socio-economic variables, tobacco use, alcohol use, and physical inactivity. If countries have the means to do so, the physical assessment of height, weight, and blood pressure is also recommended, as well as collection of information on other selected behavioural risk factors.

WHO's perspective is based on providing technical support to countries for establishing population-based, integrated, and systematic NCD risk factor surveillance systems that can be sustained over time. With attention focused on the substantial global burden due to NCDs, the need for NCD risk factor data is underscored and the urgency to collect such data is realised. At present, efforts to control the rising NCD burden are hindered because of the absence of information on the levels and trends of the major risk factors that predict these diseases. WHO's stepwise approach to NCD risk factor surveillance aims to address this shortcoming.

7. REFERENCES

Berkelman, R. L., Stroup, D. F., and Buehler, J. W., 1997, Public health surveillance, in: *Oxford Textbook of Public Health, Third Edition. Volume 2, The Methods of Public Health*, R. Detels, W. W. Holland, J. McEwen, et al., eds., Oxford University Press, New York, pp. 735–750.

Eastern Stroke and Coronary Heart Disease Collaborative Research Group, 1998, Blood pressure, cholesterol, and stroke in Eastern Asia, *Lancet.* **352**:1801–1807.

King, H., Aubert, R. E., and Herman, W. H., 1998, Global burden of diabetes, 1995–2025: prevalence, numerical estimates, and projections, *Diabetes Care.* **21**:1414–1431.

Last, J. M., ed., 2001, *A Dictionary of Epidemiology, Fourth Edition*, Oxford University Press, Oxford, UK.

McQueen, D. V., 1999, A world behaving badly: the global challenge for behavioral surveillance, *Am J Public Health.* **89**:1312–1314.

Murray, C. J. L., and Lopez, A. D., eds., 1996, *Global Burden of Disease and Injury Series, Volume 1: The Global Burden of Disease. A Comprehensive Assessment of Mortality and Disability from Diseases, Injuries, and Risk Factors in 1990 and Projected to 2020*, Harvard University Press, Cambridge, MA.

Stamler, J., Stamler, R., Neaton, J. D., et al., 1999, Low risk-factor profile and long-term cardiovascular and noncardiovascular mortality and life expectancy: findings for 5 large cohorts of young adult and middle-aged men and women, *J Am Med Assoc.* **282**:2012–2018.

University of Pittsburgh, 2001, *GlobalPAQ, Global Physical Activity Questionnaire*, University of Pittsburgh Department of Epidemiology, Pittsburgh.

Vartiainen, E., Sarti, C., Tuomilehto, J., et al., 1995, Do changes in cardiovascular risk factors explain changes in mortality from stroke in Finland? *Br Med J.* **310**:901–904.

World Health Organization, 1998, *Guidelines for Controlling and Monitoring the Tobacco Epidemic*, WHO, Geneva.

World Health Organization, 2000a, *Global Strategy for the Prevention and Control of Noncommunicable Diseases. Report by the Director-General*, Fifty-third World Health Assembly, WHO, Geneva (Provisional Agenda Item 2.11; A53/14).

World Health Organization, 2000b, *International Guide for Monitoring Alcohol Consumption and Related Harm*, WHO, Geneva.

World Health Organization, 2000c, *World Health Report 2000. Health Systems: Improving Performance*, WHO, Geneva.

World Health Organization, 2001a, *Mega Country Health Promotion Network: Mega Country Behavioral Risk Factor Surveillance Protocol*, WHO, Geneva.

World Health Organization, 2001b, *World Health Report 2001. Mental Health: New Understanding, New Hope*, WHO, Geneva.

8. APPENDIX: KEY QUESTIONS FOR PLANNING NCD RISK FACTOR SURVEILLANCE

8.1. What Are the Long-Term Objectives?

Completion of NCD risk factor surveillance should not be seen as an end in itself, but as a contribution to some other objective, such as:

- tracking the direction and magnitude of trends in risk factors,
- planning or evaluating a health promotion or preventive campaign, or
- collecting data to predict likely future demands for health services.

In all cases, the move towards regular data collection underpins planning NCD health promotion and disease prevention programmes and policies. Furthermore, compared with repeat surveys, the initial planning and development of an ongoing surveillance system represents an economy of scale and returns better and more consistent data quality.

8.2. Which Risk Factors Will Be Measured?

WHO recommends including core risk factors in any given survey. In addition to demographic questions and questions about height and weight, these risk factors include tobacco and alcohol use, physical inactivity, and high blood pressure, where feasible. Each country can also identify additional priority questions to measure.

8.3. How Will the Risk Factor Measures Be Obtained?

Designing a good questionnaire or interview schedule is much harder than would first appear. Thus, much can be said for using standard, validated instruments to avoid having to develop and validate one's own. This strategy is also likely to enhance comparability of the new data with results of other, more established surveys. Additional data should be collected only after careful consideration of the potential benefits and the additional cost involved.

Any new questions and any modifications that are made to "standard" questions need to be tested carefully in pilot assessments to ensure they yield valid and reliable data. Consideration of maintaining consistently worded questions for analysis of trends over time must be carefully weighed against the need for changes in wording to ensure a question is working appropriately to provide useful data.

8.4. What Is the Sample for the Survey?

Surveying the entire population of a country is usually impracticable. Instead, NCD risk factors are assessed in a sample of the population. The critical issues are that the sample selected for participation is representative of the whole population and that the persons who actually participate are representative of those invited. Satisfying these criteria requires a clear definition of the population from which the sample will be drawn (i.e., the sampling frame), a valid technique for selecting the sample, and the maximum possible level of participation among those selected to take part.

8.5. How Big Must the Sample Be?

Expert statistical advice should be obtained early in the process for selecting a sample. Factors affecting sample size include:

- level of variation around parameters, such as average blood pressure or proportion of current smokers,
- likely size of the differences anticipated to exist between particular sub-groups or between two points in time, and
- likely extent of non-response.

However, for those seeking to detect trends in the framework of the surveillance system, a rough guide of the sample size is 200 individuals for each 10-year age-and-sex group in the age range of 25 to 64 years. This is the recommended minimum to estimate the means of the variables included in STEPS with a high level of precision, and it will be just sufficient to estimate prevalence of tobacco use. Wherever possible, a wider age range is recommended to better suit the local context, such as including younger ages or better reflecting an ageing population structure (e.g., expanding the age range to 15 to 74 years).

8.6. Will the Data Be Trusted?

Answering this question involves a judgement about whether the answers provided by the data are likely to be correct, which in turn will depend on how the data were originally collected and how they were analysed. Relevant aspects of collection of the data include:

- response rates (as a broad rule, response rates of 80% or more are good, while those of 60% or less are inadequate),
- valid and reliable instruments for making the measurements, and
- attention to calibration of instruments, training of staff, and monitoring of the quality of measurements themselves.

Potential criticism and scepticism towards the survey results will be minimised if all of these issues are carefully documented. The quality of the surveillance process needs to be continually checked as the data are collected, and re-calibration or re-training must be undertaken if necessary.

8.7. How Will the Data Be Handled and Analysed?

Data collected from NCD risk factor surveys represent a large investment of time, effort, and money. Therefore, great care needs to be taken in the handling, storage, and analysis of data. These concerns include physical handling, transport, and storage of paper forms and entry and storage of the data on electronic media. Entering all records twice, as well as developing computer programmes that automatically check for improbable data values and internal inconsistencies, can reduce data entry errors.

8.8. What Will the Project Cost?

Careful planning and preparatory work should simplify preparation of a budget and of applications for funds to support NCD risk factor surveillance. Budgetary items may include the following:

- staff (e.g., costs of advertising, selection, training, workers' compensation or other insurance, provision for holidays and sick leave, and subsistence allowances),
- communication, including advertising and publicity,
- printing, post, and stationery,
- interpreters and translation of forms,
- data entry,
- statistical analysis and computing,
- preparation and dissemination of reports,
- long-term storage of data, paper forms, and specimens,
- hire of venues for surveillance administration,
- equipment and its maintenance,
- transport of survey teams and specimens,
- laboratory costs, and
- other miscellaneous expenses (e.g., snacks and drinks for participants, or laundry and cleaning).

8.9. What Ethical Approval Is Required?

All surveillance staff must be aware of their responsibilities to respect and protect the confidentiality of surveillance participants. Without the assurance of confidentiality to all surveillance participants, the quality of the data obtained cannot be trusted.

Arrangements and requirements for formal approval of the surveillance protocol by one or more ethics committees will vary between settings and with the content of the survey itself. For example, interviews or questionnaires without potentially sensitive personal or medical information may not require ethical clearance in some jurisdictions and may be conducted on the basis of verbal consent alone. The same could even apply to surveys that include only simple, non-invasive physical examinations such as measurements of height, weight, and girth. Blood pressure is more medically significant, however, and most ethical committees would require written consent.

Preparing and obtaining approval for submissions to ethics committees can take weeks and even months, depending on how often committees meet and their own rules of operation. Therefore, early identification and contact with relevant committees are imperative.

8.10. Is Everything Ready To Start?

Teams beginning the NCD risk factor surveillance process for the first time are well advised to begin compiling, from very early in the process, their own carefully indexed manual of operations. Such a document contributes directly to uniformity and therefore precision of measurements and helps avoid solving the same problems repeatedly. It is only by attempting to run the entire system as an integrated whole that one can identify problems, system incompatibilities, or oversights in need of correction.

Even for a team that has conducted surveillance of several large surveys before, it takes several months of preparatory work before a new surveillance cycle or survey can begin. Recurrent tasks include:

- preparation of budgets and applications for funds,
- modification, testing, and printing of questionnaires and supporting documents,
- applications for ethical clearance and access to sampling frames,
- hiring and training of staff,
- location and negotiation for use of suitable venues,
- re-calibration of equipment,
- arranging for supplies of single-use items, and
- negotiations with laboratories about assays and quality control systems.

8.11. How Will Oversight and Quality Control of the Surveillance System Be Managed?

To be able to trust surveillance results, it is crucial that surveillance systems include quality control measures for all key surveillance functions. These functions include ensuring that common questions are used by all participating locations, that data collection procedures are adhered to so that results will be valid, and that data are analysed consistently across all locations. Participation in a global or regional network such as STEPS, which includes guidelines and training materials, will enhance standardised data collection.

8.12. How Is Surveillance Infra-Structure Being Built and Maintained?

The design of surveillance systems requires ongoing commitment and resources, including personnel and technology for communication and data use. Efficiencies are gained by building infra-structure for surveillance, rather than conducting a series of repeat surveys in which new staff and new administrative and procedural guidelines must be developed.

As the team begins planning to conduct surveillance across more locations and on a more ongoing basis, a central or lead agency should be identified to co-ordinate the surveillance activities and ensure quality control. A partnership that receives input from all participating agencies and locations to help develop, maintain, and expand the surveillance system will allow all participants, whether at a national or local level, to share ownership of the system and the surveillance information produced.

CHAPTER 4

PARTNERSHIPS, STRATEGIES, AND ALLIANCES FOR GLOBAL SURVEILLANCE

Vivian Lin[*]

1. INTRODUCTION

Global risk factor surveillance requires comparable systems operating at local and national levels. For a global system to work, the twin issues of infra-structure and content must be addressed at each level. Insofar as surveillance is concerned with continuous monitoring of risk factors that feeds into public health action, infra-structure and content are inseparable. These issues are not solely technical questions about information science or epidemiology, however. The key concerns are, ultimately, meaningful use and sustainable systems.

Surveillance systems require investments of human and financial resources to develop, implement, and maintain. Like most other information systems, the resources required to continually provide reliable and valid data may be more substantial than many decision-makers imagine or desire. But if the necessary investments are not made, the surveillance system cannot be sustained. For decision-makers, the questions are what are the returns from the investment, and for whom do the returns accrue? These are questions about what uses are made from the surveillance data, by whom, and for what end results. Thus, the issues of meaningful use and a sustainable system are not inseparable. Yet in global approaches and adaptations to different systems and environments, these two dimensions must be considered independently.

This chapter is concerned with how to secure the conditions necessary for sustainable surveillance systems and their meaningful use (i.e., the partnerships needed and how they can be formed), especially as they pertain to information infra-structure and content insofar as partners may have different priorities. Potential users of and partners in surveillance systems are defined, then potential strategies for developing partnerships and alliances are considered. Practical lessons from risk factor surveillance systems in China and Australia are discussed, and the critical issues for global development are elucidated in the concluding section.

---

[*] La Trobe University, Melbourne, VIC 3086, Australia.

2. USERS AND PARTNERS

Risk factor surveillance systems, at the local level, require collaboration between technical staff (system designers, data collectors, and information analysers) and users of survey data. Users are most likely to be those who design, implement, and evaluate intervention programmes to change the levels of risk factors in the surveyed population, but depending on the intervention programmes, the users may include policy-makers in government, industry, and civil society organisations. Other possible users of survey data are members of a surveyed community who want to better understand their own health and well-being.

At the local level, the major tension is likely to exist between staff, who aim for "perfect" data, and those potential users who focus on community programmes and getting action on the ground. These users, with different professional backgrounds and a more immediate time frame, are more concerned with timeliness of the data and whether the data are received in easily comprehensible forms. Many potential users have performed their duties over the years without any surveillance data, so they will be looking to see how the data can add value to what they do; their interest will be on informational content.

At the national level, the dynamics become more complex. The specifics will vary by how the national system for health administration is configured (e.g., whether a country has a federalist or unitary system), but we can reasonably expect tensions to exist between different levels of government and between the functional or programme areas within the health sector. In a federalist or a de-centralised health system, for example, the development and maintenance of a national surveillance system depend on the partnership between the epidemiologists, information system managers, and data analysts at the different levels. There are also myriad other interests among the users. Governments represent one user group, insofar as they invest in both surveillance systems and health promotion programmes and could make policy decisions based on the surveillance information. Other users who represent more diffuse interests but may be influential are academic researchers, industry marketing personnel, and members of health professional organisations.

A national government will likely aim for consistency in information and efficiency in infra-structure, whereas state or provincial governments will likely be interested in local applications and variations across communities. The extent to which persons on the ground are most familiar with local circumstances and needs will be debated, as will information requirements. There will be concerns about the roles of different levels of government in running the surveillance system, and therefore the timing and feedback of information versus data quality control. And there may well be underlying issues of control, if not sovereignty. Forging a partnership among those who work on the surveillance system at different levels is often a major challenge.

At the global level, these local and national tensions are replicated, with more complexity but with less sense of urgency for action. Agreement on core data sets and definitions becomes more difficult when the cultural contexts, patterns in health care practise, and technical capabilities are different. Concerns may arise about dominance by particular countries or multi-lateral organisations or by particular disciplines or programme areas.

With all the possible tensions between key players, it is tempting to dispense with any partnerships and to focus simply on the technical aspect of perfecting an information system for epidemiological surveillance. Yet, any system beyond the local level will require collaboration among the persons responsible for the surveillance system at different levels and among technical staff and users. Besides, the very aim of risk factor surveillance is to engender preventive action, and the continued existence of the surveillance system itself requires visible application and user support. Using information for action and taking this action to make a difference is the ultimate challenge of system sustainability. So developing partnerships between those who work on surveillance systems and those who work on health promotion strategies is critical.

3. STRATEGIES FOR PARTNERSHIP DEVELOPMENT

The notion of "partnership" has become fashionable in the health sector in recent years. Terms such as "strategic alliance," "joint venture," "public-private partnership," "co-ordinated service delivery," and "joint planning" are all now in common use in the managerial and political vocabulary (Huxham, 1996). The notion is also consistent with contemporary health promotion ideology and practise, which stress inter-sectoral collaboration as well as community participation and ownership. But in different worlds, the term takes on different meanings: in business it usually means "joint commercial ventures," for development assistance programmes it can mean "mixed-funding packages," and for governments it can be a code for "shared responsibility" (R. Tennyson, The partnership-building process, working paper for the Fourth International Conference on Health Promotion, 1997, Jakarta, Indonesia).

The ready adoption of the term "partnership" by persons in public health suggests the confluence of a number of perspectives (Wilson and Charlton, 1997):

- most societal problems have multiple causes, are multi-dimensional, and require complementary efforts for their resolution,
- emerging concepts of communitarianism and a stakeholder society reflect the increasing level of demand for participation by all affected interests, and
- increased scarcity of and competition for resources mean partnerships are becoming an instrumental approach to achieving shared objectives.

Partnerships form when organisations share similar goals but have insufficient capacity to resolve problems, when boundary problems in areas of responsibility lead to communication and co-ordination difficulties, when unintended negative consequences occur for fraternal organisations, or when there is benefit in sharing skills, knowledge, and resources (Human Resources Development Unit, 1998).

Regardless of the philosophical position of proponents and participants, partnerships formed for mutual benefit work when synergies are created and maintained. Common forms of partnership—along a continuum—include (Himmelman, 1996)

- network (organisational links that facilitate the exchange of information for mutual benefit),
- co-ordination (organisational mechanisms or processes that require altering some common activities to achieve a common purpose and mutual benefit),

- co-operation (organisational commitment to share resources for a common purpose and mutual benefit), and
- collaboration (risks, responsibilities, resources, and rewards are shared by organisations, resulting in enhancing the capacity of each partner to achieve defined objectives).

The form of partnership that develops depends on a range of factors (Figure 1). For risk factor surveillance, a partnership with users is ideally not driven solely from the instrumental objective of gaining user support for a surveillance system to be established and funded. Rather, the partnership would be more productive with a shared vision of effective public health action. The purely instrumental approach may focus on periodic dialogues and, if managed well, may lead to trust, integrative ideas, and increased legitimacy for all partners. If not well managed, however, a partnership based purely on utilitarian considerations may lead to disputes about whether responsibilities have been fulfilled and to an underlying level of distrust. In contrast, the partnership based on shared vision could move from mutual assistance in planning activities to collectively strengthening public health infra-structure and achieving health gains.

Successful partnerships rest on some pre-conditions as well as on the hard work of building and maintaining relations. Six factors have been identified as critical conditions for an effective partnership (Harris et al., 1995):

- necessity (agreement that a partnership is useful),
- opportunity (receptivity for a partnership to occur),
- capacity (organisational ability to carry through),
- relationship (clear definition of organisational links for achieving the purpose of the partnership),

MOTIVATING FACTORS		EXPECTED OUTCOME	
		INFORMATION EXCHANGE	JOINT AGREEMENT
	Shared Vision	Assisted Planning	Collective Strategies
	Conflict Resolution	Dialogues	Negotiated Settlement

Figure 1. Factors determining type of partnership desired. Adapted from Huxham, C., ed., 1996, *Creating Collaborative Advantage,* Sage Publications, London, with permission from Sage Publications.

- planned action (agreement on clear roles, responsibilities, and activities), and
- sustained outcomes (a system exists to monitor progress and achievements).

Conversely, six variables that may hinder the success of building and sustaining a partnership are (Challis et al., 1988)

- people in structures (leaders are not able to search for mutual benefit or focus on problem solving),
- turf (professional defensiveness and concern for administrative domains),
- structural complexity (number of organisations involved, and asymmetry in resources and power),
- product diversity (large variation in the volume and range of activities or services),
- policy congruence (divergence in basic objectives), and
- planning capacity and philosophy (disparities in skill level and timetables, and differing emphases on strategic versus operational issues).

Forging partnerships requires a certain element of risk taking, and some autonomy and control must be relinquished. The needs, agendas, and styles of other parties must be accepted rather than judged. Different professional values, language, interests, and skills need to be brought into complementary alignment. Each party must endorse the roles and contributions of the others. These are particular challenges for bringing together the surveillance system designers, owners, and the users; it is unlikely that such partnerships will spontaneously occur. Rather, an inter-active working process must be engineered to achieve consensus about the vision and to establish shared ownership of the enterprise. The principles of equity, transparency, and mutual benefit need to be visited frequently in these processes.

If achieving local partnerships between persons working on health surveillance and persons working on health promotion is a challenge, then national and global partnerships represent another degree of difficulty. Typically, inter-governmental collaboration occurs to resolve problems of boundary overlap (either the task is duplicated, or no one does it because it is assumed someone else will do it), resolve policy disputes, speed decisions, or develop consensus on new policies and programmes (Gray, 1989).[†] Differences in policies, programmes, and practises between levels of government reflect different contexts for their development, and reaching agreement may require not only relinquishing control but also overcoming history and culture.

A partnership between government and civil society, while a crucial ingredient for successful public health action, is even more difficult to achieve because of imbalances. Governments traditionally have financial resources, extensive information, and administrative authority, and sharing these with non-governmental organisations is necessarily a learned behaviour.[‡] Building multi-lateral collaboration at the global level between

---

[†] The Australian National Public Health Partnership, while aiming for whole-of-system co-ordination of the national public health effort, was built from the platform of reform of functional responsibilities across governments (Lin and King, 2000).

[‡] The success of the Australian HIV/AIDS strategy has been attributed in part to the partnership established between governments and the affected community. Elaborate structures and processes were needed to bring together researchers, community activists, states and territories, and the federal government. Joint decision making in all activities—research, information, interventions, and policies—was often preceded by lively debates. The partnership approach is now seen as a model for other public health strategies.

governments and non-governmental organisations will require not only participation structures and resources, but also a shared understanding about global inter-dependence and trust.

Complex partnerships—which inter-governmental and global partnerships necessarily are—will require processes for negotiating the common ground and for defining both the problems to be addressed and the agenda for action. These steps typically require a convenor or a facilitator who is deemed neutral, non-threatening, trustworthy, and credible by the parties involved (Gray, 1996). The convenor's role is carried out within a defined process for systematic management of inter-organisational relations. The theory is simple, yet the reality is often great distrust—by state or provincial governments about the national government, or by World Health Organization Member States about multi-lateral organisations—and difficulty in identifying the intermediary, or "glue," who can keep the dialogue moving and is without the imperative to dominate or control the agenda.

In unavoidably complex partnerships, such as at national or global levels, network arrangements may be more acceptable and achievable than highly organised systems. As a form of inter-action between organisations to use their talents and resources for mutual benefit, networks are increasingly common in the business world, particularly in light of new information technology and uncertainty in the external environment (Castells, 1996; S. Clegg and S. Porras, Trust as networking knowledge, paper presented at Trust in the Workplace Conference, 2000, Newcastle, UK). A global network for risk factor surveillance may be more feasible than one standardised system, because the former allows for different types of partnerships at different levels and for incremental negotiated agreements. A network forms the basis for long-term development of a relationship (to share resources and expertise and to achieve negotiated actions for joint objectives) that will deliver benefits over time.

A partnership with such long-term objectives as risk factor surveillance and effective interventions to improve the health of populations requires parties at various levels to commit to a vision of public health action. It also requires a credible convenor; agreement about roles and contributions of the parties; and a process that prevents dominance by any particular party, supports local innovation, and invites contribution by multiple leaders. A mature partnership allows co-existence of different views and positions where they do not impinge upon the common goal, and it requires partners to put aside objectives or actions that undermine the partnership.

4. LESSONS FROM THE GROUND

4.1. China (Top-Down Partnership)

Under the Health Promotion Project (known as World Bank Health VII), in 1995 the China Ministry of Health adapted the Behavioral Risk Factor Surveillance System (BRFSS) of the U.S. Centers for Disease Control and Prevention for implementation in eight cities (ranging from large cities like Shanghai and Beijing to provincial centres like Liuzhou and Weihai). The project consisted of four components: policy reform and institutional development, human resources development, surveillance, and community-based interventions. At the time, mortality and hospital morbidity data were neither sufficient nor appropriate for health promotion interventions, and it was thought that the risk factor surveillance system would provide more timely planning and evaluation of the interventions in the eight communities. Annual intervention plans were required of the participating cities to ensure consideration and reflection of empirical evidence.

The adapted BRFSS was planned and piloted in 1995 and implemented in 1996. Because of the limited availability of telephones to the populace, the Chinese system used household interviews; otherwise, almost no changes were made to the BRFSS questionnaire. Data analysis was completed centrally, in Beijing. Extensive training and manuals were provided to surveillance personnel, who were located within the Epidemic Prevention Stations of the municipal health bureaux.

The implementation was largely positive. Data collection, analysis, and reporting were achieved smoothly. The adaptation of the BRFSS to Chinese conditions was shown to be possible. Even so, several years later a number of issues have arisen, as reported by Prof. Wang Rutao and Prof. Yang Gonghuan at the September 1999 conference "Global Issues and Perspectives in Monitoring Behaviors in Populations: Surveillance of Risk Factors in Health and Illness" in Atlanta, Georgia:

- Should the survey questions have been altered more, to suit local priorities and adapt to Chinese culture and societal conditions?
- How can greater and more meaningful use of the data be ensured, particularly at the local level and by persons involved in intervention design?
- Would a less centralised arrangement for data management and analysis engender greater ownership by local organisations? If so, what level of epidemiological skills is required locally?

The annual supervision missions from the World Bank and the China Ministry of Health also identified insufficient use of the survey data for intervention planning. A gulf between persons who worked on the surveillance system and those who worked on health promotion programming existed in institutional structures and in professional language and practise. Local workers expressed concerns that the centrally analysed data were not fed back soon enough for intervention planning and that not all questions were relevant. In other words, all the expected dynamics were observed. The system had been developed, but a true partnership between data analysers and data users had yet to emerge.

The 1996 implementation efforts centred on getting a surveillance system in place; 6 years later, focus is on the survey content insofar as the behavioural risk factor surveillance system is a key element of non-communicable disease prevention and control efforts. Indeed, this system was chosen as part of an explicit decision not to invest, for the purposes of health promotion, in collection of hospital morbidity data regarding non-communicable diseases nor in surveys of biomedical risk factors. The Chinese now see having more relevant content as one approach to securing better application and use of the surveillance system—although it may be open to debate as to whether "relevant" means cultural appropriateness, reflection of local interests and priorities, or more involvement of local people in determining content. If there is to be greater local involvement in determining how the system might evolve, to what extent will the local users and other decision-makers be involved?

For China, at the moment, attention probably needs to shift to achieving the appropriate infra-structure so that whatever content modifications will be required can be implemented. By the time the health promotion project concludes, the Chinese will need to decide whether this information infra-structure will be maintained and how. Additionally, the Chinese are increasingly concerned about developing an appropriate system to monitor risk factor behaviour for issues such as sexually transmitted diseases and human immuno-deficiency virus infection. How should the behavioural risk factor surveillance system relate to other surveillance systems or other systems for data collection and management?

Other infra-structure issues must be considered in the future development of the behavioural risk factor surveillance system. As the Chinese move to de-centralise data analysis and thus increase ownership and use at the local level, further consideration will need to be given to the level of skills required locally for epidemiology and data analysis. And given the organisational barriers between users and current owners of the data system, what mechanisms and processes need to exist at the local level to ensure continued dialogue between the two groups?

The experience of introducing a modified BRFSS in China has shown that while it is possible to drive a top-down process to develop a surveillance system, and indeed necessary to address local capacity issues, the longer term maintenance of the system will require more attention to local ownership and to links between national and local levels. Additionally, where design capabilities for programme interventions are weak at the local level, the partnership between those who operate the surveillance system and its users should be facilitated by persons who understand well the potential applications of the information. A strong partnership at the local level will be important to assure sustainability of the Chinese behavioural risk factor surveillance system.

4.2. Australia (Bottom-Up Partnership)

Australia, with eight states and territories with unique histories and vastly different approaches to structuring health administration, is a microcosm for global issues (or at least the European Union issues). Unlike the top-down, organised approach of China in developing and implementing a behavioural risk factor surveillance system, the Australian states and territories have taken individual initiatives, at different times and for different reasons, to develop and implement health surveys. These efforts arose in part from concerns that national health survey arrangements were not providing timely data nor data relevant to local public health.

Where possible, the states and territories have adopted computer-aided telephone interviewing (CATI) technology and have aimed for a system that provides continuous monitoring of key health issues. Small population size and remote locations have made CATI infeasible in some jurisdictions. The content of the surveys vary—some cover the standard behavioural risk factors; some cover issues related to health services access, use, and satisfaction; and some focus on population sub-groups of concern, such as youth. Still others have ventured into sensitive social issues, such as gambling and domestic violence.

Cross-jurisdictional communication began as an ad hoc professional liaison. Under the development of the National Public Health Partnership, national processes for collaboration have been instigated. Co-ordination has focused on infra-structure (methodology and systems) rather than content. Consistent with the framework for health information management, set out in the Australian National Health Information Agreement, a work programme exists to ensure that common definitions, common data standards, and national minimum data sets can be developed and adopted over time.

Because state and territory survey programmes have different origins and histories, wide variation in their content has made national co-ordination difficult. Developing a national public health strategy, such as a strategy on preventable chronic disease, has been virtually impossible. Some have argued, however, that the infra-structure has allowed for new issues to be picked up as needed, particularly in identifying possible cohorts in future investigations. New topics and uses, such as community perceptions of genetically modified food and the investigation of food-borne illnesses, are some of the recent activities that have been built upon this infra-structure.

The CATI surveys have arisen from local need, relied on local input and innovation, and depended on local political will for investment and support. Some states, such as South Australia, have been running the system from subscriptions, but sustainability of the infra-structure is a major concern in many jurisdictions. The flexibility and usefulness of the infra-structure have been successfully demonstrated to decision-makers in some jurisdictions, but the jury is still out among users in other states.

The discussion in Australia is now evolving from survey methods to a surveillance system. Work is under way to define core modules that can be used by all jurisdictions. As such, emphasis on content has increased, particularly in relation to chronic diseases. The impetus has come in part from such related developments as a national health performance framework, reporting on progress on national health priorities (including cardio-vascular disease, cancer, and diabetes), and a national chronic disease prevention strategy. Questions remain, however, about the extent to which the focus should be on health conditions or risk factors and about links to other forms of health surveys (such as a system for monitoring biomedical risk factors). Achieving co-ordination on content remains a challenge for a federal system, as does co-ordination on other aspects of a national health information infra-structure.

The Australian experience suggests that building a national surveillance system from diverse local systems requires not only patience but trust between government levels. The sustainability of the system at both local and national levels will require greater ownership by the users, because of the relatively small size of the health promotion workforce. In other words, the information generated from the surveillance system must be capable of adding value to public health strategies and programmes. Brokerage of the partnership will similarly require people at all levels who are able to traverse the language and imperatives for surveillance and intervention.

5. ISSUES FOR GLOBAL DEVELOPMENT

A surveillance system comprises both content and information infra-structure. It also involves the data designers, collectors, and analysts and the users of those data.

Whether the system exists at the national or global level, co-ordination is complex, especially when local and national systems have been developed for different purposes and through different histories. In this regard, the Australian Constitution offers a useful lesson for leadership in co-ordination. The principle of subsidiarity holds that responsibility for services should be vested with the level closest to the community; thus, any efforts in a global network should be based on mutuality and involve the users in partnership with the technical people.

The participants at the September 1999 conference "Global Issues and Perspectives in Monitoring Behaviors in Populations: Surveillance of Risk Factors in Health and Illness" represented potentially strong collaborators across countries on many conceptual and technical matters: numerous experts are doing surveillance work and are concerned with methodology, system design, scientific validity, and other issues. The involvement of practitioners and policy-makers, who are or should be the immediate beneficiaries of the information collected, still has to be engineered. If information is be translated into meaningful action—whether that action is designing interventions or policies and whether it is at the local, national, regional, or global level—stakeholder participation is needed.

In a global approach, a balance must be struck between content issues and infra-structure issues. From the viewpoint of content, harmonisation (a concept familiar to Australians and European Union members) might be more appropriate than standardisa-tion. Harmonisation could occur with coverage of topics, that is, the shared priority areas; common measurement tools might be possible. This approach recognises diversity of cultures and contexts.

In terms of the specific content of surveillance systems, moving beyond the current focus on standard individual behavioural risk factors is valuable in picking up risk con-texts and issues in a variety of settings. At the same time, however, the trap of focusing on any one particular hot research topic (such as the current interest in social capital) must be avoided. A surveillance system is concerned with observations in natural set-tings and can serve as the basis for particular investigations, but it should not become locked into a research project and thereby contribute to what Bernard Choi (personal communication, "Global Issues and Perspectives in Monitoring Behaviors in Populations: Surveillance of Risk Factors in Health and Illness," planning question-answer session, September 1999) terms "hot stuff bias."

Additional questions need to be explored more globally, such as the extent to which health behaviour is universal or is specific to context or culture. Does a theoretical model underlie the BRFSS based on "Western" perspectives that may not be entirely applicable to other settings?

In relation to the infra-structure of surveillance systems, the key inputs to be consid-ered include people, skills, money, technology, and legislative framework:

- How de-centralised should it be?
- What legislative framework might be required in contemplating issues of pri-vacy, confidentiality, and links?
- What co-ordination is required with other data systems?
- What technology can be brought to bear?
- What level of training is required, not only of the data collectors, managers, and analysts, but of the users as well?
- What are the partnership structures required that would allow sharing of meth-ods and innovations?

This type of infra-structure is not limited to those risk factors assumed to be related to non-communicable diseases. Use of the system in South Australia for investigating outbreaks of food-borne disease illustrates how the system can be a practical tool for urgent public health action. At the same time, it is important to recognise that the information infra-structure is only one tool and offers a particular type of information. Decision-makers and programme planners may need other forms of information not captured by a risk factor surveillance system. Indeed, risk factor surveillance must be complemented by qualitative methods and more in-depth investigations at the local level, in particular settings and with particular population groups, that will help build local action.

Funding and people are both important for system sustainability. Meaningful use is the ultimate test, however. If a surveillance system can help a range of key users and demonstrate its usefulness, it is much more likely to last and to have supporters and advocates.

6. REFERENCES

Castells, M., 1996, *The Rise of the Network Society*, Blackwell Publishers, London.

Challis, L., Fuller, S., Henwood, M., et al., 1988, *Joint Approaches to Social Policy: Rationality and Practice*, Cambridge University Press, Cambridge, UK.

Gray, B., 1989, *Collaborating: Finding Common Ground for Multiparty Problems*, Jossey Bass, San Francisco.

Gray, B., 1996, Cross-sectoral partners: collaborative alliances among business, government, and communities, in: *Creating Collaborative Advantage*, C. Huxham, ed., Sage Publications, London, pp. 57–79.

Harris, E., Wise, M., Hawe, P., et al., 1995, *Working Together: Intersectoral Action for Health*, Australian Government Publishing Service, Canberra.

Himmelman, A. T., 1996, On the theory and practice of transformational collaboration, in: *Creating Collaborative Advantage*, C. Huxham, ed., Sage Publications, London, pp. 19–43.

Human Resources Development Unit, 1998, *Partnership Framework*, Tasmania Department of Community and Health Services, Hobart.

Huxham, C., ed., 1996, *Creating Collaborative Advantage*, Sage Publications, London.

Lin, V., and King, C., 2000, Intergovernmental reforms in public health, in: *Health Reform in Australia and New Zealand*, A. Bloom, ed., Oxford University Press, Melbourne.

Wilson, A., and Charlton, K., 1997, *Making Partnerships Work: A Practical Guide for the Public, Private, Voluntary and Community Sectors*, Joseph Rowntree Foundation, York, UK.

CHAPTER 5

ANALYSIS AND INTERPRETATION OF DATA FROM THE U.S. BEHAVIORAL RISK FACTOR SURVEILLANCE SYSTEM (BRFSS)

Deborah Holtzman[*]

1. INTRODUCTION

The Behavioral Risk Factor Surveillance System (BRFSS) is a unique, state-based surveillance system currently active in all 50 states, the District of Columbia, and three territories of the United States (hereafter, all referred to as "states"). For almost two decades, the U.S. Centers for Disease Control and Prevention (CDC), in collaboration with state health departments, has conducted telephone surveys of the civilian, non-institutionalised adult population (persons aged 18 years or older) as a part of this system to estimate the prevalence of behaviours linked to specific health problems.

For many states, the BRFSS is the only source of this population-based health behaviour data. The usefulness and success of the system are evident by its longevity and continued growth. As the number of participating states, interviews, and years have increased, so have the complexity and detail of data analysis and interpretation. To understand how the data have been analysed and interpreted, it is first necessary to understand the development and characteristics of the surveillance system.

2. THE SYSTEM

2.1. DEVELOPMENT OF THE BRFSS

By the early 1980s, it was evident from scientific research that personal health behaviours play a major role in premature morbidity and mortality (Anderson et al., 1988). Although estimates of such behaviours among U.S. adult populations had been periodically obtained through national surveys (e.g., the National Health Interview Survey), these data were not available at the state level—a critical gap, because the role of targeting resources to reduce behavioural risks and their consequent illnesses falls

---

[*] Centers for Disease Control and Prevention, Atlanta, Georgia 30341, USA.

primarily on state health agencies. Moreover, national data may not be relevant for any given state, even though participation by state and local agencies is important in achieving national health goals.

About the same time the role of personal health behaviours in morbidity and mortality received wider recognition, telephone surveys emerged as an acceptable method for determining the prevalence of many health risk behaviours among populations (Groves and Kahn, 1979). In addition to their relatively low costs, telephone surveys were especially desirable at the state and local levels, where the expertise and resources necessary for conducting area probability sampling for in-person household interviews were generally not available. As a result, telephone surveys were developed and implemented to monitor state-level prevalence of the major behavioural risks associated with premature morbidity and mortality among adults. The basic philosophy was to collect data on actual behaviours (rather than attitudes or knowledge) and behaviours related to premature morbidity and mortality (i.e., from chronic disease and injury, or non-communicable rather than communicable disease). Such behavioural data were thought to be especially useful for planning, implementing, monitoring, and evaluating health promotion and disease prevention programmes.

To determine the feasibility of behavioural surveillance, initial point-in-time surveys were conducted in 29 states from 1981 through 1983 (Gentry et al., 1985; Marks et al., 1985). In 1984, the BRFSS was formally established by CDC, with 15 states participating in monthly data collection. The surveillance system was designed to collect state-level data, but a number of states stratified their samples to allow them to also estimate prevalence for smaller geographic areas within their respective states.

A standard, "core" questionnaire was developed by CDC to generate data that could be compared across states. Except for physical activity, for which there were no standard questions available at the time, the survey included existing questions from current national surveys such as the National Health Interview Surveys on cigarette smoking, diet, and alcohol consumption and the National Heart, Lung, and Blood Institute surveys on hypertension. The initial questionnaire was designed to last no more than 10 minutes so that states could add their own questions to the survey, but keep the interview to a reasonable length.

2.2. Sampling Procedures

Each month, a representative sample of persons aged 18 years or older is selected for interview. The sampling procedure has varied by state and over the years. States were initially encouraged to use cluster designs based on the method of Waksberg (1978), but even for the initial 29 point-in-time surveys, nine states used simple random samples. Data collection is directed by states, and some variability in sampling methodology has continued. Over time, the majority of states moved to disproportionate stratified sampling (DSS), which is more cost-effective.

2.3. Joint Venture

Although designed as a co-operative federal-state venture, most decisions about the BRFSS during the first several years were made by CDC staff, primarily because the resources and expertise in survey methodology, questionnaire development, and data analysis were limited at the state level. As a result, the questionnaire was designed by CDC staff with informal input from interested state health department personnel. Throughout the 1980s, most modifications to the core questionnaire were made by individuals or groups at CDC with interest and expertise in certain subjects or with specific research agendas.

As participating states became increasingly involved in survey operations and new states entered the system, development of the questionnaire became a more co-operative federal-state effort. In 1990, this partnership was formalised with the creation of the BRFSS Working Group, which comprises selected BRFSS state representatives and CDC staff and meets regularly during the year. States are now actively involved in discussions concerning proposed changes to the BRFSS questionnaire. The ultimate authority on questionnaire content and wording, however, is still CDC.

2.3.1. State Responsibilities

At the state level, all BRFSS programmes are located within the state health department. The state programme oversees all aspects of data collection, including hiring appropriate staff, ensuring interviews are conducted according to protocol, and training and evaluating interviewers. Other duties include editing data, forwarding data to CDC for processing, and working to achieve CDC quality assurance goals. States also are expected to demonstrate how they have analysed and disseminated BRFSS data, which may include publication of state reports or other documents incorporating BRFSS data.

2.3.2. Federal Responsibilities

At CDC, responsibility for the BRFSS lies with the Behavioral Surveillance Branch, which is located in the Division of Adult and Community Health in the National Center for Chronic Disease Prevention and Health Promotion. The Behavioral Surveillance Branch is responsible for purchasing randomly generated telephone number samples, programming the states' questionnaires for computer-assisted telephone interviewing (CATI), editing monthly data files, re-formatting data to adhere to a common CDC standard, generating quality control reports to facilitate monitoring activities, and computing annual weighting factors. From the beginning, CDC has had primary responsibility for processing the data, both as a way to ensure receiving the data and as a service to participating states. The Behavioral Surveillance Branch produces data sets for analysis, prepares annual tabular summaries of BRFSS data for each state (including median estimates, ranges, and cross-tabulations by demographic variables), and prepares annual summary prevalence reports that reflect estimates across states for selected variables. Additionally, the Branch collaborates and provides assistance to states for data collection, analysis, interpretation, and use and coordinates and facilitates the exchange of technical information among states.

The tasks of analysing data from the BRFSS and of encouraging and promoting analysis of the data rest primarily with the Behavioral Surveillance Branch. Staff are responsible for developing research initiatives, establishing priorities and tracking progress, and consulting or collaborating with state health departments, other centres and divisions within CDC, and organisations outside CDC (other federal agencies, national and international health agencies, voluntary health agencies, and universities) that have an interest in analysing data from the BRFSS.

2.4. Expansion

2.4.1. Number of States, Interviews, and Years

Additional CDC funding allowed the BRFSS to expand to 50 states by 1993 and to gradually increase the overall number of completed interviews to an average of almost 2,300 per state in 1995. Since 1995, the number of interviews has increased further in most states. In 2000 alone, more than 175,000 interviews were completed nationwide. Because the surveillance system is continuous and many questions have been comparable over time—some for as many as 17 years—within a few years BRFSS data for certain states and certain topics could be combined across states and over time for more detailed analyses.

2.4.2. Number of Topics and Questions

Because of its ability to obtain state-level data and the absence of comparable surveillance systems, by the late 1980s the BRFSS was recognised as a unique mechanism for obtaining health data from the general population of U.S. adults. As a result, several programmes within CDC, as well as state health departments, became interested in using the BRFSS to obtain other types of information, although still with a focus on health behaviour, clinical preventive practices, and selected health conditions related to chronic disease and injury. Gradually, the size of the questionnaire increased as new subject areas were added. Currently, the BRFSS core questionnaire, asked by all participating states, contains questions on HIV/AIDS, cancer screening and other clinical preventive services, diabetes, and tobacco-related topics. In addition to changes to the core questionnaire, CDC-supported modules (one or more questions on a single topic) were offered to states beginning in 1988. Although selection of new subject areas for the BRFSS is now based on input from states and CDC about priority topics, as well as financial support from other divisions and centres at CDC, these modules have almost always been the result of other CDC centres or divisions within the National Center for Chronic Disease Prevention and Health Promotion proposing a set of questions on a subject of interest. This activity has grown substantially; in 2000, 19 modules were offered to states.

Over the years, states and CDC generally agreed that the BRFSS core questionnaire would not exceed 80 questions so that states could continue to include their own questions without the interview becoming overly long. By the early 1990s, there was no room for additional expansion of the BRFSS core. In 1992, the BRFSS Working Group proposed a long-term plan which covered the years 1993–2000 and included development of a "rotating core." Under this arrangement, questions on certain topics would be asked every other year (Table 1). The plan also added up to five "emerging core" questions to the questionnaire. This option allowed questions in new subject areas to be tested; if these questions were found useful, they could eventually be added to the core questionnaire or a CDC-supported module. Emerging core questions are allowed to stay on the core for 1 year, although the questions can be extended for an additional year.

Table 1. BRFSS questionnaire plan, 1993–2000

Fixed core		Rotating core I (odd years)		Rotating core II (even years)	
Topic	No. of Questions	Topic	No. of Questions	Topic	No. of Questions
Health status	4	Hypertension	3	Physical activity	10
Health insurance	3	Injury control	5	Fruit and vegetable	6
Routine checkup	1	Alcohol use	5	consumption	
Diabetes	1	Vaccinations	2	Weight control	6
Smoking	5	Colorectal cancer screening	4		
Pregnancy	1	Cholesterol screening	3		
Women's health	10				
HIV/AIDS	14				
Demographics	14				
Total Men	42	Total	22	Total	22
Women	53				

In CDC's ongoing efforts to improve BRFSS data quality, a policy was established and instituted in 1998 that required all new or substantially revised questions (core and module) to undergo formal cognitive testing. This testing primarily checks the wording and structure (for clarity, intent, comprehension, etc.) of questions through interviews with a small number of individuals who are characteristic of the BRFSS target population. Consequently, results from the cognitive testing are a factor in selection of questions. Since 2000, questionnaire planning has been carried out from year to year; planning for 2003 is currently under way. Another long-term plan will likely be developed for 2005 through 2015.

3. ANALYSIS AND INTERPRETATION OF BRFSS DATA

As the BRFSS has evolved and expanded, so have analyses and interpretation of the collected data. Analysis is guided, of course, by the characteristics of the system, none more visible than the content of the questionnaire. As mentioned, the BRFSS was designed to collect information on the health behaviours, health conditions, and preventive health practices of U.S. adults that contribute to the major causes of morbidity and mortality from chronic disease, injury, and preventable infectious disease. Other system characteristics that guide analysis and interpretation are questionnaire flexibility, sample design, and quality of the data. Obviously, to be useful the BRFSS data must be accessible to states, public health professionals, and other individuals and agencies. Depending on their goals, states analyse and interpret data in numerous ways, as do CDC and other agencies.

3.1. Questionnaire Flexibility

All participating states are asked to use the core questionnaire; however, one important feature of the BRFSS is its flexibility. States can add questions of their own design and CDC-supported modules that may be of interest. CDC has supported up to 19 modules annually, but it is not feasible for a state to use them all at one time; states must be selective with their choices to keep the questionnaire a reasonable length. (Across states the total number of questions for a given year ranges widely, from about 90 to more than 150.) New questionnaires are implemented in January and usually remain unchanged throughout the year, but additions of, changes in, and deletions of state-added questions at any time during the year are allowed, notably for emerging issues. The final version of the questionnaire for any year determines the analytic content at the state (or aggregate) level for that year.

3.2. Sample Design

The target population in the BRFSS is the non-institutionalised civilian population aged 18 years or older in each participating state. Respondents in households are identified through telephone-based methods. By definition, persons in households without telephones are not included in the BRFSS, but telephone coverage in the United States is quite high (U.S. Bureau of the Census, 1994) so this limitation creates relatively little bias for most analyses. Moreover, although the BRFSS uses no direct method of compensating for non-telephone coverage, post-stratification weights (by age-race-sex or age-sex categories) serve to partially correct for any bias caused by non-telephone coverage.

To ensure representativeness of the samples, the BRFSS surveys in each state employ random-digit-dialing methods of sampling. As mentioned, specific sampling designs have varied among states; currently, all but two (Guam and the Virgin Islands) use DSS. Interviews are conducted each month of the year, usually during a 2-week period. Because the sample is scientifically drawn and each state has a target number of interviews, results can be inferred to the populations on which they are based. For example, in 1999 interviews ranged from about 100 to 425 per month, yielding annual state samples from about 1,200 to 5,100—large enough to produce stable estimates for most behaviours and major demographic sub-groups within states.

Various statistical methods can be employed to analyse BRFSS data. Importantly, the BRFSS uses a complex design to obtain a representative sample of respondents in each state. Consequently, the analyst should use an analytic package that accounts for this design when any type of statistical testing is conducted.

3.3. Data Quality

Central to analysis and interpretation of the BRFSS data is the credibility of the data, as evidenced by reliability and validity. In a study of the reproducibility of responses obtained through telephone interviews with respondents to the Massachusetts BRFSS, reproducibility of demographic characteristics was extremely high and generally good across risk factors (Stein et al., 1995). In another study of the reliability of BRFSS measures among U.S. women aged 40 years or older, behavioural risk factors, including physical inactivity, were generally consistent across two interview periods (Brownson et al., 1999). More recently, a validity study comparing BRFSS estimates with those from medical records for chronic diseases and receipt of preventive clinical services found good concordance between the two (Martin et al., 2000). Several other studies have looked at the reliability and validity of data from the BRFSS or measures similar to those on the BRFSS. To assess the extent of such research and to provide information to persons who analyse and use BRFSS data, the quality of the core BRFSS measures for the years 1993–2000 was addressed in a comprehensive summary of reliability and validity studies; most measures on the questionnaire were found to be at least moderately reliable and valid, and several were highly reliable and valid (Nelson et al., 2001).

3.4. Accessibility of Data

Analysis and interpretation of BRFSS data are possible only if the information is accessible. A policy of the Behavioral Surveillance Branch is to provide timely access to BRFSS data to as diverse an array of public health professionals as possible while ensuring data quality and respecting the needs of participating states. Each year, the Branch provides BRFSS data collected in the prior year that have been edited and are ready for statistical analysis with weights and uniform variable formats. Priority is given to participating states for access to their own BRFSS data. After each state has an opportunity to review its own data, the BRFSS data for all states are made available for analysis—a process that now takes approximately 4 months after the end of the year. To both encourage and facilitate use, several years of data have been made available on CD-ROM. In addition, data from as far back as 1995 can be easily down-loaded from the BRFSS web site (http://www.cdc.gov/nccdphp/brfss/) by any user.

3.5. Use of BRFSS Data by States

An important aspect of the BRFSS is how the data are used by the states. Major uses are to estimate the prevalence of important behaviours that contribute to morbidity and mortality, identify demographic variations in health-related behaviours, accurately target health programmes and services, address emergent and critical health issues, guide health legislation and policy, and measure progress towards state and national health objectives. During the 1990s, a number of topics on the BRFSS were linked to specific national health objectives set forth in the *Healthy People 2000* initiative (U.S. Department of Health and Human Services, 1991). Current questionnaires are linked to *Healthy People 2010* objectives (U.S. Department of Health and Human Services, 2000); in fact, 7 of the 10 leading health indicators for 2010 can be measured by BRFSS data. Such use of the BRFSS provides state policy-makers with informed options for public health decisions, helps in designing public health intervention strategies, and allows evaluation of an intervention's impact on the state's population.

Not only must the data be analysed and reported, but the information must be disseminated. All BRFSS-participating states prepare reports or fact sheets to educate the public, the health professional community, and state legislators about the current status and trends in lifestyle patterns in their state. Examples of BRFSS data applications at the state level are provided in Table 2.

Use of BRFSS data to address specific health issues has varied from state to state. For example, following the passage of a bicycle helmet law in Oregon, the state used the BRFSS questionnaire to evaluate the effect of the legislation on helmet use. BRFSS data have been used to support tobacco control legislation in most states, particularly in California, where the data were influential in supporting the passage of Proposition 99 Tobacco Tax legislation, which generated millions of dollars in state funds to support health

Table 2. How BRFSS data have been used by state health departments

Guide health policies

Determine priorities and plan long-range strategy

Monitor progress towards state or national health objectives

Guide minority health programme initiatives

Monitor the effectiveness of prevention programmes

Propose and support legislation

Assess and document needs

Develop point-in-time studies

Document state-specific prevalence of selected behaviours

Monitor programme goals

Guide educational interventions

Develop community surveys

Increase public awareness

Influence physician adherence

Prepare proposals for funding

Guide resource allocation

Serve as models for other surveys

education and chronic disease prevention programmes. With passage of the National Breast and Cervical Cancer Mortality Prevention Act by Congress in 1990, funds became available to state health departments to establish breast and cervical cancer control programmes. Data from the BRFSS on use of mammography and Papanicolaou tests provide critical information to states about baseline cancer screening levels and a means to monitor the impact of breast and cervical cancer control programmes. In Illinois, two successful legislative initiatives—an act requiring no-smoking areas in public buildings and one requiring the inclusion of mammography screening in all health insurance coverage—were supported by data on the prevalence of smoking and mammography screening. In Nevada, BRFSS data documenting the state's high rates of chronic and binge drinking were used to support legislation to place a wholesale per-gallon tax on distilled alcohol. Because of its tremendous morbidity and mortality burden, cardiovascular disease continues to be the focus of state health promotion and risk reduction efforts; BRFSS data provide a continuous way to monitor changes in cardiovascular-related health behaviours in the population and to assess the effectiveness of risk reduction initiatives in many states. Numerous additional examples of how state BRFSS programmes have used the data are available (CDC, 2000a).

3.6. Use of BRFSS Data by CDC and Other Agencies

Similar to the states, analysis and use of BRFSS data at the federal level include estimating the prevalence of important behaviours that contribute to morbidity and mortality, identifying demographic variations in health-related behaviours, targeting programmes and services, addressing emergent and critical health issues, guiding health legislation and policy, and measuring progress towards health objectives. Because researchers at the federal level have ready access to BRFSS data from all participating states and because more years of data are available (states entered the system at different times), however, these analyses are often at the regional or national level.

Essentially every topic area covered by the BRFSS has been analysed and reported— from summary reports of each variable across states (see for example Bolen et al., 2000; Holtzman et al., 2000) to reports on a single behaviour or practice that contributes to disease or injury (see for example Nelson et al., 1996; CDC, 2000b; Ebrahim et al., 2000; Li et al., 2000). To date, there have been well over 500 BRFSS-related publications and at least four times as many presentations of the data.

Because the BRFSS has been in operation for nearly two decades and many items on the questionnaire have remained unchanged, most trends are easily monitored. Numerous reports have looked at BRFSS data over time. For example, Mokdad et al. (1999) used BRFSS data to document the growing epidemic of obesity among U.S. adults over the past decade. Another advantage in aggregating the data over place and time (i.e., yielding larger samples) is that select sub-groups of the population can be analysed. For example, older adults (Janes et al., 1999; Mack and Bland, 1999; Powell-Griner et al., 1999) or persons of specific racial or ethnic groups, such as American Indians and Alaska Natives (Denny and Taylor, 1999), have been examined in several reports. Furthermore, scientists can combine states that have used the same CDC-sponsored modules to obtain larger samples and conduct more in-depth analyses (see for example Saaddine et al., 1999; Holtzman et al., 2001).

International consultation and collaboration is also an activity of the BRFSS. One collaboration involved modifying the BRFSS for use in seven municipalities in China, which is discussed in detail in Chapter 14. Other countries have also undertaken BRFSS-type surveys, including Australia, Canada, and Russia. Most recently, Brazil and Argentina have consulted CDC about establishing behavioural surveillance for chronic disease and injury.

4. CONCLUSION

Despite the range of applications of BRFSS data, it is important not to lose sight of what the BRFSS cannot do. As with many survey systems, especially large-scale surveillance systems, the BRFSS does not cover any topic in great depth (so as to include as many behaviours related to chronic disease and injury as possible). Consequently, few items measure, for example, determinants of behaviour. The length of the interview and the increasing competition for space on the BRFSS also constrain the number of questions that can be asked on any one topic. Moreover, even though the system is quite broad, it covers only certain main topics (related primarily to chronic disease and injury), so other areas one may be interested in would have to be found in another system. Furthermore, the system was not designed with a theoretical framework to answer specific research questions.

The analyst also must be aware of other characteristics of the BRFSS that affect generalisation. As a telephone survey, the BRFSS obviously does not include households without telephones and thus likely under-represents the nation's indigent population and other select groups; for example, an estimated 23% of American Indian households do not have a telephone—a much higher percentage than for other racial or ethnic groups in the United States (Denny and Holtzman, 1999). Moreover, persons not in households (e.g., institutionalised or homeless) are excluded. In addition, persons with poor health habits may be more likely to refuse to be interviewed. Finally, because the data are self-reported and not confirmed by other means (e.g., medical record review), some behaviours may be subject to under- or over-reporting.

Conversely, such a system offers several advantages. The BRFSS is flexible, new questions can be added in a timely manner, and it is relatively inexpensive to operate. Standardised procedures facilitate comparability. States can compare their data with those from other states, a region, or the nation. Importantly, the system provides prevalence estimates of behaviours that are useful in evaluating relevant state programmes and in guiding relevant legislation. Thus, states have their own data on which to base programmatic and policy decisions, yet the data can be easily combined to produce regional or national estimates (Battelle, 1999). Emerging health issues can also be examined in this system. Once established, the system can be adapted for other uses, other topics, other populations, and other countries. Many of the same data are collected continuously with a standard methodology, which makes the BRFSS ideal for monitoring trends. This same structure also allows for a very large amount of data that enables even small sub-groups or low-prevalent behaviours within a population to be analysed and to yield relatively stable estimates. Furthermore, many of the measures on the BRFSS are at least moderately reliable and valid. Finally, although data from the system can be aggregated to provide national or regional prevalence estimates, in many cases the BRFSS is the only source of population-based, state-level behavioural data for chronic disease in the United States. As such, its importance cannot be over-stated.

So, what can we conclude about analysis and interpretation of BRFSS data? The BRFSS yields representative, state-specific estimates for the general population of U.S. adults for health behaviours and preventive health practices primarily related to chronic disease, injury, and preventable infectious disease. Sample size is generally sufficient to produce stable estimates for most measures, both for the total population and for major demographic sub-groups. Standard methods of data collection across participating states enable the data to be aggregated across place as well as time. Furthermore, when states or years are combined, estimates for even finer breakdowns in the population can generally be obtained. Various types of statistical procedures can be employed in analysis of the data. The quality of the data from the BRFSS is relatively good, the data are widely available for analysis, and multiple uses of the data have been demonstrated.

The BRFSS has grown and matured to a point that it is now barely recognizable from the system initiated in 1984. The diversity of programmes of which BRFSS is a part, interest in the system from both within and outside of CDC, and widespread use of the data are clear evidence of its successful evolution. The next few decades must continue to expand data analysis and use. The challenge is to make the data even more useful, widely available, and timely and to adapt the system as necessary to ensure continued receipt of high-quality, representative data.

5. ACKNOWLEDGEMENT

I acknowledge the contributions of Mike Waller and Craig Leutzinger of CDC, who provided information on the history and operation of the BRFSS.

6. REFERENCES

Anderson, R., Davies, J. K., Kickbusch, I., et al., eds., 1988, *Health Behaviour Research and Health Promotion,* Oxford University Press, Oxford, UK.

Battelle, 1999, *Evaluation of the Behavioral Risk Factor Surveillance System (BRFSS) as a Source for National Estimates of Selected Health Risk Behaviors: Final Report,* Battelle, Baltimore.

Bolen, J. C., Rhodes, L., Powell-Griner, E., et al., 2000, State-specific prevalence of selected health behaviors, by race and ethnicity—Behavioral Risk Factor Surveillance System, 1997, *Mor Mortal Wkly Rep CDC Surveill Summ.* **49**(SS-2):1–60.

Brownson, R. C., Eyler, A. A., King, A. C., et al., 1999, Reliability of information on physical activity and other chronic disease risk factors among US women aged 40 years or older, *Am J Epidemiol.* **149**:379–391.

Centers for Disease Control and Prevention, 2000a, *BRFSS in Action: Tracking Health Objectives,* National Center for Chronic Disease Prevention and Health Promotion, Atlanta.

Centers for Disease Control and Prevention, 2000b, Prevalence of leisure-time physical activity among overweight U.S. adults—United States, 1998, *Mor Mortal Wkly Rep.* **49**:326–330.

Denny, C. H., and Holtzman, D., 1999, *Health Behaviors of American Indians and Alaska Natives: Findings from the Behavioral Risk Factor Surveillance System, 1993–1996,* Centers for Disease Control and Prevention, Atlanta.

Denny, C. H., and Taylor, T. L., 1999, American Indian and Alaska Native health behavior: findings from the Behavioral Risk Factor Surveillance System, 1992–1995, *Ethn Dis.* **9**:403–409.

Ebrahim, S. H., Floyd, R. L., Merritt, R. K., et al., 2000, Trends in pregnancy-related smoking rates in the United States, 1987–1996, *JAMA.* **283**:361–366.

Gentry, E. M., Kalsbeek, W. D., Hogelin, G. C., et al., 1985, The behavioral risk factor surveys: II. Design, methods, and estimates from combined state data, *Am J Prev Med.* **1**:9–14.

Groves, R. M., and Kahn, R. L., 1979, *Surveys by Telephone: A National Comparison with Personal Interviews,* Academic Press, New York.

Holtzman, D., Bland, S. D., Lansky, A., et al., 2001, HIV-related behaviors and perceptions among adults in 25 states: 1997 Behavioral Risk Factor Surveillance System, *Am J Public Health.* **91**:1882–1888.

Holtzman, D., Powell-Griner, E., Bolen, J. C., et al., 2000, State- and sex-specific prevalence of selected characteristics—Behavioral Risk Factor Surveillance System, 1996 and 1997, *Mor Mortal Wkly Rep CDC Surveill Summ.* **49**(SS-6):1–39.

Janes, G. R., Blackman, D. K., Bolen, J. C., et al., 1999, Surveillance for use of preventive health-care services by older adults, 1995–1997, *Mor Mortal Wkly Rep CDC Surveill Summ.* **48**(SS-8):51–88.

Li, R., Serdula, M., Bland, S., et al., 2000, Trends in fruit and vegetable consumption among adults in 16 states: Behavioral Risk Factor Surveillance System, 1990–1996, *Am J Public Health.* **90**:777–781.

Mack, K. A., and Bland, S. D., 1999, HIV testing behaviors and attitudes regarding HIV/AIDS of adults aged 50–64, *Gerontologist.* **39**:687–694.

Marks, J. S., Hogelin, G. C., Gentry, E. M., et al., 1985, The behavioral risk factor surveys: I. State-specific prevalence estimates of behavioral risk factors, *Am J Prev Med.* **1**:1–8.

Martin, L. M., Leff, M., Calonge, N., et al., 2000, Validation of self-reported chronic conditions and health services in a managed care population, *Am J Prev Med.* **18**:215–218.

Mokdad, A. H., Serdula, M. K., Dietz, W. H., et al., 1999, The spread of the obesity epidemic in the United States, 1991–1998, *JAMA.* **282**:1519–1522.

Nelson, D. E., Grant-Worley, J. A., Powell, K., et al., 1996, Population estimates of household firearm storage practices and firearm carrying in Oregon, *JAMA.* **275**:1744–1748.

Nelson, D. E., Holtzman, D., Bolen, J., et al., 2001, Reliability and validity of measures from the Behavioral Risk Factor Surveillance System (BRFSS), *Soz Praventivmed.* **46**(Suppl 1):S1–S42.

Powell-Griner, E., Bolen, J., and Bland, S., 1999, Health care coverage and use of preventive services among the near elderly in the United States, *Am J Public Health.* **89**:882–886.

Saaddine, J. B., Venkat Narayan, K. M., Engelgau, M. M., et al., 1999, Prevalence of self-rated visual impairment among adults with diabetes, *Am J Public Health.* **89**:1200–1205.

Stein, A. D., Courval, J. M., Lederman, R. I., et al., 1995, Reproducibility of responses to telephone interviews: demographic predictors of discordance in risk factor status, *Am J Epidemiol.* **141**:1097–1105.

U.S. Bureau of the Census, 1994, *Phoneless in America*, U.S. Department of Commerce, Bureau of the Census, Washington, DC (Statistical Brief 94-16).

U.S. Department of Health and Human Services, 1991, *Healthy People 2000: National Health Promotion and Disease Prevention Objectives. Full Report, With Commentary*, U.S. Department of Health and Human Services, Public Health Service, Washington, DC (DHHS Publication No. (PHS) 91-50212).

U.S. Department of Health and Human Services, 2000, *Healthy People 2010, Second Edition, With Understanding and Improving Health and Objectives for Improving Health*, 2 vols., U.S. Government Printing Office, Washington, DC.

Waksberg, J., 1978, Sampling methods for random digit dialing, *J Am Stat Assoc.* **73**:40–46.

CHAPTER 6

SURVEILLANCE SYSTEMS AND DATA ANALYSIS: CONTINUOUSLY COLLECTED BEHAVIOURAL DATA
British and American Examples

Stefano Campostrini[*]

1. INTRODUCTION

Many public health initiatives are concerned with making behavioural changes happen at a population level (e.g., community-wide initiatives to change sexual practices to reduce the threat of HIV infection, or physical activity and nutrition campaigns to reduce the number of people who are overweight). The need for a surveillance system to monitor and track changes at this level is clear. In this chapter I discuss how data analysis should contribute to such a system and help make it responsive to the needs of those who use behavioural surveillance data.

1.1. Behavioural Risk Factor Surveillance Systems

A system that monitors behavioural risks related to non-communicable diseases could involve one or more kinds of surveillance. Different characteristics can define the kind of surveillance, but the presence or absence of some peculiar characteristics allow us to recognise a system as "surveillance" at all. These characteristics are

- time, a fundamental aspect around which the data collection must be organised,
- the focus on non-communicable diseases and on the risk behaviours that can determine them (the link to a theory), and
- attention given to all the processes of data management: collection, analysis, interpretation, and use.

These characteristics are not discussed in great detail in this chapter; they are taken for granted. However, before introducing the analytic issues of chief concern in a behavioural surveillance system, I would like to briefly discuss what would be an ideal system from the perspective of analysis, which is so important in a surveillance system.

[*] University of Pavia, 27100 Pavia, Italy.

If we acknowledge that, in any surveillance system, data analysis and interpretation are embedded in the whole systemic process, then the output of analysis and interpretation is determined by the type of analysis undertaken. And if we accept the importance of the output of data analysis (and also that of data use [i.e., feedback from stakeholders]), we cannot think this output has little or no influence on data collection. Finally, if a core of data—collected in a stable way over time—is absolutely important (for several reasons, some of which will be discussed later in this chapter), we can't see any objection to data collection being partly modified by factors that develop during the surveillance process, or even by the knowledge that the system itself has produced. From this perspective, we could think of a surveillance system as a learning system.

1.2. Peculiarities of Data from Surveillance Systems

Several large behavioural risk factor surveys, such as Lifestyle and Health (LAH) in Great Britain and the Behavioral Risk Factor Surveillance System (BRFSS) in the United States, have collected data for many years. These two survey systems have collected data nearly continuously and over an extended period, separating them from the more usual one-shot or periodic survey often found in official data collection systems of health agencies internationally. The BRFSS started in the early 1980s and now collects monthly some thousands of interviews in all the American states. It is undoubtedly the largest set of time-based data in the world that is continually collected. Yet despite the quantity collected, most analyses of BRFSS have tended to use methods appropriate to the analysis of point-in-time cross-sectional surveys, thus missing the opportunity to learn about the dynamics of behavioural change captured by the data.

The notion of continuously collected data (CCD) (see McQueen et al., 1992a; Campostrini, 1996) requires elaboration. Continuous data are actually data collection points on a continuum, with a time interval between data points. No collection of behavioural data can realistically be continuous; there will always be gaps of time when no data are being collected. For example, even if we interviewed a sample every day, one could argue that during the night no data were collected, thus producing a break in continuity. Even a seismograph cannot, in practise, continuously monitor the Earth's movements, because the digital input operates at some hertz cycle of input that is broken in time, even if it is only one-sixtieth of a second between data points. Time may be theoretically continuous, but any mechanism to measure it or record events over time will be interrupted. Thus, we can have only a concept of CCD. The continuity is given more by the "sufficient" proximity among the observations (i.e., the repeated surveys on independent samples) than by the actual continuity of the data collection.

Although CCD cannot be truly continuous, frequent collection of information can create a continuous stream of data. For some stable population behaviours monthly or even quarterly data collection can produce sufficient data points to pick up subtleties in behavioural change, whereas some very unstable variables could require day-in, day-out observation. Nonetheless, stable and unstable behaviours may be bundled in a way that makes them time dependent on each other. The important point is that the data stream is ongoing, over an extended time, without any long periods of interruption. Thus a time-based data stream is produced. Such data may be characterised as dynamic rather than static, as usually produced by the typical cross-sectional survey. This chracteristic is how we define continuous data as used in behavioural surveillance.

⎣In this chapter I discuss possible ways to solve problems of analysis that arise in dealing with CCD. My purpose is not to give a complete, ultimate list of methods that must be used in the different scenarios, but to emphasise the richness of the CCD approach.⎦ Presented are typical substantial questions that could arise when CCD are available, and possible appropriate methodologies to address the situations.

2. SAMPLE GOALS AND APPROACHES

Some research goals and possible approaches that use CCD in a scheme are presented in Table 1. I cannot present and discuss all the methodological aspects; that would be well beyond the scope of a single chapter and involve extensive scientific literature. Instead, for each of the six goals listed I present three components: why problems of changes over time arise in health promotion and disease prevention, how these data could inform the situation, and what the proposed methodological approach could be. I then illustrate each schema by reviewing work (most already published) done within the surveillance system described above, seeking more to clarify the approach than the sophistication or the relevance of the application itself.

2.1. Simple Trend Estimates

Every country's public health agency has always placed great importance on tracking disease trends. This interest has historically been dominated by a concern with changes in infectious disease trends, but the rise of the awareness of the global burden of chronic diseases has generated interest in tracking non-infectious diseases as well. In the later half of the 20th century there arose increasing interest in following and exploring the so-called "real" causes of most chronic diseases, namely behavioural risk factors. In health promotion and public health planning, such trends are viewed as basic information.

Tracking behaviour has usually relied on rather simplistic estimates of trends. Commonly, behaviours are compared from year to year, based on large data sets. This approach is very rough and at best provides only very general direction as to changes over time. We want to discover not only whether trends are moving up or down, but also the dynamic characteristics of the trends. Are they slowing down, speeding up, wobbling, etc.? These are the kinds of questions typically asked in econometrics and financial trend reporting, but seldom considered in public health. CCD allow for a more appropriate and dynamic approach to understanding such trends. Simple regression techniques that do not take into account possible auto-correlation effects could give biased estimates (and, particularly, testing) of the real trend. Auto-regressive integrated moving average (ARIMA) and similar models solve this and similar kind of problems, offering better estimates.

In an analysis of data from the LAH study, the aim was to determine whether a trend was detectable in some AIDS-related variables describing behaviours and attitudes, to better understand possible links among changes in these variables (Table 2) (see also Section 2.4). Once auto-correlation was checked through the Durbin-Watson test, a simple regression (logistic, because of the dichotomous dependent variable) was run to determine which variables seemed more promising to study.

Table 1. Possible approaches to analysing continuously collected data over time

Goal	Approach	Data type	Reference	Why
Simple trend estimates	Time series analysis	Series of monthly estimates	Box & Jenkins (1970), McCleary & Hay (1980), Scott et al. (1977), Smith (1978)	Improve the quality of the estimates, smooth trends, take out seasonality (if any), and forecast future values.
	Regression techniques	All the raw data	Johnston (1984), Ostrom (1990)	As above, but there is no control on seasonality, so forecasting can be less precise.
"Sophisticated" trend estimates (and inter-action among variables)	Dynamic linear models	Series of monthly estimates	West & Harrison (1989)	Take maximum advantage of the continuous data stream.
Deconstruction of change	Composite estimation	All the raw data	Holt & Skinner (1989)	Decompose an observed change into effects due to net differences within domains and to effects due to changing domain composition.
Trends and changes in the association among variables	Log-linear analysis	All the raw data	Hagenaars (1990), Payne et al. (1993)	Deal with categorical variables, when more interested in finding out the association among them and how this evolves over time.
Evaluation and intervention analyses	Interrupted time series analysis	Series of monthly estimates	Box & Tiao (1975), McDowell et al. (1980)	As in first row, but also estimate if a change has occurred at a given point.
	Impact analysis	Raw data	Heckman & Hotz (1989)	Not as interested in the trends as in the net effect of the intervention.
	Impact analysis using pseudo-panel	Series of estimates for cohorts	Deaton (1985), Moffitt (1993), Piazzetta et al.*	As above, also taking maximum advantage of the structure of the data.
Estimate of the change point over time	Change-point analysis	Series of monthly estimates	Siegmund (1985), Campostrini & Pallini (1991)	When the change happened isn't known; non-parametric perspective.

* Frederico Piazzetta, Enrico Rettore, and Stefano Campostrini, Department of Statistical Sciences, University of Padua, Italy, 1998.

Table 2. Trends of some AIDS-related variables among persons in Scotland aged 18–40 years, Lifestyle and Health survey, 1987 and 1992

Variable	1987 (n = 3,000)	1992 (n = 3,000)	Beta[a]
Changed anything in your daily life because of AIDS			
Have changed	12%	21%	.021[b]
Will change	8%	8%	NS
No change	80%	70%	−.016[b]
Talk about AIDS with your friends			
Often	25%	22%	−.008[b]
Seldom	62%	63%	NS
Never	12%	15%	.009[b]
Condom use			
No use	39%	27%	−.020[b]
Former use	40%	39%	NS
Using	12%	16%	.009[b]
Using as protection	8%	15%	.036[b]
Number of partners			
0	5%	5%	NS
1	61%	60%	NS
2 or 3	19%	23%	.006[b]
4–10	14%	13%	NS

NS = not significant.
[a] Comparison of estimated slope co-efficients from a logistic regression in which time (month of observation; 400 cases each month for 60 months) was considered an independent variable.
[b] Hypothesis of beta = 0 rejected at $p < .01$.
Source: Research Unit in Health and Behavioural Change, Edinburgh.

2.2. "Sophisticated" Trend Estimates (and Inter-Action among Variables)

A simple comparison of a variable at two points in time provides basic information, but the real desire in data analysis is to understand and model more subtle trends over time. There has been an increasing recognition of the complexity of behavioural data, especially the idea that behavioural changes are set in a multi-variate context that needs to be considered. CCD analysis allows for much more consideration of the rich possibilities of interpretation of data. Recent statistical studies have shown how the classic regression problem could be revised considering the parameters as random components. This randomness could be used to interpret both the dynamic of the data and the behavioural processes we wish to observe.

Another consideration, perhaps more subtle from a methodological point of view, is critical in promoting studies of the application of dynamic analyses to CCD. Very few studies have been done so far. It is certainly possible and correct (Smith, 1978) to use the standard time series tools to analyse trends in CCD-based survey systems; nevertheless, we usually analyse monthly means (or weekly or whatever, depending on the data collection strategy) (see Figure 1) but we cannot take into consideration the monthly observed variability around those means. Quite often, this variability is not relevant for the substantial problem we want to analyse (this is the case of the analysis shown in Figure 1), but when we need more—when we want to understand what is behind a process, and not only whether it had taken place—perhaps we would like to use all the information possible (i.e., including the monthly observed variability).

2.3. Deconstruction of Change

Quite often, we will observe a change in a variable over time (e.g., percentage of smokers in a certain area) and wonder whether this has been caused by a real change or simply by a change in the population's demographic composition. By deconstructing change, we can study the "net" change over the variable of interest, once changes in other domains have been removed. This approach is useful in decomposing an observed change into effects due to net differences within domains and to effects due to changing domain composition. Realistically, only CCD can accurately monitor these changes and only then when it is analysed appropriately and dynamically.

2.4. Trends and Changes in the Association among Variables

Particularly when we are dealing with "global" measures (e.g., the level of a population's perceived health status), our interest is in determining which of the other variables observed has influenced a detected (broad) change, rather than in observing relatively small changes in single variables. The availability of data over time is essential to answering this kind of question, because time could be used as proxy for many other unobservable measures and because time itself could play an important role in explaining the relationship between the variables considered. For example, quite often we might wish to explain the association among observed *changes* in some variables and not the *levels* of the same variables.

Logit and log-linear models are essential tools in analysing the association among categorical variables. When time is considered a variable, these models can help unveil associations among the other variables through standardising by the time (i.e., time is confounding) or through observing how this association changes over time (i.e., time is interacting). An example of the application of this approach to some of the data in Table 2 is presented in Table 3. This was the question: "An increase in condom use has

Table 3. Comparison of the goodness of fit for three log-linear models of AIDS-related variables among persons in Scotland aged 18–40 years, Lifestyle and Health survey, 1987–1992 (N = 14,666)

Model	Degrees of freedom	Likelihood ratio	p Value
CAY (saturated)			1.00
CA, AY, CY	4	3.22	.521
CY, AY	5	369.07	.000

A = declared change because of AIDS; C = current use of condoms; Y = time by year of interview (from July to June).
Source: Research Unit in Health and Behavioural Change, Edinburgh.

been observed; could this be attributable to changes in AIDS-related knowledge and attitudes?" This kind of analysis offers this possible answer: "The third model suggests that the association between each two variables is identical when the third is held constant. For example, the association between condom use and declared changes is the same for all periods considered (i.e., the association is stable over time). Thus, the declared intention to change something because of AIDS and the actual change in behaviour (i.e., the use of condom) was significantly related over time, both when the declared changes involved only a small percentage of population (12% in 1987) and when this proportion had almost doubled (21% in 1992)."

2.5. Evaluation and Intervention Analyses

Has the programme or intervention produced the expected outcome? Are the observed changes attributable to (only) the programme? These and similar questions arise often in health promotion activities, particularly when we are dealing with global programmes targeted to the general population. When this is the case, experimental data are difficult to collect. Even when data collection is feasible, substantial problems such as attrition or selection bias could arise. The quasi-experimental design could be an appropriate solution to address causality questions and to study the (net) impact of an intervention. CCD could offer a good quasi-experimental set.

There are several possibilities for appropriate techniques for analysis once CCD are collected; these techniques take into account time trends, building on multiple observations. More than 7 years of BRFSS data for one state, regarding the prevalence of drinking and driving, are presented in Figure 1. Here the question to be analysed is fairly simple: Did the change in the law regulating driving under the influence of alcohol affect people's behaviour? Using these BRFSS data and interrupted time series analysis, we can demonstrate that a simple change in the law reducing the percentage of alcohol allowed

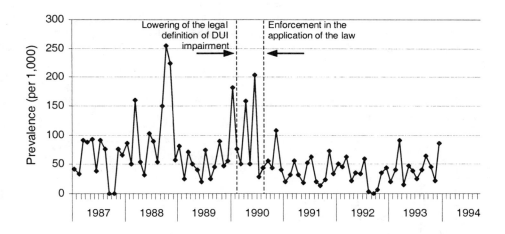

Figure 1. The time series: monthly average estimated number of episodes of driving under the influence (DUI) in California, per 1,000 persons, Behavioral Risk Factor Surveillance System, January 1987–January 1994 (N = 20,006).

in the blood did not produce a significant change, whereas increased law enforcement (immediate suspension of the driving license) substantially affected Californians' drinking and driving behaviours. It is interesting to note that these results are also found with time series analysis of motor vehicle accidents among drunk drivers.

2.6. Estimate of the Change Point over Time

When did a change occur? Is there a specific point in time in which a change can be detected? Can a change observed in one variable be related to the ones observed (possibly in different time points) in other variables? CCD on several specific variables can offer the opportunity to answer these questions. To have a system running and collecting data on the major health problems can help answer questions which are now not crucial but could be tomorrow.

The parametric estimation can be difficult in this kind of problem. Statistical researchers have found reasonable ways to answer these questions, using CCD, through non-parametric estimation methods and combinations of dependent tests. An example is a study conducted at the University of Edinburgh using data from the LAH survey (Campostrini and Pallini, 1991). Here the problems were detecting and analysing the significance of the links among possible changes in AIDS-related variables. Two were methodological problems. The first was the necessity for an exploratory technique to detect changes difficult or impossible to situate in a specific time point. Such changes in AIDS-related attitudes can be the result of an organised intervention (e.g., a public health campaign) for which quite often the effects are not immediate and can be delayed over an unforecastable period of time, or the result of a non-organised event (e.g., a pop star's death because of AIDS) that is, by definition, unforecastable. The second problem was finding a way to estimate the overall significance of the observed changes, which can be dependent but not necessarily simultaneous. As I stated previously, changes in knowledge, attitude, and behaviours can happen at different times.

With the availability of a data stream, the first problem has been solved by using the so-called change-point test (James et al., 1987); the second problem has been addressed through a non-parametric combination of several dependent tests (Pesarin, 1991). The main results of the study are summarised in Table 4. The period of observation was

Table 4. Change-point tests and the minimum time needed to estimate change in several AIDS-related variables, persons in Scotland aged 18–40 years, Lifestyle and Health survey, 1988–1991

	Change-point test (p value)	Minimum no. of months needed to estimate change
Variable		
How often do you talk about AIDS?	.107	2
How concerned are you about getting AIDS?	.007	34
Knowledge index	.209	4
Risk index	.065	27
Combined test statistics	.062	

Source: Research Unit in Health and Behavioural Change, Edinburgh.

3 years (1988–1991) and the variables examined were two attitude assessments, one index summarising the level of knowledge about AIDS, and one index summarising the level of risk of infection from sexual behaviours. It is interesting to notice how the association among the observed changes was significant ($p = .062$), although the single observed changes were significant to different extents ($.01 < p < .21$).

3. CONCLUSION

As the field of evaluation in health promotion enters the 21st century, there are many challenges. Much of health promotion evaluation will be concerned with issues regarding participatory interventions, where qualitative approaches are most appropriate. However, there will always be an important place for sound quantitative approaches to the evaluation of interventions, particularly at the population level. Policy-makers will continue to want and rely on numerical data for decision making. Nonetheless, routine analyses of point-in-time surveys of the type which have become all too commonplace in health promotion provide a less than adequate understanding for the complexity of health promotion interventions and behavioural changes in a population. Only when the full analytic advantages of CCD are realised will interventions be better understood and results more useful to decision-makers.

4. REFERENCES

Agresti, A., 1990, *Categorical Data Analysis*, John Wiley & Sons, New York.

Box, G. E. P., and Jenkins, G. M., 1970, *Time Series Analysis: Forecasting and Control*, Holden-Day, San Francisco.

Box, G. E. P., and Tiao, G. C., 1975, Intervention analysis with applications to economic and environmental problems, *J Am Stat Assoc*. **70**:70–79.

Campostrini, S., 1996, Dynamic approaches to the study of behaviour: the continuous collection of data in comparison with panel surveys, *Stat Applicata*. **8**:695–708.

Campostrini, S., and McQueen, D. V., 1993, Sexual behavior and exposure to risk of infection: estimates based on an index for the general population, *Am J Public Health*. **83**:1139–1143.

Campostrini, S., and Pallini, A., 1991, Analysis of change for AIDS-related variables: a non-parametric combination of dependent tests, Università di Padova, Italy (Working Paper del Dipartimento di Scienze Statistiche No. 10).

Deaton, A., 1985, Panel data from time series of cross-sections, *J Econometrics*. **30**:109–126.

Escobedo, L. G., Chorba, T. L., Remington, P. L., et al., 1992, The influence of safety belt laws on self-reported safety belt use in the United States, *Accid Anal Prev*. **24**:643–653.

Goodman, L. A., 1972a, A general model for the analysis of surveys, *Am J Sociol*. **77**:1035–1086.

Goodman, L. A., 1972b, A modified multiple regression approach to the analysis of dichotomous variables, *Am Sociol Rev*. **37**:28–46.

Hagenaars, J. A., 1990, *Categorical Longitudinal Data*, Sage, Newbury Park, CA.

Hastie, T., and Tibshirani, R., 1993, Varying-coefficient models, *J R Stat Soc B*. **55**:757–796.

Heckman, J., and Hotz, J., 1989, Choosing among alternative nonexperimental methods for estimating the impact of social programs, *J Am Stat Assoc*. **84**:862–874.

Holt, D., and Skinner, C. J., 1989, Components of change in repeated surveys, *Int Stat Rev*. **57**:1–18.

James, B., James, K. L., and Siegmund, D., 1987, Tests for a change-point, *Biometrika*. **74**:71–83.

Johnston, J., 1984, *Econometric Methods, Third Edition*, McGraw-Hill, New York.

McCleary, R., and Hay, R. A., 1980, *Applied Time Series Analysis for the Social Sciences*, Sage, Beverly Hills, CA.

McDowell, D., McCleary, R., Meidinger, E., et al., 1980, *Interrupted Time Series Analysis*, Sage, Newbury Park, CA (Quantitative Applications in the Social Sciences Series).

McQueen, D. V., Bellini, P., and Campostrini, S., 1992a, Measuring behaviour and behavioural change: the continuously collected data approach, Research Unit in Health and Behavioural Change, Edinburgh (European Sciences Foundation Network on Household Panel Studies, Working Paper Series, No. 34).

McQueen, D. V., Uitenbroek, D. G., and Campostrini, S., 1992b, Implementation and maintenance of a continuous population survey by CATI, Proceedings of the 1992 Bureau Census Research Conference, Washington, DC.

Moffitt, R., 1993, Identification and estimation of dynamic models with a time series of repeated cross-sections, *J Econometrics.* **59**:99–123.

Nelson, D. E., Thompson, B. L., Bland, S. D., et al., 1999, Trends in perceived cost as a barrier to medical care, 1991–1996, *Am J Public Health.* **89**:1410–1413.

Ostrom, C. W., 1990, *Time Series Analysis: Regression Techniques*, Sage, Newbury Park, CA (Quantitative Applications in the Social Sciences Series).

Payne, C., Payne, J., and Heath, A., 1993, Modelling trends in multiway tables, in: *Analysing Social and Political Change: A Casebook of Methods*, R. Davies and A. Dale, eds., Sage, London.

Pesarin, F., 1991, A resampling procedure for a nonparametric combination of several dependent tests, *J Ital Stat Assoc.* **1**:87–101.

Scott, A. J., Smith, T. M. F., and Jones, R. G., 1977, The application of time series methods to the analysis of repeated surveys, *Int Stat Rev.* **45**:13–28.

Siegmund, D., 1985, *Sequential Analysis,* Springer-Verlag, New York.

Smith, T. M. F., 1978, Principles and problems in the analysis of repeated surveys, in: *Survey Sampling and Measurement*, N. K. Namboodiri, ed., Academic Press, New York, pp. 206–216.

Spall, J. C., ed., 1988, *Bayesian Analysis of Time Series and Dynamic Model*, Marcel Dekker, New York.

West, M., and Harrison, J., 1989, *Bayesian Forecasting and Dynamic Models*, John Wiley and Sons, New York.

CHAPTER 7

FINBALT HEALTH MONITOR
Monitoring Health Behaviour in Finland and the Baltic Countries

Ritva Prättälä, Ville Helasoja, and the Finbalt Group[*]

1. INTRODUCTION

Finland and the Baltic countries are geographically close (Figure 1) and have many cultural ties. However, the countries are going through different stages of economic and social development. Thus, the Baltic Sea region provides a unique opportunity for the study of any phenomena related to social changes. Public health situations in Estonia, Finland, Latvia, and Lithuania are very different. Life expectancy at birth is 5 to 10 years higher in Finland than in the Baltic countries. During the last decades life expectancy in Finland has increased relatively steadily, while in the Baltic countries the development has been less favorable (Zvidrins and Krumins, 1993; Puska et al., 1995). The latest statistics, however, show an increase in life expectancy also in the Baltic countries (Nordic Medico-Statistical Committee, 1998; World Health Organization [WHO] Regional Office for Europe, 2001a).

The Finbalt Health Monitor is a collaborative system for monitoring health behaviour and related factors in Estonia, Finland, Latvia, and Lithuania (Prättälä et al., 1999). The origins of the project are in Finnish health promotion activities related to prevention of chronic conditions (Puska et al., 1995). The Finnish system, launched in 1978, consists of an annual mailed questionnaire, the Health Behaviour among Finnish Adult Population (AVTK) survey. As the title indicates, the AVTK survey acquires information on adult Finns. Smoking, food habits, and other health-related factors (e.g., alcohol consumption, physical activity, subjective health, and symptoms), as well as socio-demographic and psycho-social factors associated with these, have been included in the survey (Helakorpi et al., 1998).

[*] Ritva Prättälä and Ville Helasoja, National Public Health Institute, 00300 Helsinki, Finland. Principal investigators of the Baltic countries: Anu Kasmel, Estonian Centre for Health Promotion, 10130 Tallinn, Estonia; Jurate Klumbiene, Kaunas University of Medicine, 3007 Kaunas, Lithuania; Iveta Pudule, Health Promotion Centre, 1010 Riga, Latvia.

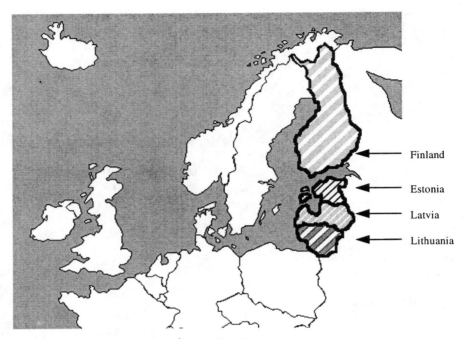

Figure 1. The Finbalt countries.

In collaboration with the National Public Health Institute of Finland (KTL), a monitoring system similar to the Finnish one was launched in Estonia in 1990. Lithuania joined the system in 1994, and Latvia in 1998. A biennial health behaviour survey directed to a random sample of adult population forms the basis of the system.

The Finbalt Health Monitor has both practical and theoretical purposes. The system serves public information, programme planning, and evaluation needs of the individual countries. In addition to its practical purposes, the system produces a databank which can be used in comparative research on health behaviour and related factors.

In this chapter we aim to give relevant background information of the Finbalt system to researchers and health administrators working in health-related international projects. Development of the questionnaire is described, and reliability of results evaluated. Finally, we discuss the limitations and advantages of the system. We hope the details presented here help in interpreting the results of the Finbalt project and in planning and evaluating similar projects.

2. ESTONIA, FINLAND, LATVIA, AND LITHUANIA: NATIONS AND POPULATIONS

Situated between Eastern and Western Europe, Finland and the Baltic countries have tumultuous histories. The Baltic Sea has provided an important economic and cultural link between the countries. The countries are influenced by both the Scandinavian and

Central European culture and politics, and also by Anglo-American ideologies. All countries also have historical ties with Russia and the Soviet Union. Trade and politics, as well as linguistic relations and religions, have all contributed to the interaction between the countries. Denmark, Germany, Poland, Sweden, Russia, and the Soviet Union have by turns ruled considerable parts of the region. Until 1809 Finland was part of Sweden, then an autonomous province of Russia. German influence has been strong in Estonia and Latvia since the Middle Ages. Later Denmark and Sweden held large parts of Estonia. Lithuania was more influenced by Poland than by the other Baltic countries.

Latvian and Lithuanian belong to Baltic languages, Estonian and Finnish to the Fenno-Ugrian family. Estonia and Finland have been Lutheran Protestant since the 16th century, Lithuania is Roman Catholic, and in Latvia there are both Roman Catholics and Protestants (WHO Regional Office for Europe, 1996a, 1996b, 1996c).

Finland reached independence from Russia in 1917 and identified with Western economy, culture, and everyday life. After World War II the country experienced a rapid transition from an agrarian society into a modern Scandinavian welfare state. Integration of Finland with other European countries has strengthened during the last 5 years: Finland joined the European Union in 1995 and the European Monetary Union in 1998.

All the Baltic countries had a period of independence between 1920 and 1940; thereafter they were incorporated into the Soviet Union. After World War II the centralised Soviet rule lead to re-orientation of the economic structure. Industrial plants re-shaped the economy, in particular in Estonia. Lithuania remained more agricultural than the other two Baltic countries. Lithuania became independent in 1990; Estonia and Latvia in 1991.

The process of political, economic, and cultural transition is in a different phase in each Baltic country. Estonia has proceeded further than the other two, at least in the reform of the economy. In Estonia and Latvia, the establishment of a market economy has pushed aside social policy issues. The process in Lithuania seems to have been less dramatic and more emphasis has been laid on social security (Simpura, 1995). The material living standard differs between Finland and the Baltic countries. For example, in Finland the real gross domestic product (measured in PPP$) was about three times higher than those in the Baltic countries in the mid-1990s (WHO, 2001).

The population of Estonia is 1,5 million, of which about 65% are Estonians and 30% Russians (Statistical Office of Estonia, 1997). In Finland there are 5,1 million inhabitants. The country is ethnically very homogenous. Over 90% of Finns have Finnish as their native language, and about 6% Swedish (Statistics Finland, 1997). Of the 2,4 million inhabitants of Latvia, only 56% are Latvians. The largest ethnic group is the Russians (32%); the others include Belarussians, Ukrainians, Poles, and Lithuanians (WHO Regional Office for Europe, 2001a). Lithuania is ethnically the most homogenous Baltic country; of its 3,7 million inhabitants, 81% are Lithuanians; the rest are Russians, Poles, and other nationalities (WHO Regional Office for Europe, 2001b).

Birth rates have declined in all the countries. In the Baltic countries the decline was especially steep, from 16 to below 10 live births per 1,000 habitants in a decade. Between 1990 and 1993 birth rates in all Baltic countries dropped below the Finnish level. At the turn of the century the lowest number was observed in Latvia and the highest in Finland (8 and 11 live births per 1,000 inhabitants, respectively) (WHO, 2001). In the Baltic countries the population has, because of high migration and mortality rates, decreased. The decrease has been larger in Estonia and Latvia than in Lithuania. Migration was especially extensive in Estonia and Latvia in 1992 (21,9 and 17,8 persons per 1,000 inhabitants, respectively) (Nordic Medico-Statistical Committee, 1998).

3. CONDUCTING THE FINBALT HEALTH MONITOR

3.1. Origins and History of the Finbalt Project

The sharp contrast in health conditions around the Baltic Sea in the early 1990s—the increase in life expectancy in Finland versus the decrease in the Baltic countries—was the starting point of the Finbalt Health Monitor. The project focuses on health-related lifestyles (e.g., smoking, alcohol consumption, food habits, and physical activity) because cardiovascular diseases, alcohol-related violent deaths, and cancer are the major causes of mortality. To plan health promotion and disease prevention programmes, information on health lifestyles and their social and cultural determinants is necessary.

The collapse of the Soviet system had social and economic consequences not only in the Baltic countries but also in Finland. The social and economic changes were much more dramatic in the Baltic countries, but Finland experienced an economic depression as well. Great social change may influence the health and lifestyle of individuals. Therefore, following trends in health behaviour was considered important right from the start of the Finbalt project.

Finnish health authorities and public health scientists have successfully implemented health promotion programmes aimed at preventing non-communicable diseases. This experience was used in planning the Finbalt Health Monitor. The origins of the Finbalt system are in the Finnish North Karelia project, a demonstration programme for prevention of cardiovascular diseases (Puska et al., 1995). In that project various evaluation and information procedures were developed, one of which was a health behaviour questionnaire. In 1978 the questionnaire was transferred to the national level because it was considered a useful instrument for health professionals and administrators in evaluating the effectiveness of national health policy and health promotion activities. Since then the national cross-sectional questionnaire has been carried out every year by KTL and supported by the Finnish Ministry of Social Affairs and Health.

In collaboration with KTL, the health behaviour monitoring system was launched in Estonia in 1990 (Lipand et al., 1995). The first survey coincided with a Finnish–Estonian smoking cessation programme. In Lithuania the first national health behaviour survey was carried out in 1994 (Grabauskas et al., 1997) and thereafter, similarly to Estonia, every second year. Latvia joined the project in 1997. The survey was carried out simultaneously in all Baltic countries and Finland for the first time in the spring of 1998.

3.2. Administration of the Finbalt Project

The Finbalt Health Monitor is funded from different sources, of which KTL and the Finnish Ministry of Social Affairs and Health are the most significant. The Finnish funding enabled the hiring of one full-time researcher/data analyst beginning in 1998. In addition to this, the funding provides a half-time co-ordinator, regular meetings of the project group, and printing of the national reports. The research centres in Estonia, Latvia, and Lithuania finance the collection and analyses of their national data.

The Finbalt Health Monitor organisation consists of (1) a steering committee, (2) a co-ordinating centre, and (3) national monitoring centres. KTL co-ordinates the comparative project. Each participating country has a national research centre with a responsible researcher and other members of the study team. The steering committee has a representative from each national centre and the Finnish co-ordinating centre. Each national centre owns its own data and carries out the national analysis independently. The general principles of analyses, as well as the structure of the national reports and joint publications, are discussed and agreed on in project meetings. The steering committee, the co-ordinator, and two to four members of each national research team have met twice a year. The meeting places rotate among the national centres. To harmonise principles of data entry, organise files, and plan the analyses, statisticians and researchers from the Baltic countries have paid separate visits to the Finnish co-ordinating centre (Prättälä et al., 1999).

3.3. Development of the Finbalt Questionnaire

The predecessor of the Finbalt questionnaire was used in 1972, before the initiation of the North Karelia project. A baseline survey on risk factors and health behaviour was needed before the planned health promotion activities could be implemented in the demonstration area. The effects of the project were evaluated by repeating the baseline survey, a mailed questionnaire on health behaviour and risk factors. In 1978 the idea of the repeated cross-sectional surveys grew into a national monitoring system, which used the AVTK survey. The Finnish health authorities considered it important to increase information on the trends and prevalences of risk factors of major diseases in the whole country. There was a lack of information especially concerning smoking and other dimensions of health behaviour. In addition to the example of the North Karelia project, some other countries' systems, like the U.S. National Health Interview Survey (U.S. Department of Health, Education, and Welfare, 1975) and the Canadian health survey (Woods, 1977), influenced the Finnish health behaviour monitoring system. The Finnish national monitoring system, which started in 1978, focused on health behaviour and subjective health, not on mortality, morbidity, environmental, or biological risk factors. Since the focus was on health behaviour, the system could be carried out with the help of a mailed questionnaire and its costs could be kept relatively low (Rose and Blackburn, 1968; Puska, 1978).

Before every Finbalt monitoring survey, an English-language version of the questionnaire is prepared and agreed on in project meetings involving experts from all participating countries. In the project group there are medical, nutritional, and social science researchers, as well as health administrators. The working language of the team is English, but the Estonian and Finnish participants can also communicate in Finnish and the Baltic participants in Russian.

In the English-language version there are usually about 100 questions. When planning the English version, the project steering committee decides on the importance of each question to the system: the questions are collectively classified into "obligatory," "recommended," or "optional." The obligatory questions deal with socio-demographic background, health (i.e., health services, diseases, subjective health), smoking, food habits, height, weight, and physical activity. To allow comparisons between the countries, the obligatory questions and most of the recommended questions are included in the national questionnaires in an identical form. The number and formulations of the optional questions may vary among the countries. Because of differences in local conditions (e.g., in food selection), some questions are relevant only in one country. Therefore, each country may also have its own questions based on local interests.

In some cases it has been necessary to include local response categories even to the obligatory questions. If local categories are added, they have to fall clearly into one of the shared categories.

The multi-disciplinary expertise of the project team is extremely valuable when decisions are made on the concepts and formulations used in the questionnaires. Because of practical reasons a great majority of the questions are structured. This means that all the relevant options from which a respondent may choose an answer have to be known to the project team in advance. Thus, planning the questionnaire requires a good knowledge of the culture, living conditions, and health problems of the target groups.

The questionnaires have been mailed to respondents in April and May. The completed forms are expected to be returned within 1 to 2 weeks. Those who do not answer the questionnaire are reminded once, whereafter still another reminder with a new form may be sent out. The number of reminders varies from one to three in the different countries. The countries have used a similar type of cover letter, which describes the purpose of the survey and guarantees anonymity. Filling out the survey is considered to imply informed consent. In Latvia and Lithuania the first page of the questionnaire form has been the cover letter. The size of the questionnaire leaflet/booklet has been either A4 or A5; since 2000 all the countries have used the larger A4 size. No material incentives have been offered in any country except Latvia, where a lottery with small prizes was organised for the respondents.

In all the countries there are ethnic groups that do not speak the main language of the country. Efforts have been made to allow the respondents to answer in their native language. In Finland the languages are Finnish and Swedish, and the Swedish-speaking Finns have been identified on the basis of the population register. In the Baltic countries it is not possible to identify the native language of the respondents from registers. Therefore, in Estonia the native language, Estonian or Russian, has been identified on the basis of the person's name and place of residence. A similar procedure was used in Latvia during the first survey. In unidentified or unclear cases, respondents were informed that they could ask for an Estonian-, Latvian-, or Russian-language questionnaire. During the first reminder all respondents were informed that they could ask for a new questionnaire in the other language. The number of those asking for the new questionnaire was very low—5 to 10 persons. In Lithuania mainly the Lithuanian-language version has been used, but in 1998 a Russian version of the questionnaire was used in some cases: if a non-respondent had a Russian name, a Russian-language form was mailed. The Russian versions used in Estonia and Latvia have been cross-checked, although they are, because of differences in the local questions, not identical.

In modifying and translating the Finnish questionnaire to be suitable for the Baltic countries, detailed face-to-face discussions in the project team have been the most effective way to avoid mis-interpretations. Translation procedures have not been completely identical in each country, and professional translators have not been used in all cases. The original Finnish questions were first translated into English by the Finnish researchers. The first Estonian and Russian translations were made as a team by the Estonian and Finnish researchers; later, translation-back-translation procedures were adapted. In Lithuania the English version has been translated by two independent translators into Lithuanian. Both translations have been analysed by a third person, after which an agreement of the final version of the questionnaire has been achieved.

3.4. Main Domains of the 1998 Finbalt Questionnaire

The annual questionnaires have been kept as similar as possible in each country. Some modifications and corrections have, however, been necessary because of changing conditions (e.g., introduction of new margarines into the market) and observed problems in comparability. Because of the similarity of the questionnaires during the years 1990–1998, only the 1998 version will be described here.

The shared part of the Finbalt questionnaire of 1998 had 65 questions (Table 1). Similar to the earlier rounds, each of the participating countries included some additional questions of local interest. Almost all these questions dealt with personal attributes and behaviours of the respondents. Only three of the shared questions were attitude- and belief-oriented. The questions can be classified into six domains according to their substance: background information (8 questions), health services and health status (15), smoking (17), food habits (12), alcohol consumption (2), and other questions, such as height, weight, physical activity, and traffic safety (11). Most of the questions were close-ended with either unordered or ordered response choices. There were no fully open-ended questions. Partially close-ended questions were used to provide respondents with more alternatives and also to obtain quantitative information, such as year of birth. The majority of the questions consisted of only one item, but questions on diseases, symptoms, medication, and use of common foods comprised series of separate items.

3.4.1. Background Information

The questionnaire began with obligatory questions on sex, year of birth, and marital status. The question on education, "How many years altogether have you gone to school or studied full-time in your life?" was also obligatory. Questions on family size and type of work were classified as recommended.

Education was the only obligatory variable measuring socio-economic status in the Finbalt Health Monitor. Compared with other measures of socio-economic status, such as occupation or income, education has advantages (Mackenbach and Kunst, 1997). Each economically active or inactive person can be classified according to his or her

Table 1. Summary of the 1998 Finbalt questionnaires

	Common	Estonia	Finland	Latvia	Lithuania
Size of questionnaire form (mm)	Not specified	152*210	210*304	152*210	152*210
Language	English	Estonian Russian	Finnish Swedish	Latvian Russian	Lithuanian
Total no. of questions	65	77	125	87	88
Background information	8	11	9	10	9
Health services and health status	15	17	22	21	28
Smoking	17	11	27	13	17
Food habits	12	11	20	14	14
Alcohol consumption	2	3	4	8	5
Height, weight, and physical activity	5	5	9	5	6
Traffic safety	4	6	6	4	4
Others	2	13	28	12	5

education. Occupation is a comprehensive indicator of socio-economic status but difficult to measure.

The educational systems as well as the general level of education vary in Estonia, Finland, Latvia, and Lithuania. Therefore, the project team has not found a question which could measure the different educational levels comparably. A question on the number of school years has been considered the best alternative. The duration of compulsory schooling is 9 years in all countries.

3.4.2. Health Services and Health Status

Health-related questions were focused on major public health problems, especially cardiovascular diseases. There were altogether 15 obligatory or recommended questions on health status and the use of health services. The first questions asked about visits to the general practitioner and absence at work due to sickness. The group of questions on health and illness included a list of common diseases and symptoms, as well as evaluation of the respondent's general state of health, mental well-being, use of medication, and some aspects of preventive behaviour (e.g., blood pressure and cholesterol checkups).

Self-rated health was used as the main measure of health status in the Finbalt system because of its simplicity. It has also been recommended by WHO for monitoring population health (de Bruin et al., 1996). Self-rated health has been found to be a strong predictor of morbidity and mortality (Idler et al., 1990).

3.4.3. Smoking

Questions on smoking form a significant part of the Finbalt questionnaire because of the importance of smoking as a risk factor. Their inclusion follow the guidelines of WHO expert groups (Rose and Blackburn, 1968; WHO, informal consultation on Tobacco Control Guidelines, Geneva, 1995) to facilitate monitoring of the tobacco epidemic and comparisons between countries. Especially in Finland, the system has been used in the evaluation of several anti-smoking and health promotion campaigns. The 1998 version of the questionnaire included 17 individual questions on smoking which followed the terms suggested by WHO. "Do you smoke daily, occasionally, or not at all?" and "How many of the following items do you smoke per day (...)?" are the two key questions recommended by WHO. In addition to these questions, a series of questions dealing with previous smoking, exposure to smoke at home or in the workplace, willingness to quit, and concern about harmful effects of smoking and a group of questions measuring nicotine dependence (Fagerstrom, 1978) belong to the core of the Finbalt questionnaire.

3.4.4. Food Habits

In a broad questionnaire covering several dimensions of health behaviour, detailed measures of food consumption cannot be included. Therefore, the survey does not provide quantitative information on food consumption and nutrient intake. The data can, however, be used in identifying extreme groups, such as "high" and "low" users of certain foods.

The original Finnish food questions designed in the late 1970s were based on the contemporary knowledge of healthy and unhealthy diets. When the Finnish system started, the use of butter on bread was a good indicator of high intake of saturated fats (Räsänen and Pietinen, 1982). However, recent studies have shown that the predictive value of this particular question has decreased especially among women (Roos et al., 1995). In the Baltic countries no studies on the validity of short survey questions concerning food habits have been carried out.

In 1994, the questionnaire included 30 separate food-related questions. The obligatory questions dealt with cooking fats, bread spreads, fruits, vegetables, coffee, tea, sugar, and bread. The 1990–1996 questionnaires omitted many usual food items like meat, potatoes, cheese, rice, and pasta. In the 1998 version the section of food habits was modified and a new type of food question including several items was added. The respondent was asked to mark the frequency of 17 common food items: "How often during the last week have you consumed the following foods and drinks?" The respondent could choose one of the following: never, 1 to 2 days a week, 3 to 5 days a week, or 6 to 7 days a week. Questions on fruits and vegetables, which previously were asked separately, were included in this larger question. The former obligatory questions on cooking fats, bread spreads, meats, coffee, tea, sugar, and bread were unchanged.

The new food frequency question was based on the 1997 Dietary Survey of Finnish Adults (National Public Health Institute, 1998) and the survey Health Behaviour among Finnish Adult Population (Helakorpi et al., 1997), but it has not been validated against other dietary survey methods. However, preliminary or pilot surveys showed that moving the earlier individual questions on the use of fruits, vegetables, and sweet pastries into items of the food frequency series did not influence the results significantly.

With respect to the obligatory questions on food habits, deviation from the common English version of the questionnaire has been necessary in some places. For instance, food availability in the individual countries has been taken into account when offering alternatives from which the respondent can choose an answer. To give an example, some common fats used in Finland are not available in Estonia or Lithuania and vice versa (Table 2).

3.4.5. Alcohol Consumption

In the 1998 questionnaire there were two obligatory alcohol-related questions. The first one asked, "How many glasses (regular restaurant portions) or bottles of the

Table 2. Example of local categories[a] in an obligatory question in the 1998 Finbalt questionnaires: What kind of fat do you mostly use for food preparation at home?

Common	Estonia	Finland	Latvia	Lithuania
Vegetable oil (1)	Vegetable oil (1)	Vegetable oil (1)	Vegetable oil (1)	Vegetable oil (1)
Margarine (2)	Margarine (2)	Low-fat spread (2)	Margarine (2)	Margarine (2)
Butter or product with mainly butter (3)	Butter or product with mainly butter (3)	Benecol (2)	Butter or product with mainly butter (3)	Butter (3)
		Soft margarine (2)		Lard (4)
		Hard margarine (2)		No fat at all (5)
Lard or other animal fat (4)	Lard or animal fat (4)	Mix of butter and oil (3)	Lard or animal fat (4)	
No fat at all (5)	No fat at all (5)	Butter (3)	No fat at all (5)	
		No fat at all (5)	I don't know	

[a] Corresponding common categories are shown by number in parentheses.

following drinks have you had during the last week (7 days)? If you have not had any, mark 0." The drinks and possible answers were medium strong or strong beer (__ bottles), free-mixed highballs (__ bottles, strong alcohol), spirits (__ restaurant portions of 4 cl.), and wine or equivalent (__ glasses). This period-specific, normal-week method has been found to be more suitable than the quantity-frequency method in countries where alcohol consumption is concentrated on weekends and where food does not accompany alcohol consumption (Romelsjo et al., 1995).

The second obligatory question on alcohol measured the frequency of strong alcohol use: "How often do you usually have strong spirits?" Answer options were daily, 2 to 3 times a week, once a month, a few times a year, and never.

3.4.6. Physical Activity

Physical activity is not measured in detail in the questionnaire. The main aim has been to classify respondents into broad categories according to their long-term habits (Rose and Blackburn, 1968). The three questions in the 1998 questionnaire dealt with leisure-time exercise, physical activity at work, and the journey to work. Similar types of questions have been applied in Finnish risk factor surveys (Vartiainen et al., 1993).

4. EVALUATION OF THE FINBALT MATERIAL

4.1. Data Collection

To date Finland has carried out the national health behaviour questionnaire 23 times, Estonia 6 times, Lithuania 4 times, and Latvia twice. Table 3 presents the sample sizes and response rates of the Finbalt surveys from the years 1994, 1996, and 1998. The sample sizes have been determined by practical reasons; the number of cases per cell allows classification of the respondents by the central socio-demographic characteristics and health behaviours.

All countries have nationally representative population registers for sampling purposes. In Finland all the samples have been drawn from the national population register by Statistics Finland. In Estonia, in 1990 the sample was drawn from the national voting register and in 1992 from the State Address Bureau. In 1994, 1996, and 1998 the National Address Bureau of Estonia was used. The Latvian sample of 1998 was drawn from the national population register. The Lithuanian sample was drawn in 1994 from the national voting register and in 1996 and 1998 from the national population register.

The national registers cover basically the whole populations and allow the use of individuals as sampling units. The register data can be linked with questionnaire data provided that the anonymity of each respondent is guaranteed. Information on age, gender, place of residence, occupation, or other socio-demographic characteristics can be obtained from the registers, but especially in the Baltic countries access to register data is more limited for legislative reasons. In all countries a simple random sample has been drawn from specified age groups: 15 to 64 years in Finland, 16 to 64 years in Estonia and Latvia, and 20 to 64 years in Lithuania.

The response rates in the Finbalt surveys have generally been high, with the lowest ones observed in Lithuania (62%). In Estonia response rates have decreased from 83% to

Table 3. Sample sizes and response rates to the Finbalt questionnaires

	Estonia	Finland	Latvia	Lithuania
1994				
Sample size (no.)	1,500	5,000		3,000
Respondents (no.)	1,243	3,500		1,864
Response rate (%)	83	70		62
1996				
Sample size (no.)	2,000	5,000		3,000
Respondents (no.)	1,507	3,597		2,021
Response rate (%)	75	72		67
1998				
Sample size (no.)	2,000	5,000	3,002	3,000
Respondents (no.)	1,362	3,505	2,318	1,874
Response rate (%)	68	70	77	62
Total				
Sample size (no.)	5,500	15,000	3,002	9,000
Respondents (no.)	4,112	10,602	2,318	5,759
Response rate (%)	75	71	77	64

68%. In Finland a similar decreasing trend is visible if the current response rates are compared with those obtained in the late 1970s. However, between 1994 and 1998 no decrease took place. In 1998 the response rates were still above 60% in all countries (Table 3). Reasons for the relatively high response rates are difficult to estimate. Self-administered mailed questionnaires require a high degree of literacy of the respondents, an up-to-date address register, and a reliable postal system. These requirements are met in Finland and the Baltic countries.

To increase the response rates, one to three reminders have been sent in every country to persons who do not answer the first questionnaire. In Finland, Latvia, and Lithuania, information on responders answering at the different questionnaire rounds is available. In 1998, the highest response rate without reminders was in Lithuania (Table 4). In Latvia the proportion of persons answering after the first reminder was clearly higher than those in Finland and Lithuania. The differences are evidently related to variations in the circumstances in each country. In Lithuania the questionnaire is short (see Table 1). Furthermore, the share of ethnic minorities is lower in Lithuania than in Latvia. A more detailed statistical analysis of late response and non-response has been published (Helasoja et al., 2002).

In Estonia, Latvia, and Lithuania the questionnaires are, in addition to the national language, translated into Russian, but it is not easy to find out the native language of each

Table 4. Sample sizes and response rates, by round, in the 1998 Finbalt questionnaires

	Estonia	Finland	Latvia	Lithuania
Sample size (no.)	2,000	5,000	3,002	3,000
Response rate (%)				
Round 1	(no data)	47	48	51
Round 2	(no data)	22	46	24
Round 3	(no data)	16	20	
Round 4	(no data)	14		
Total	68	70	77	62
Respondents (no.)	1,362	3,505	2,318	1,874

respondent. In Finland non-response cannot in effect be associated with language problems, because a great majority speak Finnish and the Swedish-speaking Finns can easily be identified from population registers. Decreasing response rates have been a consistent trend in all mailed surveys in Finland since the late 1970s, when the health behaviour monitoring system was launched.

In all the countries the proportion of late responders is slightly higher among men than women. In Finland younger men are more reluctant than average to answer. In Lithuania the youngest age group responds earliest. In Latvia no systematic variation by age can be observed. In all the countries respondents with a high educational level answer more actively. Late response is somewhat more common among Finnish men in the countryside and among Latvian women in the cities. Otherwise the differences between urban and rural areas are small. All in all, differences in the characteristics of early and late responders are not significant. Comparisons of non-respondents and respondents have not been carried out because in the Baltic countries legislation does not allow the use of information on non-respondents in dropout analyses.

4.2. Quality of the Data

The amount of missing data can be used as an indicator of the feasibility of a questionnaire. It is probable that a question does not give reliable information on the studied phenomenon if the proportion of respondents who do not answer it is high. Not all questions in the shared questionnaire of 1998 can be used in the analysis of item non-response. Only the questions in which an empty field cannot be interpreted to indicate zero are included. For example, a question like "How often did you see a doctor during the last year?" cannot be included. At least one indicator from each of the six domains (background information, health services and health status, smoking, food habits, alcohol consumption, and others) has been used in the analysis of missing data.

The total proportion of missing information per question is on average less than 10%. The proportion has varied somewhat among the countries and is the lowest in Finland. Gender differences in the total percentage of missing data are small. Men and women belonging to older age groups and with a lower educational level seem to have more difficulties filling in the forms, as the proportion of missing data is higher in these sub-groups (Helasoja et al., 2002).

Answering the questions dealing with food habits has been difficult in all the countries, especially among men (Figure 2). Among Estonians the question on consumption of strong spirits is often left unanswered by women (15%). The highest proportions of missing data are observed in the items measuring the frequency of the use of cereals, boiled vegetables, and soft drinks (Prättälä et al., 1999).

5. DISCUSSION

The Finbalt Health Monitor was put into action in 1990 to disseminate information and expertise among the countries in order to serve national health policy and health promotion and to carry out comparative studies related to major public health problems. The latest monitoring surveys took place in spring 2000. The Finbalt project is administrated by a steering committee, which includes the principal investigators of the national

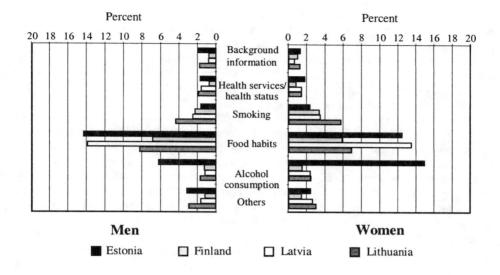

Figure 2. Missing items in the main domains of the 1998 Finbalt questionnaires.

research teams and researchers of the Finnish co-ordinating centre. Each country is responsible for its own survey, but the principles of data collection and reporting are decided in project meetings which take place about twice a year.

Formulating the joint version of the Finbalt questionnaire is one of the core activities of the steering committee. In addition to the collectively accepted obligatory, recommended, and optional questions, the participating countries may add questions of local interest. The first draft of the common questionnaire was an English translation from the Finnish questionnaire. The English version was then translated into the major languages of the participating countries.

The mailed questionnaire used in the Finbalt Health Monitor has important advantages over interviews and other methods. Planning of the questionnaires and interpreting the results require professional researchers in every country, but the data can be collected without a staff specialised in health and lifestyle research. Furthermore, increasing the sample size does not increase labor costs as it does in interviews. The layout of the forms, the principles of data entry and management, and the format of basic tabulations and reports have been relatively easy to transfer from one country to another. The questionnaire is low enough in cost to be repeated at regular intervals in the participating countries. On the other hand, all stages of the Finbalt system have been observed to include some risks of biases and errors. Neither the sampling procedures nor the questionnaires have been completely identical in every country.

A typical problem faced with every new monitoring survey is the contradiction between new and old questions in the joint questionnaire. To follow trends the old questions need to be repeated. On the other hand, the availability of foods, tobacco, and alcohol products change with time, as do many other phenomena measured in the survey. It is sometimes necessary to change the questions even if trends are lost.

In regard to alcohol and food consumption there are problems related to ordinary portion sizes. Consumption figures cannot be compared in a straightforward manner because the size of the normal bottles, glasses, plates, and cups differ among the countries. Similarly, certain food items or drinks can be very common in one country but practically unknown in another. For example, in the 1994 survey the use of lard could not be asked in Finland, nor butter–vegetable oil mixture in Lithuania, because these fats were not used in the respective countries.

In the optimum case a mailed questionnaire should be validated against more exact survey methods. The scarcity of validation studies in the Finbalt Health Monitor makes direct comparisons among the countries unreliable. Instead of absolute differences, patterns of variation and direction of changes can be compared. Therefore, data from the individual Finbalt countries have been analysed separately without weighting them (e.g., according to sample sizes). Comparisons focus on socio-demographic variation of health behaviours in the participating countries. Comparing differences between sub-groups is more reliable than comparing the absolute prevalence of the studied phenomena. In addition, the Finnish experience has shown that repeating the cross-sectional survey regularly can give relevant information on overall changes in different population groups (Prättälä et al., 1992). The Finbalt trend data on the use of vegetable oils are in line with consumption statistics of the respective countries, whereas data on alcohol consumption and smoking seem to be less reliable (Puska, 2000).

The amount of missing data has been small except in some food frequency questions belonging to the set of 17 items. The higher proportion of missing data might be caused by the somewhat unclear layout of the 17-item question. The items asked were considered relevant and common by the research team, but it is possible that the respondents did not recognise them, or indeed, did not use them at all. It can be expected that a respondent who does not know or use a food item leaves the question unanswered. Further analyses on the association between the proportion of missing data and the frequency of the use of individual food items are needed to interpret the reasons for missing data in the food frequency questions.

6. CONCLUSIONS

On the basis of practical experience and analyses carried out until now, the following conclusions can be offered:

1. Collecting data by a common mailed questionnaire in Finland and the Baltic countries is feasible. An important prerequisite is the multi-disciplinary and multi-lingual project team and the regular project meetings organised in turn by the participating countries. Face-to-face contacts before and after every monitoring round are crucial for checking the wording in the questionnaires and other details of data collection.

2. There is no evidence of serious response bias in the Finbalt questionnaires. Response rates have been satisfactorily high in all the surveys, and late responders have not differed from early responders. If some differences have been observed, they have been consistent in all countries and have not, therefore, disturbed comparisons among the countries. In addition, the proportion of missing data has been low (with the few exceptions concerning food-related questions).

3. The Finbalt data can be used in comparing time trends and patterns of health behaviour, but comparisons of absolute prevalences among the countries need to be treated with caution.

The Finbalt data are appropriate primarily for estimating the prevalence of common health behaviours in the general population. They are not suitable for analysing rare or sensitive phenomena, such as illegal drug abuse or alcohol problems, because persons involved in these types of behaviour are often non-respondents.

The unavoidable bias caused by cultural differences can be leveled off if, instead of national averages, patterns of variation in selected habits are compared. When the limitations of the data are known and results are interpreted in the light of information from other studies, health policy reports, statistics, mass media, and the like, comparative analyses will provide new information on social factors influencing health behaviour.

7. REFERENCES

de Bruin, A., Picavet, H., and Nossikov, A., eds., 1996, *Health Interview Surveys: Towards International Harmonization of Methods and Instruments*, WHO Regional Office for Europe, Copenhagen (WHO Regional Publications, European Series No. 58).

Fagerstrom, K. O., 1978, Measuring degree of physical dependence to tobacco smoking with reference to individualization of treatment, *Addict Behav.* 3:235–241.

Grabauskas, V., Klumbiene, J., Petkeviciene, J., et al., 1997, *Health Behaviour among Lithuanian Adult Population, 1994*, National Public Health Institute, Helsinki.

Helakorpi, S., Uutela, A., Prättälä, R., et al., 1997, *Health Behaviour among Finnish Adult Population, Spring 1997*, National Public Health Institute, Helsinki.

Helakorpi, S., Uutela, A., Prättälä, R., et al., 1998, *Health Behaviour among Finnish Adult Population, Spring 1998*, National Public Health Institute, Helsinki.

Helasoja, V., Prättälä, R., Dregval, L., et al., 2002, Late response and item non-response in Finbalt Health Monitor, *Eur J Public Health.* 12:1–6.

Idler, E. L., Kasl, S. V., and Lemke, J. H., 1990, Self-evaluated health and mortality among the elderly in New Haven, Connecticut, and Iowa and Washington counties, Iowa, 1982–1986, *Am J Epidemiol.* 131:91–103.

Lipand, A., Kasmel, A., Tasa, E., et al., 1995, *Health Behaviour among Estonian Adult Population, Spring 1994*, National Public Health Institute, Helsinki.

Mackenbach, J. P., and Kunst, A. E., 1997, Measuring the magnitude of socio-economic inequalities in health: an overview of available measures illustrated with two examples from Europe, *Soc Sci Med.* 44:757–771.

National Public Health Institute, 1998, *The 1997 Dietary Survey of Finnish Adults*, NPHI, Helsinki (NPHI Publication No. B8/1998).

Nordic Medico-Statistical Committee, 1998, *Nordic/Baltic Health Statistics 1996*, NOMESCO, Copenhagen.

Prättälä, R., Berg, M.-A., and Puska, P., 1992, Diminishing or increasing contrasts? Social class variation in Finnish food consumption patterns, 1979–1990, *Eur J Clin Nutr.* 46:279–287.

Prättälä, R., Helasoja, V., and the Finbalt Group, 1999, *Finbalt Health Monitor: Feasibility of a Collaborative System for Monitoring Health Behaviour in Finland and the Baltic Countries*, National Public Health Institute, Helsinki.

Puska, P., 1978, *Health Behaviour among Finnish Adult Population, Spring 1978*, National Public Health Institute, Helsinki.

Puska, P., 2000, Nutrition and mortality: the Finnish experience, *Acta Cardiol.* 55:213–220.

Puska, P., Tuomilehto, J., Nissinen, A., et al., eds., 1995, *The North Karelia Project: 20 Year Results and Experiences*, National Public Health Institute, Helsinki.

Räsänen, L., and Pietinen, P., 1982, A short questionnaire method for evaluation of diets, *Prev Med.* 11:669–676.

Romelsjo, A., Leifman, H., and Nystrom, S., 1995, A comparative study of two methods for the measurement of alcohol consumption in the general population, *Int J Epidemiol.* 24:929–936.

Roos, E., Ovaskainen, M.-L., and Pietinen, P., 1995, Validity and comparison of three saturated fat indices, *Scand J Nutr.* 39:55–59.

Rose, G., and Blackburn, H., 1968, *Cardiovascular Survey Methods*, World Health Organization, Geneva.

Simpura, J., 1995, Social policy in transition societies: the case of the Baltic countries and Russia. An introduction, in: *Social Policy in Transition Societies. Experience from the Baltic Countries and Russia*, J. Simpura, ed., Finnish International Council for Social Welfare Committee, Finnish Federation for Social Welfare, Helsinki.

Statistical Office of Estonia, 1997, *Estonia in Figures*, Statistical Office of Estonia, Tallinn.

Statistics Finland, 1997, *Finland in Figures*, Statistics Finland, Helsinki.

U.S. Department of Health, Education, and Welfare, 1975, *Health Interview Survey Procedure, 1957–1974*, DHEW, Rockville, MD (DHEW Publication No. (HRA) 75-1311).

Vartiainen, E., Jousilahti, P., Tamminen, M., et al., 1993, *FINRISKI '92 Implementation and Basic Results of the Study*, National Public Health Institute, Helsinki.

Woods, D., 1977, Canada health survey should provide useful information if carefully used, *Can Med Assoc J.* **116**:1302–1303.

World Health Organization, 2001, HFA Statistical Database (September 2001); http://www.who.int/whosis/.

World Health Organization Regional Office for Europe, 1996a, *Health Care Systems in Transition: Estonia*, WHO, Copenhagen.

World Health Organization Regional Office for Europe, 1996b, *Health Care Systems in Transition: Latvia*, WHO, Copenhagen.

World Health Organization Regional Office for Europe, 1996c, *Health Care Systems in Transition: Lithuania*, WHO, Copenhagen.

World Health Organization Regional Office for Europe, 2001a, Highlights on Health in Latvia (April 2001); http://www.who.dk.

World Health Organization Regional Office for Europe, 2001b, Highlights on Health in Lithuania (March 2001); http://www.who.dk.

Zvidrins, P., and Krumins, J., 1993, Morbidity and mortality in Estonia, Latvia and Lithuania in the 1980's, *Scand J Soc Med.* **21**:150–158.

CHAPTER 8

TOWARDS A EUROPEAN HEALTH MONITORING SYSTEM
Results of a Pilot Study on Physical Activity

Alfred Rütten, Randall Rzewnicki, Heiko Ziemainz,
Wil T. M. Ooijendijk, Frederico Schena, Timo Stahl,
Yves Vanden Auweele, and John Welshman[*]

1. INTRODUCTION

The relationships between physical activity (PA) and a wide variety of health and well-being outcomes have been well established in the last decade. Regular PA reduces the risk of premature death and disability from many medical conditions, including coronary heart disease, diabetes, colon cancer, and osteoporosis. There is also evidence for a positive relationship with well-being, particularly in alleviating depression and anxiety. Reduction of the large public health burden associated with a sedentary lifestyle has become a priority in many countries and is endorsed by the World Health Organization.

Changes in the approach of public health officials have included considerable modification in the focus of public health recommendations for PA. Previous recommendations focused on multiple discrete bouts of vigorous sports and exercise which required much time and effort. Newer recommendations focus on those types of PA that are much more common and easily integrated into daily life, such as brisk walking, working in and around the house, and recreational PA. The current research consensus is that a very wide range of moderate PA can provide health benefits (U.S. Department of Health and Human Services, 1996).

One of the main challenges of current research in this area is measuring the frequency, duration, and intensity of such wide-ranging PA, which includes activities that

* Alfred Rütten and Heiko Ziemainz, Friedrich-Alexander University of Erlangen-Nürnberg, D-91058 Erlangen, Germany; Randall Rzewnicki and Yves Vanden Auweele, Catholic University of Leuven, 3001 Heverlee, Belgium; Wil T. M. Ooijendijk, TNO Prevention and Health, 2301 CE Leiden, The Netherlands; Frederico Schena, Centro Interuniversitario di Recerca in Bioingegneria Scienze Motorie, Rovereto, Italy; Timo Stahl, University of Jyväskylä, FIN-40351 Jyväskylä, Finland; John Welshman, Lancaster University, Lancaster LA1 4YT, United Kingdom.

respondents may or may not recognise and report as relevant to health. A wide variety of measures of PA have been used for public health. At one time, over 30 different measures were reported to have been used for the assessment of PA in populations (Laporte et al., 1985). Many of them adequately obtained reports on leisure-time PA. However, there is now a wide range of other kinds of PA which are recommended but are not covered by those measures, including transportation, occupational PA, and housework.

Assessment of the PA of a population is a complex procedure that has lacked standardisation (Ainsworth et al., 1993). Standardised approaches to collecting and analysing PA data are essential for public health surveillance, policy making, and communication. "Valid comparisons between states (populations, or countries) or years simply cannot be made without standard definition of terms and compatibility between public health recommendations and the collection and analysis of surveillance data" (Brownson et al., 2000, p. 1916).

1.1. Background: Relevance of a European Community Approach to Health Monitoring

The planned European Health Monitoring System is designed to provide high-quality, comparative information on health status, trends, and determinants throughout the European Union (EU). This information will help the EU carry out its overall responsibility in the field of public health (e.g., in planning, monitoring, and evaluating EU programmes and action) as well as help EU countries in their own public health responsibilities (e.g., in providing adequate health information to make comparisons and support their national health policies). In particular, such a system will help to overcome major problems of the current situation: because health monitoring in Europe has been conducted by many different organisations and the various initiatives have not been co-ordinated in any important way, there are large gaps in the data available. Data and information are often of medium or poor quality and of limited comparability among countries, and many efforts are unnecessarily duplicated.

1.2. The Health Monitoring Programme

Against this background, the EU has been conducting a programme on health monitoring (from 1997 through 2002) which is intended to contribute to the establishment of an EU health monitoring system. Due to the current lack of co-operation, the general aim is to concentrate the efforts of the different actors in European health monitoring to improve its quality and value. More specifically, the programme aims to develop an EU-wide network for sharing and transferring health data, establish EU health indicators, and develop methods and tools for analysis and for reporting on health and the effects of health policies.

The programme should work by making use of the expertise which had been built up in the EU countries and acts as a co-ordinating force between them. Because future efforts in the field of European health monitoring must be based on data and available expertise, particularly at the national but also the international level, the programme especially insists on not adding to but instead reducing the burdens of reporting, meanwhile improving the quality of information and data exchanged.

According to the specific aims of the programme, most projects subsidised by the European Commission within this framework critically review existing health data and indicators to prepare the collection of progressively comparable health data needed to establish EU health indicators. For example, one project generates a computerised database of methods and contents of existing and planned health surveys in the EU to provide insight into the coverage of areas relevant for health monitoring in Europe. Other projects are more topic specific, dealing with problems of quality and comparability of data and indicators in a diversity of areas (e.g., alcohol consumption, mental health, death statistics, and health care). A few projects focus mainly on data analysis (e.g., monitoring socio-economic differences in health indicators in the EU).

The Health Information Exchange and Monitoring System (HIEMS) project, which is part of the European Health Monitoring Programme, aims specifically to establish a European health data network. This project has helped to set up a technical infra-structure (telemetric network), which already could provide public health administrations and other users with comparative information on health in the EU—when such data are available. Other projects selected by the programme face particular challenges related to their potential impact on policy making. These targets are expected to feed information into HIEMS as soon as possible, but this information has to be of high quality (e.g., valid and comparable), effectively analysed, and appropriately presented to policymakers. To strengthen such impact, the EU has asked projects to focus on improving three areas: comparability of data sets between EU countries, indicator definitions to be used in an EU indicator set, and availability of (comparable) data from EU countries for use in HIEMS.

In conclusion, one may say that the current situation in Europe is fraught with major problems related to the lack of co-operation between countries. The different national institutions and initiatives related to PA, if they exist at all, have not been co-ordinated in any meaningful way. The result is that, viewed from the European level, although some efforts are duplicated, there are large gaps in the data on PA available for the different countries. The data which are available are often of modest or poor quality, and usually cannot be compared with other countries in the EU. On the other hand, the EU is at an ideal conjuncture as it begins to encourage and assist its members to work together towards the generation of an international database of health data that includes measures of PA.

1.3. Demonstration Project: The European Physical Activity Surveillance System

The European Physical Activity Surveillance System (EUPASS), a demonstration project, is designed to contribute to a European health monitoring system and its methodological foundations. It is focused on developing and testing a surveillance system for PA as a major behavioural determinant of health. According to the current discussion on global health monitoring, the term "surveillance" particularly refers to "the creation of a data system for changing the public health" (McQueen, 1999, p. 1313). Thus, surveillance can be described as a complex organised effort to continuously collect data (e.g., monitor long-term changes in behaviour risk factors), analyse these data, and feed back results of analysis to potential users (e.g., public health policy-makers). The specific goals of EUPASS are related to investigating implementation structures of health monitoring in the EU, providing a valid and cross-nationally comparable list of core indicators and optional indicators for PA, and testing selected PA indicators by employing different survey methodologies.

The development of a comparable set of PA indicators for health monitoring at the EU level must be based on detailed information from previous and ongoing PA surveillance activity throughout the EU. Thus, an inventory of PA surveillance was planned as a logical first step of EUPASS.

Investigating the quality and comparability of existing national indicators as well as of new indicators developed by co-ordinated international efforts is a crucial step for improving the health monitoring structure in the EU. Thus, the primary aims of EUPASS are to test:

- the reliability of PA indicators used in surveillance systems in the EU countries to date, new and comparable indicators of PA behaviour, and new and comparable sets of psycho-social determinants of PA (Rütten et al., 2000);
- the comparability of extant and new PA indicators;
- the predictive power of the different sets of PA indicators with regard to health status; and
- the quality and feasibility of different survey methods in participating countries (e.g., the effects of two telephone interview methods, panel versus continuous, were compared with a mail questionnaire on sampling procedures and response rates).

The EUPASS network of researchers encompasses the project group of research institutions from eight EU countries (Belgium, Finland, France, Germany, Italy, the Netherlands, Spain, and the United Kingdom), counterparts in the national health surveillance institutes of participating countries, and co-operation partners of EU countries not directly included in the project group. In addition, the EUPASS network has established co-operation with other relevant research activities. For example, close contact was established with an international consensus group developing the International Physical Activity Questionnaire (IPAQ). Regarding surveillance systems, experts from the U.S. Centers for Disease Control and Prevention have been involved. Of course, the international group working on PA questions within the Health Interview Survey in Europe as well as the general health monitoring project of this survey have also been contacted. Thus, the EUPASS project has taken very seriously the approach of the EU Health Monitoring Programme requiring that all new action must take into account the methodology and activities which have been developed to date in other institutions.

As the first step to improve comparability of data sets between EU countries, EUPASS conducted an investigation of health-related PA surveys, data sets, and indicators used in the EU. As a result, an inventory of national PA surveillance systems has been generated. The logic of this inventory is represented by a matrix in which information, ordered by countries, is included on the policy environment for PA surveillance, surveys conducted, and PA indicators used.

In the second step to improve the indicator definitions to be used in an EU indicator set, surveys in the participating EU countries included new indicators for PA behaviour and determinants. In particular, indicators developed by the IPAQ Standardisation Group have been employed. These new indicators appeared to be especially relevant for the development of an EU indicator set both in terms of harmonisation of international standards and because of their validity and reliability. In addition, a set of psycho-social determinants indicators has been tested.

The steps mentioned (inventory, and tests comparing existing and new indicators) will help improve the availability of comparable data sets at the EU level. In addition, the data to be gathered in the indicator test surveys in the participating EU countries can be combined into a data set made available for use in HIEMS.

Beyond their impact on key policy issues of the health monitoring programme, the indicator test surveys in the EUPASS project will help identify methodological frames appropriate for health monitoring in Europe. For example, it tested the adequacy and feasibility of computer-assisted telephone interviewing (CATI) in various EU countries and compared this method with postal surveys. Moreover, different forms of data collection (e.g., panel or continuous) have been tested for participating countries. This feature of EUPASS appears to be especially relevant for preparing an EU surveillance system (e.g., related to health behaviour risk factors in general).

2. INVENTORY OF PHYSICAL ACTIVITY INDICATORS, SURVEYS, AND SURVEILLANCE STRUCTURES

The development of a comparable set of PA indicators for health monitoring at the EU level must be based on detailed information from previous and ongoing PA surveillance activity throughout the EU. Thus, an inventory of such surveillance was planned as a logical first step of EUPASS. Here we explain what it is that the EUPASS researchers wanted to know and how the information was gathered. Finally, we assess the degree to which the currently used measures for PA in the EU can be used and compared with each other in reports of PA in Western Europe.

2.1. Data and Methods

The EUPASS project aimed at co-ordinating expertise and improving the quality of relevant information. Therefore, exploratory analysis and evaluation of the available PA data sets were conducted by EUPASS researchers to guide the work on the inventory. In this context, the EUPASS group developed four basic questions to gather information:

1. What institutions are involved in health surveillance, and in what function?
2. How long has PA been part of health surveillance, and how frequent is it?
3. How is the monitoring of PA conducted (i.e., survey and non-survey methods)?
4. Which specific surveys are used for PA in the surveillance systems?

On this preliminary basis the EUPASS research team, as well as researchers and public health officials from other EU countries, provided information on PA surveys in 17 countries (Austria, Belgium, Czech Republic, Denmark, Finland, France, Germany, Greece, Ireland, Italy, Luxembourg, the Netherlands, Poland, Portugal, Spain, Sweden, and the United Kingdom).

2.1.1. Survey

Taking the outcomes of the reports as the starting point for further investigation, the EUPASS research team conducted a survey to collect additional information about all EU countries by contacting a selection of institutions and non-government bodies directly involved in health surveillance. This survey was carried out between June and August 2000. All selected institutions were mailed a letter and a questionnaire. Thirty-five institutions from all 17 EU countries were contacted; 21 responded. Again, information exchange and document analysis formed the work and led to the current inventory of PA surveillance for the eight EU countries directly involved in the EUPASS project and for the nine additional EU countries.

2.2. Comparison of Existing European Union Physical Activity Surveys

2.2.1. Policy Environments and Surveys at the National Level

The first notable feature concerning the policy environment for PA surveillance in EU countries is that public health institutions, such as the national institutes of public health on one hand and statistical offices conducting programmes (e.g., micro-census surveys) on the other hand, are the key actors. Second, the data reveal a diversity of surveillance approaches and assessment instruments for PA, thus underlining the necessity for EUPASS to contribute to harmonisation in this context.

In almost all EU countries, health behaviour surveillance is not prescribed explicitly by law or by government. However, in most EU countries some specific agreements or regulations can be found with particular targets and resources that determine the conduct of regular health behaviour surveys. For example, in Finland an "annual agreement" between the Ministry of Social Affairs and Health and the National Public Health Institute has provided an appropriate framework for conducting regular studies on the health behaviour of the Finnish population over the last three decades. These studies included specific questions about PA. More recently, similar agreements have been developed in Belgium (since 1997 between the federal authorities, Flemish and French Communities, and Walloon and Brussels Regions with the Scientific Institute of Public Health–Louis Pasteur), Germany (since 1997 by the Ministry of Health with the Robert Koch Institute), Italy (since the 1980s by the Ministry of Health with the Higher Institute of Health and the National Institute of Statistics), and Spain (since the 1980s by the Ministry of Health with the National Sociological Research Centre).

In some countries, regular health behaviour surveys that include PA indicators have started only quite recently, whereas the general issue of PA has already been considered by other regular national surveys (e.g., micro-census surveys) for a much longer period of time. For example, in the United Kingdom the General Household Survey (conducted by the Office of National Statistics) started in 1971 on an annual basis, but the Health Survey for England (conducted by the Department of Health) was established only in 1991. In France, different approaches to develop a "Baromètre Santé" at the national level have been co-ordinated by the Comité Français d'Education pour la Santé since the mid-1990s, but data on PA collected by general surveys on living conditions (conducted by the Institut National de la Statistique et des Etudes Economiques) were available in the 1980s.

Beyond general household surveys and comprehensive health behaviour surveys, several countries have conducted surveys specifically on health-related PA (e.g., Finland, France, and the United Kingdom). However, these surveys generally have employed cross-sectional designs and have not collected data regularly. Only the Netherlands (TNO Prevention and Health in co-operation with Interview International and with financial support from the Ministry of Public Health, Welfare and Sport) has established a specific PA surveillance system based on continuous data collection, which commenced in 1999.

To summarise, in all of the eight EU countries participating in the EUPASS project (as well as in most of the other nine EU countries considered in the inventory), a variety of more or less regularly collected data on PA of the national population are available. However, even at the level of individual countries these data are heterogenous. There are three crucial problems regarding the issue of continuous data collection for monitoring long-term changes in PA of the population over time. (1) The different institutions involved in surveying PA (e.g., public health or general statistics institutions) often use different indicators to measure PA. Thus, in most cases the different data sets are not directly comparable. (2) Even in regular health behaviour surveys, the issue of PA has not always been considered regularly. For example, the Health Surveys for England have been conducted every year since 1991, but PA indicators have been included in only 1991–1994 and 1997. (3) Even in health behaviour surveys or more general surveys that regularly consider PA issues, the indicators used may have changed. For example, in France and Italy such changes occurred during the last few years.

2.2.2. International Comparison of Physical Activity Indicators

Because of the diversity of surveys and PA indicators at the national level, the EUPASS project had to identify one or two main national surveys or sets of indicators for international comparison. In the cases of Belgium, Germany, and Spain (each with only one adequate national survey available) and Finland (with one annual survey since 1978), the selection turned out to be easy, and in the cases of the Netherlands and the United Kingdom a selection of at least two relevant surveys appeared necessary. In contrast, in France and Italy changes in the indicators used have occurred during the last few years, making it difficult to define appropriate indicators for international comparison. It was decided to include the PA items from France's latest version of the Baromètre Santé and to use Italy's PA items from the more general survey on aspects of everyday life (continuous since 1993) instead of the indicators of that country's national health survey.

Similarities and differences between the PA indicators used in the eight EU countries participating in the EUPASS project appear in Table 1. It shows questions and items selected from the main national surveys on PA. Four dimensions of PA can be considered fundamental for measurement: type, frequency, duration, and intensity. To date no single dimension is covered by all EUPASS participants. Thus, any comparison among the eight countries regarding a PA dimension (e.g., average frequency or duration) of the national population would fail due to lack of comparable information. Even within the same dimension, the questions vary considerably between countries. In Italy frequency questions relate to sporting activities, whereas in the Netherlands the frequency of stair climbing is asked for. Spain investigates the frequency of PA of different intensities (light, moderate, vigorous). In addition, in most cases different reference periods are used to report the frequency of PA (e.g., last 7 days, usual week, last 14 days, last 12 months).

Table 1. Indicators for physical activity (PA) monitoring in eight European Union countries

	Belgium[a]	Finland[b]	France[c]	Germany[d]
Type			Which type of PA during last 7 days?	
Frequency	In last 7 days, how many days of PA intense enough to sweat?	How often leisure-time PA with light sweating for 1/2 hour? (*1* = daily, *7* = no PA because ill)		How often participate in sports? (*1* = regularly for >4 hours/week, *5* = no PA) How often engage in sports or other strenuous activities to sweat? (*1* = daily, *4* = seldom)
Duration		How many minutes spend walking, running, or cycling to work? (*1* = not working, *6* = >1 hour/day)	During last 7 days, time spent on PA (hours): • in club? • at school? • at work? • alone or with friends?	Average time spend each day on activities: • Monday to Friday? (*1* = sleeping or resting, *5* = strenuous activities) • weekend? (*1* = sleeping or resting, *5* = strenuous activities) • sports or other strenuous activities? (<10, 10–20, 20–30, >30 minutes)
Intensity	Activity during free time? (*1* = physical training, *6* = mostly sitting)	How demanding is job physically? (*1* = mainly sitting, *4* = physically very demanding) How much exercise in free time? (*1* = little movement, *4* = training)		

[a] Belgian Health Interview Survey (1997).
[b] Health Behaviour among Finnish Adults (since 1978).
[c] Baromètre Santé (1999).
[d] German Health Survey (1997).

Italy[e]	The Netherlands[f]	Spain[g]	United Kingdom[h]
What sporting activities?	What kind of PA?	During last 12 months, what kind of activity? (1 = sitting, 4 = heavy work)	Walking for 1/4 mile within past 4 weeks? (yes, no) Gardening, DIY, or building work in the past 4 weeks? (yes, no)
How many months of sporting activities last year? Consistency of sporting activities over last 12 months? (1 = 1–5 times, 6 = >120 times)	Participation in PA in last 14 days? (number of times) How often climb stairs? (times/day)	How many times a week: • light PA? • moderate PA? • vigorous PA?	On how many days walking? On how many days gardening, DIY, or building work?
	Average PA participation? (hours or minutes) In ordinary week, time spend participating (hours): • in leisure-time activities? • in housekeeping activities? • at work or school?	Time spend each day on PA at work and in leisure time?	How long usually spend walking? How long usually spend on gardening, DIY, or building work?
		Activity during free time? (1 = practically inactive, 4 = physical training)	Effort of PA sufficient to get out of breath or sweat? (yes, no)

DIY = do-it-yourself projects.
[e] MULTISCOPO/Aspects of Everyday Life (since 1993).
[f] Continuous Quality of Life Survey/Health Interview Survey (since 1990).
[g] Spanish National Health Survey (since 1985).
[h] Health Survey for England (since 1991).

Finally, many types of measurement scales have been applied (e.g., nominal scales in the Health Survey for England, ordinal scales in the German Health Survey, interval scales in the Netherlands' Continuous Quality of Life Survey/Health Interview Survey). In conclusion, the PA data in the different EU countries collected by the main surveys and indicators are not comparable. Moreover, the diversity of PA concepts and indicators applied raises the question of how valid and how reliable these various indicators are.

The diversity found in the inventory of currently used PA measures in the EU underscores the need for development of common measures. From the collection of measures, the EUPASS team selected which national measures should be included in each country's survey. The next task for the research team was to bring together the new PA indicators that would be used in all EU countries.

3. DEVELOPMENT OF NEW SURVEY INDICATORS

One of the primary goals of the EUPASS project was to develop a survey instrument containing valid and internationally comparable PA indicators. This section describes how a new collection of PA indicators was developed, including the IPAQ and measures of self-efficacy for daily PA, social motivation and support for PA, and environmental support for PA.

The results of the inventory of PA measures in the EU made clear the need for new comparable indicators for PA which could be administered in all countries. The EUPASS research team gathered at the Technical University in Chemnitz, Germany, in the beginning of 2000 to ascertain which indicators to include in the survey protocol. At this meeting, M. Sjöström, from the executive committee of an international consensus group on PA measurement (a working group attending a PA standardisation meeting hosted by the World Health Organization in Geneva in April 1998), explained the development and worldwide testing of a new PA measure, the IPAQ. There were some risks to adopting· a measure for which all the validation and reliability testing was yet to be reported. However, the balance was tipped in favour of the advantages of its worldwide testing programme, expected near-universal application, and multiple reporting options. The answers to the nine items about vigorous and moderate PA, walking, and sitting can be summed to produce an overall indicator of PA-related energy expenditure (Ainsworth et al., 1993, 2000) or the number of days in which a respondent has met various PA recommendations (e.g., 3 days of 20 minutes of vigorous PA [American College of Sports Medicine, 1975] or 5 days of 30 minutes of moderate PA [Pate et al., 1995; Jones et al., 1998]). Therefore the EUPASS group decided unanimously to adopt the IPAQ as its primary and comparable measure of PA. The team then went on to adopt several other indicators as well, and these are described next.

The EUPASS questionnaire was used in all three surveys (panel, continuous, mail) and contained four sections. Section A was different for each participating country, as it included only the PA indicators used in the main surveys for that country. For example, in Finland the four questions from the national survey Health Behaviour among Finnish Adults formed Section A of the questionnaire, whereas in Italy the nine questions from the national survey Aspects of Everyday Life were used. In contrast, Sections B, C, and D used the same indicators in all countries.

Section B consisted of the questions used in the "short, last 7 days, telephone version" of IPAQ (IPAQS7T), in which EUPASS researchers selected the last 7 days as the reference period for reporting PA behaviour. The nine questions in this version concerned the frequency and duration of vigorous PA, moderate PA, walking, and sitting. IPAQS7T was developed by an international consensus group to provide an internationally comparable measurement tool. This instrument was tested for validity and reliability. Of course, because the development of IPAQ is still in the pilot phase, the validity and reliability of the current version cannot be taken for granted (see also reliability test results in Section 5.3). Nevertheless, IPAQ appears to be the best PA survey measurement currently available in terms of international testing and comparability. Several EU countries are considering using this instrument for their national PA surveillance efforts in the future because it is internationally standardised and tested for validity and reliability.

Section C of the EUPASS questionnaire included psycho-social determinants that had been tested in earlier studies for their predictive power on PA and health. These three questions made use of a three-item self-efficacy scale based on the work of Sallis and Owen (1999) and De Bourdeaudhuij and colleagues (De Bourdeaudhuij et al., 1993; De Bourdeaudhuij and Van Oost, 1994), a five-item social support scale, and a three-item supportive environment scale. The latter two were based on items tested in a European study on health policy and health behaviour (Rütten et al., 2000, 2001; Stahl et al., 2001).

Section D contained questions mainly related to socio-demographics. The items selected included sex, age, years of education, household income, occupational status (working, unemployed, retired, student, homemaker, other), height, weight, and perceived health.

4. DESIGN AND METHODS TESTING

The EUPASS project was designed to test the quality and feasibility of different survey methods in participating countries. The effects of telephone interview versus mail questionnaire designs on sampling procedures, response rates, and other factors are investigated here.

For indicator and survey method testing, three surveys were conducted in each of the EUPASS countries (Table 2). A panel study based on CATI was designed to report PA data of a representative selected group of about 100 persons in each country at three points in time (T1, T2, and T3). Data from T1 and T2 were especially used for reliability testing.

A CATI time-series survey was carried out over 6 consecutive months with the goal of realising about 100 interviews per month (i.e., in total approximately 600 per country). These data have been used to investigate the validity and comparability of the national indicators used to date and the IPAQ indicators. The data also provided an empirical basis to test the predictive power of different sets of indicators (national, IPAQ, psycho-social).

A mail survey (N = 100) was conducted in each country to control for effects of different survey methods (telephone versus mail).

Table 2. Design of the 2000 EUROPASS surveys

	Month of interview					
	June	July	August	September	October	November
CATI panel survey (repeated measures)	x (T1)	x (T2) (1–3 weeks after T1)			x (T3) (October and November)	
CATI time-series (continuous) survey	x	x	x	x	x	x
Mail (control) survey					x (October and November)	

CATI = computer-assisted telephone interview.
All sample sizes = 100 respondents.

5. DATA, TESTING, AND RESULTS

5.1. Indicator Test Study

Investigating the quality of indicators is crucial for improving health monitoring. EUPASS tested the validity and reliability of PA indicators used in the EU to date, the IPAQ, and new comparable psycho-social determinants of PA. The EUPASS research team also tested the comparability of extant and new indicators and tested the predictive power of the different sets of PA indicators with regard to health status.

5.2. Response Rates for Telephone and Mail Surveys

The results of the field work in the eight countries reveal major differences in overall response rates for telephone and mail surveys between countries as well as in specific response rates for the telephone survey versus the mail survey (Table 3). For example, Finland reported the highest response rates for all three types of surveys (panel, 51.6%; continuous, 54.5%; mail, 58.3%), while the United Kingdom had comparatively low response rates for all surveys (panel, 14.5%; continuous, 25.5%; mail, 18.6%). In Germany the response rate for the continuous telephone survey was comparably high (50.5%), whereas the mail response was very low (19.1%). In contrast, France had a much better response rate on the mail survey (52.4%) than on the continuous telephone survey (29.1%).

Because the EUPASS project made major efforts to standardise sampling procedures and field work in the participating countries as much as possible, these differences in response rates may indicate specific challenges for conducting telephone or mail surveys in different EU countries. These challenges should be considered in the further process of developing a European Health Monitoring System. Moreover, as the actual response rates from different countries are rather low, the results of the indicator analyses have to be interpreted with caution. For the explorative purposes of this study, however, the data appear sufficient.

Table 3. Sample size and response rate of the 2000 EUROPASS surveys

	Panel survey				Continuous survey	Mail survey
	T1	T2	T3	Overall		
Belgium						
Net sample size	622	200	102	622	1,577	588
Realised sample size	202	102	79	79	611	206
Response rate (%)	32.5	51.0	77.5	12.7	38.7	35.0
Finland						
Net sample size	217	151	127	217	1,107	230
Realised sample size	151	127	112	112	603	134
Response rate (%)	69.6	84.1	88.2	51.6	54.5	58.3
France						
Net sample size	482	140	91	482	2,060	250
Realised sample size	140	91	67	67	599	131
Response rate (%)	29.0	65.0	73.6	13.9	29.1	52.4
Germany						
Net sample size	951	382	202	951	1,293	350
Realised sample size	389	223	145	145	653	67
Response rate (%)	40.9	58.4	71.8	15.2	50.5	19.1
Italy						
Net sample size	608	219	121	608	1,892	500
Realised sample size	219	121	91	91	600	148
Response rate (%)	36.0	55.3	75.2	14.9	31.7	29.6
The Netherlands						
Net sample size	324	124	95	324	1,400	426
Realised sample size	124	95	76	76	606	108
Response rate (%)	38.3	76.6	80.0	23.5	43.3	25.4
Spain						
Net sample size	276	158	128	276	1,284	300
Realised sample size	158	128	100	100	600	22
Response rate (%)	57.2	81.0	78.1	36.2	46.7	7.3
United Kingdom						
Net sample size	546	148	120	546	2,838	377
Realised sample size	148	120	79	79	723	70
Response rate (%)	27.1	81.1	65.8	14.5	25.5	18.6
All countries						
Net sample size	4,026	1,522	986	4,026	13,451	3,021
Realised sample size	1,531	1,007	749	749	4,995	886
Response rate (%)	38.0	66.2	75.9	18.6	37.1	29.3

Table 4. Test-retest reliability (Spearman co-efficients) of IPAQS7T

	Belgium (100[a])	Finland (127)	France (91)	Germany (223)	Italy (98)	The Netherlands (86)	Spain (128)	United Kingdom (98)	All countries (951)
Vigorous PA									
Days	.553	.477	.278	.508	.414	.344	.540	.469	.494
Total minutes	.442	.590	.359	.536	.530	.413	.616	.345	.509
Moderate PA									
Days	.365	.283	.181	.430	.208	.402	.381	.254	.364
Total minutes	.385	.553	.352	.536	.221	.338	.322	.431	.389
Walking									
Days	.310	.550	.358	.540	.471	.292	.372	.495	.468
Total minutes	.703	.440	.504	.328	.408	.297	.721	.310	.461
Pace	.399	.339	.453	.223	.274	.422	.679	.560	.441
Sitting									
Weekdays (total minutes)	.521	.701	.422	.642	.726	.633	.618	.552	.623
Weekend (total minutes)	.338	.640	.370	.407	.333	.454	.431	.435	.461
Sum of METs[b]									
PA	.531	.405	.294	.388	.135	.341	.576	.499	.446
Sitting	.418	.582	.417	.523	.567	.497	.504	.536	.527
Total	.561	.423	.225	.293	.297	.376	.563	.400	.419

IPAQS7T = International Physical Activity Questionnaire, short, last 7 days, telephone version. PA = physical activity. MET = energy expenditure score (1 MET = 1 kcal·kg^{-1}·hour).
[a] Number of IPAQS7T variables.
[b] Sum of METs for PA includes vigorous PA, moderate PA, and walking in last 7 days; for sitting it includes weekdays and weekend; for total it includes all items.

5.3. Results of Reliability Analysis

After the distribution of the data from panel surveys T1 and T2 were tested, a non-parametric measure (Spearman's rank correlation) was used to examine the reliability of the different PA indicators. In general, most items' correlation co-efficients in IPAQS7T ranged between .3 and .5 (Table 4). Only the question related to the duration (sum of minutes) of sitting during weekdays provided slightly better results (most co-efficients were .6 or .7). The co-efficients for the overall indicator of PA (energy expenditure score, MET) differed from .2 for France to about .6 for Spain.

The generally rather low test-retest reliability scores for IPAQS7T may result from particular methodological issues. First, IPAQS7T refers explicitly to the last 7 days as the time period to consider when answering the questions. Thus, differences in frequency or duration of PA found for one respondent between T1 and T2 (i.e., about 2 weeks later) could reflect real differences in the PA of this person (e.g., three times vigorously active in the week before T1, one time vigorously active in the week before T2). Second, the original, English version of IPAQS7T had to be translated into the languages of the participating countries, which may have influenced the understanding of single questions in some countries but would not explain the rather low co-efficients for the United Kingdom, for which no translation had to be made. Finally, results of international reliability tests of IPAQS7T conducted by the IPAQ group itself showed comparably higher test-retest reliability. Because most aspects of the methodology developed and used by the IPAQ group for the application of the instrument were also applied in the EUPASS project (e.g., translation procedures, statistical procedures for reliability testing), differences in test-retest reliability may also be due to sample issues. For example, in EUPASS the respondents were randomly selected on a nationwide basis, whereas in the international tests by the IPAQ group the instruments were given to samples with rather specific geographical and socio-demographic characteristics, including convenience samples.

As a further step in the reliability analysis, the test-retest results from IPAQS7T were compared with the test-retest co-efficients for the national indicators used in the eight countries to date, as well as with the psycho-social indicators. Test-retest co-efficients for the national indicators turned out to be similar (e.g., Germany, .3 to .6; the United Kingdom, .3 to .7) or even better (e.g., Finland, .5 to .9; Italy, .5 to .8) than those for IPAQS7T. The co-efficients for the psycho-social indicators also were slightly better for all nations, ranging from .5 to .6 for the self-efficacy scale and the social support scale and from .6 to .7 for the supportive environment scale.

5.4. Results of Comparability Analysis

On one hand, the present European Health Monitoring Programme aims to support the collection of comparable health data at the European level; several EU countries are considering using scientifically tested and internationally comparable indicators such as IPAQ for their national surveillance efforts. On the other hand, neither the European Commission nor the individual countries want to lose any information on health data that was collected in the past. Thus, the question of the comparability of old and new indicators was a crucial issue for the conduct of the EUPASS indicator test survey.

As previously mentioned, the comparability of PA indicators used in participating countries to date is very low (see Table 1). Generally, in their surveys the various countries have used different concepts of PA, focused on different dimensions, and used different scales and reference periods. Most of the national instruments show little comparability with IPAQ regarding these criteria as well.

To further investigate the comparability of each of the individual indicators, for each country all of the items from Section A (national indicators) and Section B (IPAQS7T) were subjected to correlation analyses. The results were not very encouraging regarding the double challenge of necessary change (using more comparable indicators) and desirable continuation (not losing information from data collected in the past). For example, at a correlation co-efficient of .3 or higher, in Belgium only one item (PA intense enough to make one sweat) correlated with one item in IPAQS7T (days of vigorous PA per week, .3) and in Finland only one item (how demanding is job physically) correlated with two items in IPAQS7T (duration of moderate activity, .3; duration of sitting during weekdays, .4). In Italy, correlation of the national indicators and the IPAQS7T indicators produced no co-efficients at or above .3 at all. Slightly better were the results for the United Kingdom (three old items correlated with three IPAQS7T items), Germany (four correlation co-efficients above .3), and the Netherlands (five correlation co-efficients above .3). Only one item with a correlation between the old and new indicators was above .5: in the German survey, duration of sitting from Monday to Friday correlated with the IPAQS7T item on sitting (duration weekdays, .6).

5.5. Results of Regression Analysis: Predictive Power Related to Subjective Health Status

McQueen defined the creation of "a data system for changing public health" as the key issue for health surveillance (McQueen, 1999, p. 1313). Accordingly, indicators used in surveillance should be related to major determinants of health. Behavioural indicators such as PA have been considered to be those determinants closest to health outcomes, as compared with social, environmental, or policy determinants which only may indirectly affect health status through behavioural change. However, as has been demonstrated by a recent international study, policy and environmental determinants (e.g., good opportunities and political support for PA by the general public) may have an independent main effect on subjective health status besides the effect of PA behaviour itself. Moreover, a significant interaction effect between "opportunities" and PA on subjective health has been reported in this context (Rütten et al., 2001).

Following up on this background, the EUPASS project tested indicators especially related to psycho-social and environmental determinants of PA and health. For the investigation of the predictive power of the different sets of indicators used in the study (i.e., national, IPAQ, psycho-social and environmental), hierarchical regression analyses were conducted for each country with subjective health status as the dependent variable. This variable was self-rated by respondents who selected one of five response categories (very good, good, satisfactory, not so good, bad) to the item "In general, how would you rate your health?" This type of operationalisation has been shown to be valid and predictive of health indicators in numerous studies (Idler and Benyamini, 1997).

Table 5 shows the results of hierarchical regression analysis for one country, Finland, as an example. To control for potential socio-demographic effects, indicators such

Table 5. Subjective health status[a] regressed on different sets of indicators, Finland

Predictor	Demographic			National			IPAQS7T			Psycho-social and environmental		
	β	R²	F change	β	R²	F change	β	R²	F change	β	R²	F change
Demographic												
Age	.200[d]	052	4.27[d]	.152[c]			.164[c]			.125[b]		
Gender				-.107[b]								
National												
Leisure-time PA for at least 30 minutes				.125[b]	.164	6.87[e]						
Exercise or physical exertion in free time				-.273[e]			-.301[e]			-.278[e]		
IPAQS7T												
Vigorous PA (minutes)							.172[c]	.199	3.82[e]	.154[c]		
Walking (minutes)							-.127[b]					
Sitting weekdays (minutes)							.184[c]			.197[c]		
Sitting weekend (minutes)							-.140[c]			-.185[d]		
Psycho-social and environmental												
How certain are you that you could do 30 minutes of moderate PA if you were sad or tired?										.301[e]	.329	4.66[e]
My municipality/city does enough for its citizens concerning their PA							.150[e]					

IPAQS7T = International Physical Activity Questionnaire, short, last 7 days, telephone version. β = standardised correlation coefficient.
PA = physical activity.
[a] Subjective health status was ranked from 1 to 5 (1 = very good, 5 = bad).
[b] p < .10, [c] p < .05, [d] p < .01, [e] p < .001; significance is set at p < .05.

as age, gender, education, and income were included in the first step of the regression equation. Only age turned out to be a significant predictor of subjective health. Of the four indicators used in the Finnish national PA surveillance to date, two ("How often did you do leisure-time PA with at least light sweating for at least half an hour?" and "How much exercise or physical exertion in leisure time?") were significant. By including IPAQS7T items in the third step, age and one item of the Finnish national indicators (exercise in leisure time) remained significant predictors. In addition, four out of nine IPAQ indicators were significant. Finally, by including psycho-social and environmental indicators at the fourth step, the one national item on intensity of PA (exercise or exertion in leisure time; response options ranged from "little movement" to "training for sports competition") turned out to be the strongest behavioural predictor ($\beta = -.278$), followed by three IPAQS7T indicators, the most important being duration of sitting. However, the strongest of all indicators tested was a psycho-social one, an item about self-efficacy related to PA ("How certain are you that you could do 30 minutes of moderate PA if you were sad or tired?"; responses were scaled 5 = "I'm sure I could" to 1 = "I'm sure I could not"; $\beta = .301$). In addition, one environmental and policy-oriented indicator ("My municipality/city does enough for its citizens concerning their PA"; responses were scaled 5 = "definitely true" to 1 = "not true at all") was a significant predictor of subjective health ($\beta = .150$). The particular predictive power of psycho-social and environmental determinants is underlined by the R^2 changes in the different steps of the hierarchical regression analysis. Including the respective indicators at the fourth step in the hierarchical regression procedure increased the explained variance of the overall model from about 20% to about 33% (13% increase; significant F change of 4.66).

The results of the regression analysis for Finland have been observed for other participating countries as well. For example, for Germany, the Netherlands, and the United Kingdom, indicators of self-efficacy turned out to be the strongest predictors of subjective health. Moreover, in most countries R^2 changes were highest from the third step to the fourth step (i.e., when including the psycho-social and environmental indicators related to PA).

6. GENERAL CONCLUSION

The present pilot study on developing EUPASS underlines the need for co-ordinating public health and surveillance activities within the European Community. As has been demonstrated by the comparative inventory of PA indicators, surveys, and surveillance structures of all EU countries which the EUPASS team prepared, the diversity of approaches to measure the population's PA in national surveys is enormous. Existing indicators neither relate to the same concept of health-related PA nor focus on comparable dimensions, nor do they apply similar reference periods or scales. As a consequence, available data sets on PA at the country level are not directly comparable at the European level.

One major approach to overcoming this situation is related to the efforts of an international consensus group for developing IPAQ. However, before one could recommend that EU countries use the IPAQ as a comparable instrument for national PA surveillance, two key issues have to be dealt with. First, the validity and reliability of the IPAQ instrument as well as its international and inter-cultural applicability and adequacy have to be more definitively determined. For example, as has been demonstrated by the EUPASS indicator test survey, reliability co-efficients on IPAQS7T are generally quite low for all eight participating countries (see Table 4). Second, the comparability of the old indicators and the IPAQ indicators appears to be a particularly important issue for countries such as Finland (which has maintained a high-quality PA surveillance system since the late 1970s) and the Netherlands (with its programme of continuous data collection). These countries do not want to lose the possibility of monitoring long-term PA changes in their population over time by substituting their present national indicators with IPAQ indicators, especially if the information provided by the new indicators is no longer comparable to the existing data. In this regard, the results of the current analysis are not encouraging: the correlation co-efficients between old indicators and indicators of IPAQS7T are generally quite low in all the countries investigated in this study.

In conclusion, countries with a longer tradition in PA surveillance may not wish to substitute their national indicators but instead add IPAQ indicators to their system. In other countries such as Belgium (where the main national health survey with two PA items has been conducted only once) or France and Italy (where PA items have been changed and no continuous data are yet available), adoption of an internationally comparable set of indicators (e.g., IPAQ) may be easier. Because of the further elaboration and testing necessary for the IPAQ instrument and other considerations, however, at present no final recommendation can be made regarding a comparable set of indicators for PA measurement at the EU level.

Nevertheless, at least three conclusions can be drawn from the EUPASS study to guide further activities towards the development of valid, reliable, comparable, and health-predictive PA data at the EU level:

- The value of the data on PA already available at the country level should not be under-estimated. For example, one of the indicators used in the national Finnish health survey for many years (leisure-time PA) turned out to be a stronger predictor of subjective health status than the IPAQS7T indicators. Because this indicator has not been used in other EU countries, no internationally comparable data are available. However, new methods of data conversion may be used at the EU level in the future to make such national data sets internationally comparable as well.

- The validity and reliability tests of the IPAQ instrument conducted by the IPAQ group itself have provided more promising results than the EUPASS project, but only one of four IPAQ versions has been tested in the EUPASS project. Further refinement may help to overcome the deficiencies shown by the reliability tests in this study. Thus, IPAQ still appears to be the first choice in the search for internationally comparable indicators of PA.

- The importance of psycho-social and environmental determinants for public health has been increasingly recognised in the last few years. The EUPASS indicator test survey investigated the predictive power of such indicators on subjective health in comparison with old and new (i.e., IPAQ) behavioural indicators. The psycho-social and environmental indicators turned out to be stronger predictors of subjective health than their behavioural counterparts. Thus, a country interested in creating a data system for changing public health should include psycho-social and environmental determinants. The European

Health Monitoring System also may consider using indicators related to self-efficacy and opportunities for PA as tested in the present study.

7. NEXT STEPS OF DEVELOPMENT

As a basic step in creating a system of comparable health-related data for changing public health at the EU level, the European Health Monitoring Programme aims at making the best use of existing data by putting this information into HIEMS. Of course, it must ensure that data on health-related behaviours such as PA from different countries put into the system are valid, reliable, and comparable. The EUPASS project can support this aim of the European programme in two ways: use EUPASS data as a comparable international data set for HIEMS, and use the EUPASS indicator test survey to provide all the necessary information for data conversion (i.e., create a comparable international data set out of the diverse data sets on PA available at the national level of participating countries).

Further developmental steps are related to the health data collection at the EU level in the future. In this regard, the European Health Monitoring Programme and other international efforts in the field of surveillance (e.g., IPAQ) have already had some impact on different EU countries to use more internationally comparable indicators for their national health surveillance. For example, the results of the EUPASS project are already being considered as a potential tool for future PA surveillance in Belgium, France, and Italy. In the long run, the EU may also want to set up its own European health surveillance system (e.g., related to a European Health Observatory). The experience gained from the EUPASS project may provide key information on both surveillance methodology in general (e.g., challenges for continuous data collection in different EU countries) and, more specifically, on adequate international PA indicators to use in such a system.

8. ACKNOWLEDGEMENTS

EUPASS was funded by the Health Monitoring Programme of the European Union (European Commission, Luxembourg, agreement number VS1999/5133 [99CVF3-502]). We acknowledge the support of the following individuals for their contributions to the realisation of this research: H. Chamouillet, P. Ciddo, I. De Bourdeaudhuij, A. Gatrell, P. Godin, A. Haase, R. Ireland, M. Lejeune, T. von Lengerke, D. McQueen, J. M. Oppert, N. Rodriguez Avila, J. Rodriguez Diaz, K. Schmitt, M. Sjöström, T. Stahl, M. Stiggelbout, J. Vinck, and A. Vuillemin.

9. REFERENCES

Ainsworth, B. E., Haskell, W., Leon, A. S., et al., 1993, Compendium of physical activities: classification of energy costs of human activities, *Med Sci Sports Exerc.* **25**:71–80.
Ainsworth, B. E., Haskell, W. L., Whitt, M. C., et al., 2000, Compendium of physical activities: an update of activity codes and MET intensities, *Med Sci Sports Exerc.* **32**:S498–S516.

American College of Sports Medicine, 1975, *Guidelines for Graded Exercise Testing and Exercise Prescription*, Lea & Febiger, Philadelphia.

Brownson, R. C., Jones, D. A., Pratt, M., et al., 2000, Measuring physical activity with the Behavioral Risk Factor Surveillance System, *Med Sci Sports Exerc*. 32:1913–1918.

De Bourdeaudhuij, I., and Van Oost, P., 1994, Differences in level and determinants of leisure-time physical activity between men and women in 3 population-based samples, *Arch Public Health*. 52:21–45.

De Bourdeaudhuij, I., Van Oost, P., and Mommerency, G., 1993, Daily physical activity in adolescents and young adults, *Arch Public Health*. 51:407–424.

Idler, E. L., and Benyamini, Y., 1997, Self-rated health and mortality: a review of twenty-seven community studies, *J Health Soc Behav*. 38:21–37.

Jones, D. A., Ainsworth, B. E., Croft, J. B., et al., 1998, Moderate leisure time physical activity: who is meeting the public health recommendations? A national cross-sectional study, *Arch Fam Med*. 7:285–289.

Laporte, R. E., Montoye, H. J., and Caspersen, C. J., 1985, Assessment of PA in epidemiologic research: problems and prospects, *Public Health Rep*. 100:131–146.

McQueen, D., 1999, A world behaving badly: the global challenge for behavioral surveillance, *Am J Public Health*. 89:1312–1314.

Pate, R. R., Pratt, M., Blair, S. N., et al., 1995, Physical activity and public health: a recommendation from the Centers for Disease Control and Prevention and the American College of Sports Medicine, *J Am Med Assoc*. 273:402–407.

Rütten, A., Abel, T., Kannas, L., et al., 2001, Self reported physical activity, public health, and the environment: results from a comparative European study, *J Epidemiol Community Health*. 55:139–146.

Rütten, A., Lüschen, G., von Lengerke, T., et al., 2000, *Health Promotion Policy in Europe: Rationality, Impact, and Evaluation*, Oldenbourg, Munich, Germany.

Sallis, J. F., and Owen, N., 1999, *Physical Activity and Behavioral Medicine*, Sage, London.

Stahl, T., Rütten, A., Nutbeam, D., et al., 2001, The importance of the social environment for physically active lifestyle—results from an international study, *Soc Sci Med*. 52:1–10.

U.S. Department of Health and Human Services, 1996, *Physical Activity and Health: A Report of the Surgeon General*, Centers for Disease Control and Prevention, Atlanta.

CHAPTER 9

COMPARISON OF SURVEILLANCE DATA ON METROPOLITAN AND RURAL HEALTH
Diabetes in Southern Australia as an Example

David H. Wilson[*]

1. BACKGROUND

Increasingly attention is being paid to evidence-based health policy in health services (Ham et al., 1995; Smith, 1995). Yet the evidence base for making many policy decisions is deficient, and better information systems are needed to inform the process (Tollman and Zwi, 2000). With the possible exception of the United States, national health authorities have not completely accepted the value of population-based surveillance systems that would better inform their decision making and allow them to monitor health outcomes and related cost benefit. In this chapter, I argue that traditional sources of data, provided largely from cross-sectional studies or from morbidity and mortality collections, are not in themselves adequate for planning. To effectively address health problems, a sustained source of data is necessary for health authorities to (1) identify key health problem areas that require attention, (2) analyse the underlying reasons for continuation of the problems, (3) assess the circumstances in which investment can be most effective, and (4) monitor the impact of solutions.

2. INTRODUCTION

I briefly review the Australian National Rural Health Strategy (Australian Health Ministers' Conference, 1994, 1996), a policy document on the approach to rural health in Australia, and examine the basis of its recommendations and concordance with the supporting evidence. The Strategy developers relied mainly on cross-sectional morbidity and mortality data and did not have the benefit of longitudinal or surveillance data. I examine

[*] University of Adelaide, Woodville, South Australia 5011, Australia.

the level of agreement between the Strategy's recommendations and the evidence base and discuss the general limitations of the evidence. Population surveillance data collected on diabetes are used to compare the health status of a metropolitan area and several rural areas of the state of South Australia to illustrate the value of data collected over time in a surveillance system, and to compare the conclusions reached on diabetes with those of the National Rural Health Strategy.

Many recent Australian health reports provide evidence that higher rates of disease and poorer health outcomes are more prevalent among residents in rural than metropolitan areas (Australian Institute of Health and Welfare, 1994, 1996, 1998; National Rural Public Health Forum, 1998; Strong et al., 1998; National Rural Health Policy Forum, 1999). These and similar reports over the last two decades indicate that people residing in rural areas suffer health inequities compared with their metropolitan peers. Therefore, it is reasonable to conclude that the more remote the community, the greater the prevalence of disease and the poorer the health outcomes ("sicker rural health hypothesis"). From such reports the National Rural Health Strategy developers concluded that Australia required a "unique" strategy to meet rural health care needs (Australian Health Ministers' Conference, 1999). The Strategy proposed that rural health services should be based on need, equity, and access to health care; use flexible funding arrangements; involve community participation in planning; and be sensitive to social and cultural differences. Yet it is difficult to understand why these principles would not apply to any area or population group that experiences poorer health status and, therefore, how they constitute a unique strategy for rural areas. The focus of the Strategy is also concerned more with the provision of health services and not necessarily with improved health outcomes. The recommendations are fundamental and make sense, yet it is difficult to relate them to the evidence base used, which was drawn largely from cross-sectional studies. The Strategy's rationale appears to have been based more on assumptions about the tyranny of distance (small and sparsely distributed populations, and geographic and social diversity) and on selective cross-sectional supporting information than on a substantive analysis and comparison of health issues in metropolitan and rural areas.

The bulk of the evidence used by the National Rural Health Strategy in concluding that health needs are greater in rural areas was based largely on point-in-time prevalence estimates of health problems. Any descriptive information provided was often investigator driven—rather than policy driven—and left many gaps in explaining the morbidity and mortality picture of rural communities (Peckham and Smith, 1996; Muir-Gray, 1997). Such data may be suitable for indicator development, but they are not adequate for policy and intervention planning. If national health services are to make a substantial health investment in developing solutions with the best chance of achieving cost-beneficial health outcomes, we need to confirm the policy targets from more than one cross-sectional data source and use standardised methods. For example, much of the investment and progress in recent years with cancer have been based on surveillance data provided by cancer registries (dos Santos Silva, 1999). This lesson has not been applied to other major public health problems (e.g., chronic lung disease, cardiovascular diseases, and diabetes) and was not evident in the National Rural Health Strategy.

Surveillance systems for major chronic disease issues are rare, and health planners often have to resort to traditional data collections in addition to cross-sectional studies. Traditional means have inherent limitations. Even so, using data sets with inherent limitations appears to have been a substantial part of the development of the Australian National Rural Health Strategy. In the absence of population surveillance systems for health planning, a great deal of reliance was placed on data drawn from morbidity and mortality registers. Although such registers have many positive uses, these sources can present substantial problems when used for planning. For example, hospital admission data can reflect local and temporal policies of health administrators. Australian Medicare data between 1990 and 1995 showed lower rates of hospital use in rural areas than in metropolitan areas (National Rural Health Policy Forum, 1999) and would not support the sicker rural health hypothesis on which the Strategy is based: areas with higher health needs are expected to have higher rates of hospital admissions. The difference may be explained by worse access among rural people to health services, but this issue needs further investigation using representative population interview samples.

Mortality data were used in developing the Strategy but may not truly reflect the health burdens of rural areas. Not only have cause of ill health and cause of death increasingly separated, but specifying cause of death for elderly people—an increasing proportion of the population—is not always a reliable process (Rosenberg, 1999). Further, the comparability of mortality data over time is affected by the impact of science and technology (Rosenberg, 1999) and changing causes of mortality.

Problems also exist with associated life expectancy data. Differences in life expectancy rates based on mortality data from 1994 to 1996 have been documented for metropolitan and rural Australia. People living in metropolitan areas can expect to live 1 year longer than people living in rural areas and 4 years longer than those living in remote areas[†] (Strong et al., 1998). These differences could, however, be explained by the differences in survival rates following a major event or the impact of Aboriginal mortality on the overall death rate.

Much of the data used in support of the Australian National Rural Health Strategy were comparisons between metropolitan and rural health status. In such comparisons, we have to be mindful of the demographic mix of the areas being compared. Age and sex variations between regions are obvious reasons for different health profiles and were usually controlled for in the Strategy's evidence base. However, some other important confounding variables were not controlled for. For example, differences between regions may be explained by social class (which is related to health behaviours and prevention practises [Marmot et al., 1991; Blane et al., 1993]) or by the origin of the population (in Australia the Aboriginal and Torres Strait Islander populations experience disease rates several times the non-Aboriginal population [Strong et al., 1998], and in South Australian rural regions their death rates are three times that of non-Aboriginal residents [Nguyen et al., 1996]). If rurality is related to demographic, social class, or indigenous characteristics, these associations may explain health and disease differentials and the differences may also apply to sub-populations in metropolitan areas. Because of possible and

---

[†] Metropolitan areas include state and territorial capitals as well as urban centres with a population of 100,000 or more. Rural areas have an index of remoteness (determined by population density and distances to large population centres) of 10.5 or less and include urban centres with a population of less than 100,000. Remote areas have an index of remoteness higher than 10.5 and may include urban centres of any population size. For a more detailed description of geographic classification see the Department of Primary Industries and Energy and the Department of Human Services and Health (1994).

changing variations in the demographic areas, adequate analytic controls must be considered and used in comparisons. Such controls are most likely to occur in surveillance data sets designed specifically for comparisons.

Differentials in health status may also disappear when appropriate epidemiological methods are applied to the data. Epidemiological methods, within which surveillance is a key concept, are therefore as important in health planning and policy development as they are in public health investigations. It is also important that survey sample sizes are able to meet policy requirements and provide adequate information for targeting. Even quite large cross-sectional studies may not have adequate sample sizes to support the sort of break-downs required in policy development and targeting. If we cannot target adequately, then investment in solutions will be based on serendipity rather than planning. Adequate sample sizes may best be achieved by combining data collected systematically over time in surveillance systems to provide more powerful bi-variate and multi-variate analyses.

The Australian National Rural Health Strategy, like many other policy initiatives, had access to limited information that supported the sicker rural health hypothesis, but on closer examination serious questions can be raised about the quality of the information used. From the evidence cited, the Strategy developers concluded that distance is a health problem regardless of other factors. It may indeed be that distance leads to poorer health outcomes (e.g., because of difficulty obtaining specialist services), but even these outcomes may be explained by clustering problems in particular population groups for whom solutions other than those mooted in the Strategy are required. The classic example is the Aboriginal population, whose health needs are inextricably bound with social and infra-structure disadvantages as well as their need for health services.

Many of the problems I have identified can be overcome with systematic surveillance in which the data set can be tailored to investigate health differentials and their explanatory variables. Regular surveillance of health, demography, and related data allows us not only to monitor prevalence and trend, but also to build data sets that will enable investigation of the related context of health and disease and to explain exposure issues, demographic differences, and use of health services. Surveillance systems also facilitate the development of question modules tailored to specific policy needs and that produce relevant and timely data. Repeated measures in surveillance systems permit the testing of question modules for reliability and validity, which is not always possible in other forms of data collection. Systematic surveillance can facilitate advanced analyses of variables implicated in health problems and can provide more detailed multi-variate explanations of the issues. Also, if we are really concerned about improving health outcomes, we have to measure the outcome with the same yardstick as that used to determine the original priority. Comparability of data over time is therefore important and can best be provided in surveillance systems.

The major importance of surveillance is its potential contribution to the evidence base for making policy decisions. Evidence-based approaches to developing policy should not only be concerned with prevalence estimates of disease problems, but also deal with exposure (e.g., to pathogens, risk factors, health behaviours), population structure (e.g., age and sex composition, migrant and ethnic composition, socio-economic status), access to appropriate services, and the inter-action between these variables. Surveillance systems can address this wider data context as essential policy intelligence and allow more substantial multi-variate analyses of the problems and target groups. In this chapter I use diabetes surveillance data collected in South Australia for many years to explore prevalence, exposure, and population structure variables. Whether the problem of diabetes is increasing or decreasing over time is also critical policy information for the long-term investment of health resources. Such information can be provided only by systematic surveillance systems. In policy formulation we need to be concerned about not only the present situation but also the future and the preventive or health promotion strategies that will minimise future disease impact and burden. Trend data, which are provided by population surveillance systems for diseases of interest to health planners, are the best source for this information. In the analyses that follow, I use multi-variate analyses to explore the best set of variables that explain the problem of diabetes in South Australian metropolitan and rural areas. In addition, I examine inter-actions in the data and the trend in the diabetes problem over time, then assess the need for a "unique" rural health policy for South Australia in relation to diabetes.

3. METHODS

3.1. Participants

Data were collected from respondents in the South Australian Health Omnibus Surveys between 1992 and 1998 (Wilson et al., 1992). These representative surveys of adults aged 15 years or older involved a multi-stage, systematic, clustered area sample of people living in Adelaide (a metropolitan area) or in one of many rural centres with a population of over 1,000 persons. In 1996 about 836,000 persons this age lived in Adelaide and about 292,000 in the rural regions (Australian Bureau of Statistics, 1996). Hotels, motels, hospitals, nursing homes, and other institutions were excluded from the survey. The person whose birthday was next in the selected household was interviewed at home by a trained health interviewer. There was no replacement for non-respondents. Up to six' callbacks were made in an attempt to interview the selected person, resulting in approximately 3,000 interviews being conducted each year. Response rates ranged from 70% in 1998 to 74% in 1995. The total sample size available for these analyses was 18,075 for education (which was not asked in 1993), 18,069 for cholesterol, blood pressure, and exercise (which were not asked in 1994), and 21,079 for all other variables.

3.2. Data Collection

The sample for each Health Omnibus Survey was obtained by selecting a random sample of Australian Bureau of Statistics collector districts. Within each collector district a random starting point was selected, and from this point 10 households were selected in a given direction with a fixed skip interval. Because they came from a large clustered sample, the data were weighted by age, gender, geographic region, and possibility of selection in the household to estimated resident population data so that the results were representative of the South Australian population.

The Health Omnibus Surveys were conducted during the spring of each year from 1992 through 1998. Information was collected from year to year using the same question modules on diabetes, demographics, and disease risk factors. Demographic factors included area of residence, sex, age, country of birth, post-school education, annual family income, socio-economic status, and employment status. Area of residence was derived from Australian Bureau of Statistics collector districts based on regional divisions of South Australia. Socio-economic status was derived from occupational status as determined from the Australian Standard Classification of Occupations codes (Kelley and Evans, 1988; Australian Bureau of Statistics, 1990). Disease risk factors included smoking status, weight category, asthma, last cholesterol reading, vigorous exercise in last 2 weeks, ever having high blood pressure, last blood pressure reading, and alcohol risk.

Quality-of-life data from the short-form health survey questionnaire (SF-36), a generic measure of health status encompassing eight dimensions validated for Australia with use of the scoring method of the Medical Outcomes Trust (McCallum, 1994), were obtained in 1994 and 1998. The eight dimensions are physical functioning, physical role, bodily pain, general health, vitality, social functioning, emotional role, and mental health.

I obtained mortality data from the Health Statistics Unit of the South Australian Department of Human Services through death records (Australian Bureau of Statistics, 1993–1998; Nguyen et al., 1996). Age, sex, and area of residence were provided in addition to the number of deaths between 1993 and 1998 due to diabetes.

3.3. Statistical Methods

I analysed the data using SPSS for Windows Version 10.0 (SPSS Inc., 1999) and Epi Info Version 6 (Dean et al., 1994). Changes in variables over time were assessed using the chi-square test for trends. Trends were examined both overall and separately for the metropolitan region and the rural regions; statistical significance was set at $p < 0.05$. Death rates due to diabetes for both regions were standardised by age and sex to the 1996 South Australian population. Because the number of deaths per annum was small, I combined years into 1993–1995 and 1996–1998 for comparisons.

In addition to conducting trend analyses, I aggregated the data for powerful descriptive analyses at both uni-variate and multi-variate levels. The data are an aggregation of surveys conducted over 7 years, so the aggregated data may show auto-correlation over time. I excluded this possibility after the average residuals for each year from the fitted models were tested for auto-correlation.

Diabetes was used as the dependent variable in uni-variate analyses examining the associations between this chronic condition and the other variables for the metropolitan area, the rural areas, and South Australia overall. I examined explanatory variables for collinearity and inter-actions before entering them into a multiple logistic regression analysis. No significant inter-actions were detected between the continuous variable, year, or any of the other independent variables. I entered all variables with a p value of <0.25 in the uni-variate analyses into the regression analyses (Hosmer and Lemeshow, 1989). Variables that were not significant at $p < 0.05$ were progressively omitted until I obtained satisfactory models that best explained diabetes for the metropolitan area, the rural area, and the state overall.

I compared people with and without diabetes living in Adelaide and in the rural areas by self-reported health status with use of the eight dimensions of the SF-36. Multiple linear regression was used to compute differences in the eight dimensions between groups. Mean scores for each dimension were adjusted for age, sex, and socio-economic status to account for differences in these variables between the comparison groups. Equivalence of these mean scores between groups was examined using the *t*-test. Using the method of Garratt and colleagues (1993), I then calculated standard quality-of-life scores for people with and without diabetes living in Adelaide and in the rural areas. In this computation, standard scores were calculated for each SF-36 dimension by dividing the differences between the quality-of-life scores for each area of residence and the norm of the general population by the standard deviation of the general population. The standard score for the general population was set at zero. South Australian population norms were obtained from two previous Health Omnibus Surveys (Wakefield and Wilson, 1996). In interpreting the differences in standard scores between groups according to Kazis and colleagues (1989), an effect size of 0.2 (or one fifth of a standard deviation) is described as small, 0.5 as moderate, and 0.8 as large.

4. RESULTS

The prevalence of diabetes increased significantly from 1992 through 1998 in the metropolitan area, the rural areas, and South Australia overall ($p < 0.001$ for all) (Table 1). The diabetes prevalence trend appeared to increase at a higher rate in the rural areas than in Adelaide, but the difference in the rate of increase was not significant.

The proportion of people who lived in the metropolitan area or the rural areas did not change significantly (Table 1). Many other demographic characteristics changed, however. The population aged and the proportion who were born in Australia increased significantly in Adelaide, but not in the rural regions. The percentage who have post-school qualifications rose significantly in both Adelaide and the rural areas. The proportion of the population with an annual family income of $A20,000 or less dropped significantly in both the metropolitan area and the rural regions, reflecting increasing prosperity in both areas, but this income was not adjusted for inflation and may not reflect an increase in real income. The significant increase in both areas in the prevalence of low socio-economic status may, in fact, indicate a reduction in real income. The unemployment rate dropped significantly in the city, but not in the rural regions.

Several important diabetes risk factor variables are also shown in Table 1. In both the metropolitan area and the rural areas the prevalence of obesity and asthma rose significantly, and the prevalence of a high cholesterol reading and vigorous exercise decreased significantly. The prevalence of ever having been told one had high blood pressure decreased significantly only in the rural regions, but this served only to bring the rate in line with that in Adelaide. Conversely, an alcohol risk of intermediate or high increased significantly only in Adelaide, to become comparable with the risk in the rural areas.

In both 1993–1995 and 1996–1998, the recorded diabetes death rate was higher in rural regions than in Adelaide (Table 2). The rural rate decreased significantly from 1993–1995 to 1996–1998, whereas the metropolitan rate remained stable.

In the uni-variate analyses the variables for which there was a bi-variate statistically significant association with diabetes in the metropolitan area, the rural areas, and in South Australia were female sex, age 50 years or older, post-school qualifications, annual family income of $A20,000 or less, current smoking, overweight, obese, weight not stated, cholesterol reading never measured, vigorous exercise in last 2 weeks, been told have

Table 1. Prevalence of diabetes (% and 95% CI) in South Australia, by area of residence, population structure, and diabetes risk factors, 1992–1998

Variable	Year							χ^2 trend	p
	1992	1993	1994	1995	1996	1997	1998		
Total population									
Overall	2.6 (2.0–3.3)	3.2 (2.6–4.0)	3.9 (3.2–4.7)	4.2 (3.5–5.0)	3.8 (3.1–4.6)	4.4 (3.7–5.3)	5.2 (4.4–6.1)	29.28	<0.001
Metropolitan	2.9 (2.2–3.8)	2.7 (2.0–3.6)	3.7 (2.9–4.7)	3.8 (3.0–4.8)	3.5 (2.8–4.5)	4.6 (3.7–5.7)	4.8 (3.9–5.8)	18.24	<0.001
Rural	1.8 (1.1–3.1)	4.4 (3.2–6.1)	4.3 (3.1–5.9)	5.1 (3.7–6.8)	4.3 (3.1–6.0)	3.9 (2.8–5.5)	6.3 (4.7–8.2)	11.20	<0.001
Living in rural area									
Overall	29.1 (27.4–30.8)	31.1 (29.4–32.9)	30.9 (29.2–32.7)	30.7 (29.0–32.5)	30.6 (28.8–32.3)	31.3 (29.6–33.1)	28.8 (27.1–30.5)	0.03	0.91
Male gender									
Overall	48.9 (47.0–50.7)	48.8 (46.9–50.7)	49.2 (47.3–51.1)	49.2 (47.4–51.1)	49.2 (47.3–51.1)	48.7 (46.8–50.5)	49.0 (47.1–50.9)	0.00	1.03
Metropolitan	48.3 (46.1–50.6)	48.1 (45.8–50.4)	48.5 (46.2–50.8)	48.6 (46.4–50.9)	48.6 (46.3–50.9)	47.9 (45.6–50.1)	48.3 (46.1–50.6)	0.01	0.92
Rural	50.1 (46.6–53.6)	50.4 (47.0–53.8)	50.6 (47.2–51.1)	50.6 (47.2–54.0)	50.6 (47.2–54.0)	50.4 (47.0–53.8)	50.6 (47.0–54.1)	0.02	0.94
Age ≥50 years									
Overall	31.9 (30.1–33.7)	31.8 (30.0–33.6)	32.8 (31.1–34.6)	32.9 (31.1–34.7)	33.4 (31.7–35.2)	33.8 (32.0–35.6)	34.9 (33.2–36.8)	9.24	0.002
Metropolitan	31.8 (29.7–33.9)	31.5 (29.4–33.6)	32.5 (30.4–34.6)	33.0 (30.9–35.1)	33.1 (31.0–35.3)	33.9 (31.8–36.1)	34.8 (32.7–36.9)	7.14	0.008
Rural	32.1 (28.9–35.5)	32.4 (29.3–35.7)	33.7 (30.5–37.0)	32.7 (29.5–36.0)	34.1 (30.9–37.5)	33.5 (30.4–36.8)	35.4 (32.1–38.8)	2.16	0.13

Table 1. (continued)

Variable	1992	1993	1994	1995	1996	1997	1998	χ^2 trend	p
Born in Australia									
Overall	73.7 (72.0–75.4)	75.1 (73.5–76.7)	75.1 (73.4–76.7)	75.6 (73.9–77.2)	76.9 (75.2–78.4)	77.3 (75.6–78.8)	75.5 (73.8–77.1)	7.44	0.006
Metropolitan	69.8 (67.7–71.9)	72.1 (72.0–75.4)	71.1 (69.0–73.1)	72.1 (70.0–74.1)	74.0 (71.9–75.9)	72.9 (70.8–74.9)	72.1 (70.0–74.0)	4.74	0.03
Rural	83.3 (80.4–85.7)	81.9 (79.1–84.4)	84.1 (81.4–86.5)	83.5 (80.8–85.9)	83.4 (80.6–85.8)	86.8 (84.3–88.9)	84.0 (81.2–86.5)	3.25	0.07
Have post-school qualifications[a]									
Overall	40.0 (38.2–41.9)	41.8 (39.9–43.6)	42.6 (40.7–44.4)	41.9 (40.0–43.8)	42.7 (40.9–44.6)	44.0 (42.1–45.9)	46.2 (44.3–48.1)	23.45	<0.001
Metropolitan	41.9 (39.7–44.1)	43.1 (40.9–45.4)	44.4 (42.2–46.7)	44.0 (41.8–46.3)	44.7 (42.4–47.0)	46.5 (44.2–48.7)	47.1 (44.9–49.3)	15.56	<0.001
Rural	35.5 (32.2–39.0)	38.8 (35.5–42.1)	38.3 (35.1–41.7)	37.1 (33.9–40.5)	38.3 (35.0–41.7)	38.6 (35.4–42.0)	44.0 (40.5–47.5)	7.92	0.005
Annual family income ≤$A20,000									
Overall	30.6 (28.9–32.4)	29.1 (27.4–30.8)	29.3 (27.6–31.0)	27.1 (25.4–28.8)	26.3 (24.7–28.0)	26.4 (24.8–28.1)	25.6 (24.0–27.3)	28.93	<0.001
Metropolitan	30.1 (28.1–32.2)	27.7 (25.7–29.8)	27.5 (25.5–29.6)	26.3 (24.3–28.3)	25.6 (23.7–27.7)	25.6 (23.6–27.6)	23.9 (22.0–25.8)	24.20	<0.001
Rural	31.8 (28.6–35.2)	32.0 (28.9–35.3)	33.2 (30.0–36.5)	28.8 (25.8–32.0)	27.9 (24.9–31.1)	28.2 (25.2–31.3)	30.0 (26.8–33.3)	5.39	0.02
Low socio-economic status[b]									
Overall	31.1 (29.3–32.9)	30.1 (28.4–31.9)	29.7 (28.0–31.5)	29.5 (27.8–31.3)	29.9 (28.2–31.7)	35.5 (33.5–37.5)	35.6 (33.6–37.6)	24.49	<0.001
Metropolitan	30.5 (28.4–32.7)	30.8 (28.7–33.0)	29.3 (27.2–31.5)	27.0 (25.1–29.1)	29.0 (26.9–31.1)	33.8 (31.5–36.3)	33.7 (31.4–36.1)	6.43	0.01
Rural	32.5 (29.2–36.0)	28.7 (25.7–32.0)	30.5 (27.4–33.9)	35.2 (32.0–38.5)	32.1 (28.9–35.5)	39.0 (35.5–42.7)	40.1 (36.4–44.0)	26.00	<0.001

Table 1. (continued)

Variable	1992	1993	1994	1995	1996	1997	1998	χ² trend	p
				Year					
Unemployed[c]									
Overall	5.3 (4.5–6.2)		4.7 (3.9–5.6)	4.1 (3.4–5.0)	5.1 (4.3–6.0)	3.9 (3.2–4.6)	4.5 (3.7–5.3)	3.05	0.08
Metropolitan	5.5 (4.5–6.6)		4.6 (3.7–5.7)	4.3 (3.4–5.3)	5.6 (4.6–6.8)	3.8 (3.0–4.8)	3.6 (2.9–4.6)	7.24	0.007
Rural	4.8 (3.5–6.6)		4.8 (3.5–6.6)	3.9 (2.7–5.5)	4.0 (2.8–5.6)	3.9 (2.8–5.5)	6.5 (4.9–8.5)	0.86	0.40
Current smoker									
Overall	27.0 (25.4–28.8)	25.6 (24.0–27.3)	27.7 (26.1–29.5)	27.0 (25.3–28.7)	28.1 (26.4–29.8)	26.7 (25.1–28.4)	25.8 (24.2–27.6)	0.07	0.80
Metropolitan	26.5 (24.5–28.5)	24.9 (22.9–26.9)	26.4 (24.4–28.5)	25.6 (23.7–27.6)	26.8 (24.8–28.9)	25.2 (23.2–27.2)	24.9 (23.0–26.9)	0.58	0.40
Rural	28.5 (25.4–31.8)	27.3 (24.4–30.5)	30.8 (27.7–34.0)	30.1 (27.0–33.3)	31.1 (28.0–34.4)	30.1 (27.0–33.3)	28.2 (25.1–31.6)	0.44	0.50
Obese (body mass index >30 kg/m²)									
Overall	9.8 (8.6–11.0)	11.1 (9.9–12.4)	13.6 (12.3–15.0)	13.3 (12.0–14.7)	15.0 (13.6–16.5)	15.3 (13.9–16.8)	14.8 (13.4–16.2)	53.12	<0.001
Metropolitan	8.4 (7.2–9.8)	10.5 (9.1–12.0)	12.7 (11.3–14.4)	12.2 (10.7–13.8)	14.4 (12.8–16.1)	14.2 (12.6–15.9)	13.2 (11.7–14.9)	36.88	<0.001
Rural	13.3 (8.6–11.0)	12.6 (10.3–15.2)	15.5 (13.1–18.3)	15.9 (13.4–18.8)	16.6 (14.0–19.7)	18.0 (15.3–21.0)	18.5 (15.8–21.7)	16.57	<0.001
Asthma									
Overall	9.3 (8.2–10.4)	10.2 (9.1–11.4)	9.5 (8.5–10.7)	11.4 (10.3–12.7)	11.6 (10.5–12.9)	12.2 (11.1–13.6)	11.5 (10.4–12.8)	44.96	<0.001
Metropolitan	9.0 (7.8–10.4)	9.6 (8.3–11.0)	9.0 (7.8–10.4)	10.6 (9.2–12.1)	10.5 (9.2–12.0)	11.8 (10.4–13.3)	11.0 (9.7–12.5)	11.34	<0.001
Rural	9.9 (8.0–12.2)	11.5 (9.4–13.8)	10.6 (8.7–13.0)	13.3 (11.1–15.8)	14.2 (12.0–16.8)	13.3 (11.2–15.8)	12.8 (10.6–15.4)	7.89	0.004

Table 1. (continued)

Variable	Year							χ^2 trend	p
	1992	1993	1994	1995	1996	1997	1998		
Last cholesterol reading was high[d]									
Overall	22.0 (20.0–24.2)	18.9 (17.1–21.0)		17.0 (15.2–18.8)	14.4 (12.9–16.2)	15.9 (14.3–17.7)	14.5 (12.9–16.3)	42.72	<0.001
Metropolitan	21.2 (18.8–23.8)	18.0 (15.8–20.4)		16.4 (14.4–18.7)	14.6 (12.7–16.8)	16.3 (14.3–18.5)	15.3 (13.4–17.5)	16.35	<0.001
Rural	24.1 (20.2–28.6)	21.2 (17.7–25.3)		18.0 (14.9–21.6)	14.1 (11.3–17.4)	15.0 (12.2–18.3)	12.4 (9.7–15.7)	33.76	<0.001
Vigorous exercise in last 2 weeks[d]									
Overall	39.8 (38.0–41.7)	44.9 (43.0–46.7)		25.3 (23.7–27.0)	25.6 (24.0–27.3)	25.3 (23.7–26.9)	26.6 (24.9–28.3)	311.00	<0.001
Metropolitan	40.7 (38.5–42.9)	44.3 (42.1–46.6)		26.5 (24.6–28.6)	25.6 (23.7–27.7)	26.0 (24.0–28.0)	26.2 (24.3–28.2)	228.64	<0.001
Rural	37.7 (34.3–41.2)	46.0 (42.7–49.5)		22.5 (19.8–25.5)	25.4 (22.5–28.6)	23.7 (20.9–26.7)	27.5 (24.5–30.8)	82.65	<0.001
Ever told have high blood pressure[d]									
Overall	23.0 (21.4–24.6)	24.6 (23.0–26.3)		20.1 (18.6–21.7)	22.5 (20.9–24.1)	23.9 (22.4–25.6)	21.6 (20.1–23.2)	0.92	0.30
Metropolitan	21.1 (19.3–23.0)	22.8 (20.9–24.7)		18.7 (17.0–20.6)	22.1 (20.2–24.0)	23.8 (21.9–25.8)	21.7 (19.9–23.6)	1.54	0.20
Rural	27.4 (24.4–30.7)	28.7 (25.7–31.9)		23.3 (20.5–26.3)	23.5 (20.7–26.5)	24.3 (21.5–27.4)	21.5 (18.7–24.6)	12.42	<0.001
Last blood pressure reading was high[d]									
Overall	10.3 (9.2–11.5)	10.8 (9.7–12.1)		9.9 (8.9–11.2)	10.3 (9.2–11.6)	10.1 (9.0–11.3)	10.7 (9.6–12.0)	0.01	0.93
Metropolitan	9.0 (7.7–10.4)	9.9 (8.6–11.4)		9.5 (8.2–10.9)	9.5 (8.3–11.0)	9.5 (8.2–11.0)	10.5 (9.2–12.0)	1.52	0.21
Rural	13.5 (11.2–16.2)	12.8 (10.7–15.4)		11.0 (9.0–13.4)	12.1 (10.0–14.6)	11.4 (9.4–13.8)	11.2 (9.1–13.7)	2.38	0.11

Table 1. (continued)

Variable	Year							χ^2 trend	p
	1992	1993	1994	1995	1996	1997	1998		
Alcohol risk intermediate or high									
Overall	3.5	3.6	4.8	4.6	5.8	6.2	5.1	27.22	<0.001
	(2.9–4.3)	(3.0–4.4)	(4.0–5.6)	(3.9–5.5)	(5.0–6.7)	(5.4–7.2)	(4.3–6.0)		
Metropolitan	3.1	2.7	4.3	3.9	4.9	6.0	5.0	30.35	<0.001
	(2.4–4.0)	(2.0–3.5)	(3.4–5.3)	(3.1–4.9)	(4.0–6.0)	(5.0–7.2)	(4.1–6.1)		
Rural	4.7	5.8	5.8	6.3	7.7	6.8	5.3	2.00	0.23
	(3.4–6.4)	(4.4–7.6)	(4.4–7.7)	(4.8–8.2)	(6.0–9.8)	(5.2–8.7)	(3.9–7.2)		

[a] Post-school qualifications = trade (or other) certificate or degree.
[b] As determined by occupational status (Kelley and Evans, 1988; Australian Bureau of Statistics, 1990).
[c] Employment status was not asked in 1993.
[d] Last cholesterol reading, vigorous exercise in last 2 weeks, been told have high blood pressure, and last blood pressure reading were not asked in 1994.

Table 2. Annual death rates[a] (no. per 100,000 and 95% CI) due to diabetes in South Australia, by area of residence

Area of Residence	1993–1995	1996–1998
Overall	22.2 (20.4–24.0)	23.5 (21.7–25.3)
Metropolitan	19.5 (18.5–20.5)	20.8 (19.8–21.8)
Rural	43.7 (41.1–46.4)	30.5 (28.4–32.6)

[a] Standardised by age and sex to the 1996 South Australian population.

high blood pressure, last blood pressure reading high, and alcohol risk intermediate or high (Table 3).

When the variables significant at the uni-variate stage were entered into logistic regression analyses, agreement was again good. The best set of variables that explained the prevalence of diabetes overall and in separate logistic regression analyses for both the metropolitan area and the rural areas were age 50 years or older, annual family income of $A20,000 or less, overweight, obese, or weight not stated, last cholesterol reading high, been told have high blood pressure, and alcohol risk low or none (Table 4). There was also a statistically significant increase for year as a continuous variable. In addition, in the rural areas female sex was significant, and in South Australia overall and in Adelaide vigorous exercise in last 2 weeks was significant. In 1998 the mean SF-36 scores for all eight dimensions were similar in the metropolitan area and the rural areas, and in both regions scores were usually lower among persons with diabetes than without diabetes (Table 5). The deterioration in health-related quality of life for people with diabetes was greater in Adelaide than in the rural areas (Figure 1). For people in the rural areas, the quality-of-life dimensions that comprise the mental health scale (vitality, social functioning, emotional role, and mental health) differed little between persons with or without diabetes (the effect size was generally #0.2); this was not the case for people in the city (the effect size was >0.2).

5. DISCUSSION

Surveillance systems in developed countries grew out of the need for surveillance of infectious diseases (Taylor, 1992; Catchpole, 1996). With few exceptions, similar developments have not occurred for chronic diseases. The reduction of many infectious diseases has been aided by surveillance data in addition to clinical, therapeutic, and preventive services. For chronic diseases we continue to operate without systems that would provide information for an evidence-based approach to policy development and interventions that would, in turn, minimise resource waste and optimise effectiveness. In Australia today only three states conduct regular computer-assisted telephone interviews (CATI)—an inadequate situation for national planning and policy development in chronic diseases.

Today strong theoretical reasons also support a surveillance approach to policy and planning in health. Much of the conventional risk factor approach used in the development of the Australian National Rural Health Strategy can be described by "black box"

Table 3. Uni-variate analysis of variables associated with diabetes in South Australia, by area of residence, 1992–1998

Variable	Overall				Metropolitan				Rural			
	n	%	OR (95% CI)	p	n	%	OR (95% CI)	p	n	%	OR (95% CI)	p
Area of residence												
Metropolitan	14,681	3.7	1.00	0.05								
Rural	6,399	4.3	1.16 (1.00–1.35)									
Sex												
Male	10,327	3.4	1.00		7,097	3.4	1.00	0.02	3,231	3.4	1.00	<0.001
Female	10,752	4.4	1.32 (1.15–1.53)	<0.001	7,584	4.1	1.22 (1.03–1.46)		3,168	5.2	1.55 (1.20–2.00)	
Age												
15–49 years	14,108	1.7	1.00		9,847	1.6	1.00	<0.001	4,260	2.0	1.00	<0.001
≥50 years	6,971	8.3	5.23 (4.48–6.12)	<0.001	4,833	8.1	5.47 (4.51–6.64)		2,138	8.9	4.85 (3.70–6.36)	
Birthplace												
Overseas	5,144	5.1	1.00		4,111	5.0	1.00	<0.001	1,033	5.2	1.00	0.1
Australia	15,935	3.5	0.69 (0.59–0.80)	<0.001	10,569	3.2	0.63 (0.53–0.76)		5,365	4.1	0.78 (0.57–1.06)	
Education												
No post-school qualifications	12,070	4.6	1.00		8,143	4.3	1.00	<0.001	3,926	5.0	1.00	<0.001
Post-school qualifications	9,010	3.0	0.65 (0.56–0.76)	<0.001	6,538	3.0	0.69 (0.57–0.82)		2,472	3.1	0.60 (0.45–0.79)	
Annual family income												
>$A20,000	15,227	2.5	1.00		10,764	2.4	1.00	<0.001	4,464	3.0	1.00	<0.001
#$A20,000	5,852	7.5	3.10 (2.69–3.58)	<0.001	3,918	7.5	3.36 (2.82–4.00)		1,935	7.4	2.62 (2.04–3.36)	

Table 3. (continued)

Variable	Overall				Metropolitan				Rural			
	n	%	OR (95% CI)	p	n	%	OR (95% CI)	p	n	%	OR (95% CI)	p
Socio-economic status												
Medium, high, or very high	13,433	3.8	1.00		9,487	3.6	1.00		3,946	4.2	1.00	
Low	6,172	4.2	1.12 (0.96–1.31)	0.1	4,154	4.1	1.13 (0.93–1.37)	0.2	2,018	4.6	1.08 (0.83–1.41)	0.6
Not stated	1,474	3.5	0.91 (0.67–1.23)	0.5	1,040	3.4	0.93 (0.64–1.34)	0.7	434	3.5	0.81 (0.45–1.42)	0.4
Employment[a]												
Employed or not in labour force	17,245	4.1	1.00		12,034	4.0	1.00		5,210	4.4	1.00	
Unemployed	831	2.6	0.64 (0.41–1.00)	0.04	576	2.6	0.65 (0.37–1.12)	0.1	254	2.8	0.62 (0.27–1.38)	0.2
Smoking status												
Non- or ex-smoker	15,416	4.2	1.00		10,902	4.0	1.00		4,514	4.8	1.00	
Current smoker	5,663	3.0	0.71 (0.60–0.85)	<0.001	3,778	3.1	0.77 (0.62–0.95)	0.01	1,884	3.0	0.60 (0.44–0.82)	<0.001
Weight category												
Normal	8,637	2.3	1.00		6,303	2.4	1.00		2,335	1.8	1.00	
Underweight	1,952	1.4	0.63 (0.41–0.95)	0.02	1,523	1.2	0.50 (0.30–0.83)	0.004	429	2.1	1.17 (0.53–2.52)	0.7
Overweight	6,163	4.7	2.12 (1.75–2.56)	<0.001	4,212	4.3	1.81 (1.45–2.27)	<0.001	1,951	5.4	3.14 (2.15–4.58)	<0.001
Obese	2,558	8.8	4.17 (3.41–5.11)	<0.001	1,676	9.0	3.95 (3.12–5.02)	<0.001	882	8.5	5.07 (3.39–7.60)	<0.001
Not stated	1,770	4.7	2.12 (1.62–2.77)	<0.001	968	4.2	1.77 (1.22–2.54)	0.001	803	5.4	3.09 (1.96–4.87)	<0.001

Table 3. (continued)

Variable	Overall				Metropolitan				Rural			
	n	%	OR (95% CI)	p	n	%	OR (95% CI)	p	n	%	OR (95% CI)	p
Asthma												
No	18,799	3.9	1.00		13,184	3.7	1.00		5,616	4.3	1.00	
Yes	2,280	4.1	1.06 (0.84–1.32)	0.6	1,497	3.9	1.07 (0.80–1.42)	0.6	783	4.3	1.01 (0.69–1.48)	0.9
Last cholesterol reading[b]												
Low or normal	9,251	5.0	1.00		6,515	4.9	1.00		2,735	5.1	1.00	
High	1,891	6.5	1.33 (1.08–1.64)	0.006	1,323	5.8	1.20 (0.92–1.56)	0.2	568	8.1	1.65 (1.15–2.36)	0.004
Never measured	6,927	1.8	0.35 (0.28–0.43)	<0.001	4,764	1.6	0.31 (0.24–0.40)	<0.001	2,163	2.3	0.43 (0.31–0.61)	<0.001
Vigorous exercise in last 2 weeks[b]												
No	12,426	4.9	1.00		8,625	4.8	1.00		3,801	5.2	1.00	
Yes	5,643	1.6	0.31 (0.24–0.39)	<0.001	3,977	1.3	0.26 (0.19–0.35)	<0.001	1,665	2.2	0.42 (0.29–0.60)	<0.001
Been told have high blood pressure[b]												
No	13,982	2.4	1.00		9,871	2.4	1.00		4,111	2.4	1.00	
Yes	4,087	9.1	4.10 (3.51–4.79)	<0.001	2,731	8.6	3.86 (3.19–4.67)	<0.001	1,357	10.1	4.60 (3.49–6.06)	<0.001
Last blood pressure reading[b]												
Low or normal	15,691	3.7	1.00		11,034	3.6	1.00		4,657	3.9	1.00	
High	1,814	6.9	1.93 (1.57–2.37)	<0.001	1,180	6.2	1.77 (1.35–2.30)	<0.001	634	8.2	2.18 (1.57–3.04)	<0.001
Never measured	565	0.0	0		388	0.0	0		177	0.0	0	

Table 3. (continued)

Variable	Overall				Metropolitan				Rural			
	n	%	OR (95% CI)	p	n	%	OR (95% CI)	p	n	%	OR (95% CI)	p
Alcohol risk												
None or low	19,536	3.9	1.00		13,655	3.7	1.00		5,881	4.4	1.00	
Intermediate or high	1,016	1.3	0.32 (0.17–0.56)	<0.001	628	1.8	0.46 (0.24–0.87)	0.01	389	0.8	0.17 (0.04–0.54)	<0.001
Not stated	527	7.8	2.06 (1.47–2.89)	<0.001	399	7.8	2.19 (1.47–3.24)	<0.001	128	7.8	1.82 (0.89–3.63)	0.07
Survey year												
1992	3,019	2.6	1.00		2,141	2.9	1.00		878	1.8	1.00	
1993	3,004	3.2	1.26 (0.92–1.72)	0.1	2,070	2.7	0.93 (0.64–1.37)	0.7	934	4.4	2.47 (1.33–4.63)	0.002
1994	3,010	3.9	1.52 (1.13–2.06)	0.004	2,078	3.7	1.29 (0.91–1.84)	0.1	931	4.3	2.42 (1.30–4.54)	0.002
1995	3,016	4.2	1.64 (1.22–2.21)	<0.001	2,089	3.8	1.32 (0.93–1.87)	0.1	927	5.1	2.88 (1.57–5.33)	<0.001
1996	3,010	3.8	1.48 (1.10–2.01)	0.008	2,090	3.5	1.23 (0.86–1.76)	0.2	920	4.3	2.45 (1.32–4.60)	0.002
1997	3,019	4.4	1.74 (1.30–2.33)	<0.001	2,074	4.6	1.63 (1.16–2.28)	0.003	944	3.9	2.20 (1.17–4.16)	0.008
1998	3,001	5.2	2.07 (1.55–2.75)	<0.001	2,137	4.8	1.68 (1.20–2.35)	0.001	864	6.3	3.59 (1.98–6.59)	<0.001

The total sample size available for these analyses was 18,075 for education (which was not asked in 1993), 18,069 for cholesterol, blood pressure, and exercise (which were not asked in 1994), and 21,079 for all other variables.

[a] Employment status was not asked in 1993.

[b] Last cholesterol reading, vigorous exercise in last 2 weeks, been told have high blood pressure, and last blood pressure reading were not asked in 1994.

Table 4. Multi-variate logistic regression of variables associated with diabetes in South Australia, by area of residence, 1992–1998

Variable	Overall		Metropolitan		Rural	
	OR (95% CI)	p	OR (95% CI)	p	OR (95% CI)	p
Sex[a]						
Male	1.00		1.00		1.00	
Female	2.81 (2.35–3.35)	<0.001	2.85 (2.29–3.54)	<0.001	1.45 (1.11–1.89)	0.006
Age						
15–49 years	1.00		1.00		1.00	
≥50 years		<0.001		<0.001	2.76 (2.05–3.73)	<0.001
Annual family income						
>$A20,000	1.00		1.00		1.00	
≤$A20,000	1.66 (1.42–1.94)	<0.001	1.75 (1.44–2.12)	<0.001	1.45 (1.11–1.90)	0.007
Weight category						
Normal	1.00		1.00		1.00	
Underweight	0.83 (0.55–1.24)	0.4	0.71 (0.44–1.14)	0.2	1.28 (0.60–2.72)	0.5
Overweight	1.73 (1.43–2.08)	<0.001	1.50 (1.20–1.87)	<0.001	2.63 (1.81–3.82)	<0.001
Obese	3.13 (2.56–3.84)	<0.001	2.96 (2.32–3.77)	<0.001	3.84 (2.58–5.71)	<0.001
Not stated	2.02 (1.54–2.64)	<0.001	1.66 (1.16–2.39)	0.006	2.74 (1.76–4.29)	<0.001
Last cholesterol reading						
Low or normal	1.00		1.00		1.00	
High	1.10 (0.89–1.36)	0.4	0.95 (0.73–1.24)	0.7	1.48 (1.03–2.13)	0.03
Never measured	0.65 (0.53–0.81)	<0.001	0.57 (0.44–0.75)	<0.001	0.82 (0.57–1.16)	0.3
Vigorous exercise in last 2 weeks[b]						
No	1.00		1.00			
Yes	0.64 (0.51–0.81)	<0.001	0.55 (0.40–0.74)	<0.001		
Been told have high blood pressure						
No	1.00		1.00		1.00	
Yes	2.04 (1.73–2.41)	<0.001	1.82 (1.49–2.23)	<0.001	2.48 (1.85–3.31)	<0.001
Alcohol risk						
None or low	1.00		1.00		1.00	
Intermediate or high	0.40 (0.23–0.69)	0.001	0.54 (0.29–1.00)	0.05	0.22 (0.07–0.7)	0.01
Not stated	1.48 (1.05–2.10)	0.03	1.53 (1.02–2.29)	0.04	1.27 (0.6–2.53)	0.3
Year (continuous variable)	1.08 (1.04–1.13)	<0.001	1.07 (1.02–1.12)	0.007	1.13 (1.05–1.21)	0.001

[a] Not significant at multi-variate level overall and in the metropolitan area.

[b] Not significant at multi-variate level in rural areas.

Table 5. SF-36 scores[a] for people with and without diabetes living in South Australia in a metropolitan area or in rural areas, 1998

SF-36 dimension	Metropolitan			Rural		
	Mean (SD)			Mean (SD)		
	No diabetes (n = 1,647)	Diabetes (n = 63)	p	No diabetes (n = 778)	Diabetes (n = 41)	p
Physical functioning	84.5 (18.4)	61.9 (25.6)	<0.001	83.3 (18.4)	72.4 (25.8)	<0.001
Physical role	80.8 (33.9)	49.9 (44.5)	<0.001	81.6 (33.9)	67.7 (44.7)	0.01
Bodily pain	76.8 (24.8)	61.8 (29.2)	<0.001	77.2 (24.9)	68.3 (29.4)	0.03
General health	75.0 (20.2)	49.5 (26.1)	<0.001	75.4 (20.2)	64.1 (26.2)	<0.001
Vitality	64.7 (20.2)	49.7 (23.1)	<0.001	64.7 (20.2)	66.0 (23.2)	0.7
Social functioning	87.5 (21.3)	71.9 (27.4)	<0.001	90.2 (21.3)	86.4 (27.6)	0.3
Emotional role	86.4 (29.0)	79.4 (35.9)	0.06	91.2 (29.0)	85.6 (36.1)	0.2
Mental health	79.3 (16.7)	74.4 (19.9)	0.02	82.5 (16.8)	83.0 (20.0)	0.8

[a] Controlled for age, sex, and socio-economic status.

epidemiology, also known as conventional risk factor epidemiology (Susser and Susser, 1996). This approach aims to relate individual exposure to risk factors with limited attention to the wider social context. The value of the social context is articulated well by Berkman and Kawachi (2000, p. 8): "The assessment of exposures at an environmental or community level may lead to an understanding of social determinants that is more than the sum of the individual-level measures." Policy development is best served by explaining pathogenesis and causality of disease within the social context. This context is underpinned by a social theory that explains the variable relationships and their inter-actions with health outcomes. Such contextual explanations are more complex than those provided by basic epidemiology and may also be dynamic, thus necessitating surveillance.

The analyses of data in this chapter go beyond the summary data analyses that are largely the source of current policy decisions and were apparent in the National Rural Health Strategy. The systematic collection of diabetes and related data over time has allowed the investigation of diabetes trends by region, and my multi-variate analyses have provided a more comprehensive comparative picture of diabetes in both a metropolitan region and rural regions of South Australia. The analyses also help illustrate what is possible if systematic surveillance is adopted for major health problems. I acknowledge, however, that many other influences on diabetes for which data were not collected in this data set could affect health status by region. Further, although data were collected on prevalence, exposure, and population structure variables, important health service information is still missing and needs to be added in the future. These are valid limitations of the current analyses, but because a surveillance system exists, new variables can

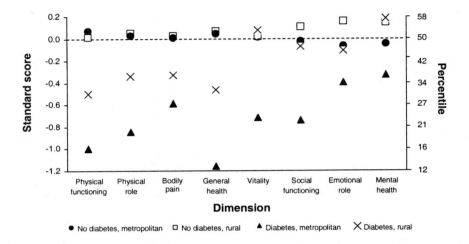

Figure 1. SF-36 standard scores for people with or without diabetes living in South Australia in a metropolitan area or in rural areas in 1998, compared with the general population. A standard score of 0.0 corresponds to the general population of Southern Australia in 1998. Scores are controlled for age, sex, and socio-economic status.

be added to the existing data set as their importance is identified. The main conclusion to draw from my analyses is that diabetes is increasing in both regions in South Australia and that agreement is high in the variables explaining diabetes in both areas.

One important explanatory variable for the increasing diabetes trend would seem to be the aging of the population in both Adelaide and the rural areas. The overall proportion of the Australian population aged 50 years or older has increased significantly over the years of data collection and will continue to do so, in line with population projections. The prevalence of diabetes will also continue to increase in the future with further aging of the population—in Australia and worldwide (King et al., 1998). In my analyses the proportion of the population aged 50 years or older did not differ significantly between the metropolitan area and the rural areas, so the policy solutions that need to be considered in relation to the diabetes trend apply equally to both. The increasing prevalence of diabetes in both regions could also be accounted for by the significant increase in prevalence of obesity and the significant decrease in vigorous exercise for the population as a whole. Taken together, this information points to the need for a health promotion policy that is consistent across regions.

A number of other population structure variables were investigated in the uni-variate analyses. The only population structure variables that remained significant in the multivariate analyses were lower income in both regions and female sex in the rural areas. The increased prevalence of diabetes among people with lower income will affect health outcomes in both Adelaide and the rural areas if people are unable to fund required lifestyle changes and medication costs. This issue also requires further investigation to better inform policy. The increased probability of diabetes among females in the rural areas means that targeting of diabetes messages should consider the female dimension in diabetes, as should all the health services in this region. Further qualitative research may also be required to explore gender differences. The increased prevalence of diabetes among women in the rural areas is consistent with other research on the global burden of diabetes identifying that more women than men have diabetes (King et al., 1998).

The diabetes-related mortality rate in the rural areas decreased throughout the 1990s but remained significantly higher than that in Adelaide. This issue requires further investigation, expecially because decreasing rural death rates occurred in the face of increasing diabetes prevalence rates. A number of possible explanations exist. The higher rural death rate may be explained by the increased diabetes mortality rate in the Aboriginal population, later diagnosis of diabetes, the need in rural areas for improved specialist care of diabetes complications and related morbidity, or differences in attributing diabetes as a cause of death. Explaining the mortality differences must be made a research priority if policy for rural regions is to be improved. Much of the information that will answer these new questions can, however, come from extending the surveillance database.

The multi-variate analyses showed some variation in both regions in the risk factors associated with diabetes. The prevalence of elevated cholesterol among people with diabetes rose significantly in the rural areas but not in the metropolitan area. This pattern was reversed in the case of vigorous exercise, in which significantly lower rates were observed in the city but not in the rural areas. These observations will have implications for health promotion strategy and diabetes management, but not for policy.

Cutting across this information about death rates and risk factors is the fact that health-related quality of life is significantly better for a number of health dimensions in the rural areas than in Adelaide. The impact of diabetes clearly affects the physical health dimensions for people in both areas, but much more in the city. In addition, there is a significant mental health impact for people with diabetes in Adelaide that is not apparent in the rural areas. Other research has shown the effect of chronic conditions on mental health (McSweeny et al., 1982), which should be considered as part of the diabetes diagnosis and treatment for people living in a metropolitan area. Quality of life should also be dealt with in the diabetes guidelines for physicians in both areas. It seems contradictory that rural areas exhibited both a higher death rate and a better overall health-related quality of life, but it may point to the need for better access by rural residents to specialist services to improve diabetes outcomes at critical stages.

Overall, the analyses conducted in this study do not provide overwhelming evidence for a "unique" health policy for rural South Australia. Of the best set of nine explanatory variables for the metropolitan area and the rural areas in the multi-variate analyses, six were common to both areas. It may still be the case that as geographic remoteness increases, diabetes management and diabetes outcomes do deteriorate. As the present database grows it will be possible to segment the rural region further and conduct these analyses, but not without a surveillance system. At this stage of knowledge of diabetes in rural areas, the case for a unique strategy is not strong. There are some subtle differences that would apply to a diabetes programme in metropolitan and rural areas, as have been discussed above. These are new insights to the targeting of diabetes in metropolitan and rural areas, and when these are dealt with the surveillance system should continue to monitor progress and outcomes from re-targeted programmes.

A comment should be made about the Australian National Rural Health Strategy basing its unique strategy on need, equity, and access. Need and equity are complex concepts that are not well understood by health service planners (Lockwood, 1988; Culyer and Wagstaff, 1993). Widespread use of these terms stems more from concern over evidence

116 D. WILSON

of growing inequalities in health care rather than any clear understanding of and agreement on the concepts (Culyer and Wagstaff, 1993). Their use in the Strategy provided no further clarification or strategic insights as to how such issues would be addressed in South Australia.

The analyses of surveillance data in this chapter illustrated the insights that can be gained from trend information and more powerful, advanced analyses of structural and exposure variables. The surveillance data have also illustrated the ability to compare target groups and identify the important exposure and population structure variables of each group. Such data are essential to targeting, policy, and strategy development, and without them positive outcomes in diabetes will be a result of guesswork rather than design.

The "evidence" in evidence-based policy needs to come from coherent and stable sources. The implicit advantage of surveillance is its comparative stability. Health authorities need to recognise the inadequacy of ad hoc data collections and recognise the need for greater investment in systematic surveillance. With burgeoning health service costs and the search for greater health service efficiency worldwide, we must not forget the need for new investment in systems that may improve outcomes and reduce the burden of disease. Surveillance is such an investment.

6. REFERENCES

Australian Bureau of Statistics, 1990, *Australian Standard Classification of Occupations, First Edition*, the Bureau, Canberra (Catalogue No. 1222.0).
Australian Bureau of Statistics, 1993–1998, *Causes of Death*, the Bureau, Canberra (Catalogue No. 3303.0).
Australian Bureau of Statistics, 1996, *Population by Age and Sex: South Australia*, the Bureau, Canberra (Catalogue No. 3235.4).
Australian Health Ministers' Conference, 1994, *National Rural Health Strategy*, Commonwealth of Australia, Canberra.
Australian Health Ministers' Conference, 1996, *National Rural Health Strategy Update*, Commonwealth of Australia, Canberra.
Australian Health Ministers' Conference, 1999, *National Rural Health Strategy Update*, Commonwealth of Australia, Canberra.
Australian Institute of Health and Welfare, 1994, *Australia's Health 1994: The Fourth Biennial Report of the Australian Institute of Health and Welfare*, the Institute, Canberra.
Australian Institute of Health and Welfare, 1996, *Australia's Health 1996: The Fifth Biennial Report of the Australian Institute of Health and Welfare*, the Institute, Canberra.
Australian Institute of Health and Welfare, 1998, *Australia's Health 1998: The Sixth Biennial Report of the Australian Institute of Health and Welfare*, the Institute, Canberra.
Berkman, L. F., and Kawachi, I., 2000, A historical framework for social epidemiology, in: *Social Epidemiology*, L. F. Berkman and I. Kawachi, eds., Oxford University Press, Oxford, UK, pp. 3–12.
Blane, C., Davey Smith, G., and Bartley, M., 1993, Social selection: What does it contribute to social class differences in health? *Sociol Health Illness.* **15**:1–15.
Catchpole, M. A., 1996, The role of epidemiology and surveillance systems in the control of sexually transmitted diseases, *Genitourin Med.* **72**:321–329.
Culyer, A. J., and Wagstaff, A., 1993, Equity and equality in health and health care, *J Health Econ.* **12**:431–457.
Dean, A. G., Dean, J. A., Coulombier, D., et al., 1994, *Epi Info Version 6: A Word Processing, Database, and Statistics Program for Epidemiology on Microcomputers*, Centers for Disease Control and Prevention, Atlanta.
Department of Primary Industries and Energy and the Department of Human Services and Health, 1994, *Rural, Remote, and Metropolitan Areas Classification, 1991 Census Edition*, Australian Government Publishing Service, Canberra.
dos Santos Silva, I., 1999, *Cancer Epidemiology: Principles and Methods*, International Agency for Research on Cancer, Lyon, France.

Garratt, A. M., Ruta, D. A., Abdalla, M. I., et al., 1993, The SF-36 health survey questionnaire: An outcome measure suitable for routine use within the NHS? *Br Med J.* **306**:1440–1444.

Ham, C., Hunter, D. J., and Robinson, R., 1995, Evidence based policymaking, *Br Med J.* **310**:71–72.

Hosmer, D. W., and Lemeshow, S., 1989, *Applied Logistic Regression*, John Wiley, New York.

Kazis, L. E., Anderson, J. J., and Meenan, R. F., 1989, Effect sizes for interpreting changes in health status, *Med Care.* **27**(3 Suppl):S178–S189.

Kelley, J. L., and Evans, M. D. R., 1988, *Using ASCO for Socio-Economic Analysis: Assessment and Conversion into Status and Prestige Indices*, Research School of Social Sciences, Australian National University, Canberra.

King, H., Aubert, R. E., and Herman, W. H., 1998, Global burden of diabetes, 1995–2025: prevalence, numerical estimates, and projections, *Diabetes Care.* **21**:1414–1431.

Lockwood, M., 1988, Quality of life and resource allocation, in: *Philosophy and Medical Welfare*, M. Bell and S. Mendus, eds., Cambridge University Press, Cambridge, UK, pp. 33–55.

Marmot, M. G., Smith, G. D., Stansfeld, S., et al., 1991, Health inequalities among British civil servants: the Whitehall study, *Lancet.* **337**:1387–1393.

McCallum, J., 1994, *The New SF-36 Health Status Measure: Australian Validity Tests*, National Centre for Epidemiology and Population Health, Australian National University, Canberra.

McSweeny, A. J., Grant, I., Heaton, R. K., et al., 1982, Life quality of patients with chronic obstructive pulmonary disease, *Arch Intern Med.* **142**:473–478.

Muir-Gray, J., 1997, *Evidence-Based Health Care: How to Make Health Policy and Management Decisions*, Churchill Livingstone, New York.

National Rural Health Policy Forum, 1999, *Healthy Horizons: A Framework for Improving the Health of Rural, Regional and Remote Australians*, National Rural Health Policy Forum and National Rural Health Alliance for the Australian Health Ministers' Conference, Canberra.

National Rural Public Health Forum, 1998, Rural public health in Australia 1997, in: *Proceedings of the National Rural Public Health Forum, Adelaide, 12–15 October 1997*, D. J. Murray and G. N. F. Gregory, eds., National Rural Health Alliance, Deakin West ACT, pp. 4–10.

Nguyen, A., McCaul, K., Carman, J., et al., 1996, *South Australia Regional Health Statistics Chart Book 1996*, Epidemiology Branch, South Australian Health Commission, Adelaide.

Peckham, M., and Smith, R., 1996, *Scientific Basis of Health Services*, British Medical Journal Publishing Group, London.

Rosenberg, H. M., 1999, Cause of death as a contemporary problem, *J Hist Med Allied Sci.* **54**:133–153.

Smith, R., 1995, The scientific basis of health services, *Br Med J.* **311**:961–962.

SPSS Inc., 1999, *SPSS Advanced Statistics 10.0*, SPSS Inc., Chicago.

Strong, K., Trickett, P., Titulaer, I., et al., 1998, *Health in Rural and Remote Australia: The First Report of the Australian Institute of Health and Welfare on Rural Health*, Australian Institute of Health and Welfare, Canberra (Catalogue No. PHE 6).

Susser, M., and Susser, E., 1996, Choosing a future for epidemiology: II. From black box to Chinese boxes and eco-epidemiology, *Am J Public Health.* **86**:674–677.

Taylor, C. E., 1992, Surveillance for equity in primary health care: policy implications from international experience, *Int J Epidemiol.* **21**:1043–1049.

Tollman, S. M., and Zwi, A. B., 2000, Health system reform and the role of field sites based upon demographic and health surveillance, *Bull World Health Organ.* **78**:125–134.

Wakefield, M., and Wilson, D. H., 1996, *SF-36 Profiles for Regions of South Australia*, Behavioural Epidemiology Unit, South Australian Health Commission, Adelaide.

Wilson, D., Wakefield, M., and Taylor, A., 1992, The South Australian Health Omnibus Survey, *Health Promot J Aust.* **2**:47–49.

CHAPTER 10

DID THEY USE IT?

Beyond the Collection
of Surveillance Information

Judith M. Ottoson and David H. Wilson[*]

1. INTRODUCTION

In the last 300 years the greatest advances in public health have been achieved by population health initiatives that have reduced or eliminated major threats or scourges to whole populations. Likewise, the future health of communities will depend on a similar population perspective that has come to be described as public health. As past successes achieved by public health practitioners depended largely on surveillance systems based on in-patient and disease registries, recording of vital events, laboratory and sentinel reporting, administrative systems, and population surveys, so too will future health status and outcomes. Information technology may change the way in which public health surveillance is conducted and information is gathered, processed, and accessed, but the fundamental concept of population surveillance will remain.

Irrespective of public health successes to date, public health practitioners at all levels have failed to take full advantage of surveillance systems. During the last 30 years the vast amount of social and behavioural data from surveys and surveillance systems has neither been fully analysed nor well used (Patton, 1988, 1997; Remington, 1988; Simpson and Weiner, 1989; Figgs et al., 2000). The pressure to change this neglect increases given the importance of research and surveillance resources and the need to optimise investments in terms of obtaining data that provide "good" evidence for policy and intervention. It will become increasingly necessary for those in control of research and surveillance systems and resources to provide value for money. How data are used will attract greater scrutiny. Increasing pressure to invest health resources more clearly on evidence-based outcomes will also involve some audit of data use. In these circumstances it should be realised that data use occurs in a sociological context that involves a number of influences often outside the control of the person collecting and the person using the

[*] Judith M. Ottoson, Georgia State University, Atlanta, Georgia 30303, USA; David H. Wilson, University of Adelaide, Woodville, South Australia 5011, Australia.

data. If surveillance systems are to have a continued and significant impact on the public's health, the use of surveillance findings needs to consider this sociological context and move from an afterthought of data collection to forethought in the planning of surveillance activity.

Even if use moves to a more prominent place in our thinking, the question remains, "What counts as use?" For example, do the scenarios below provide evidence of use?

Scenario 1: Surveillance data from a well-designed and implemented system are collected and analysed. Recommendations are made in a written report delivered on a pre-determined date to the local public health officer.

Scenario 2: A public health advisor changes the programme direction on the basis of all the surveillance data she received 2 days previously, and the action taken aligns exactly with the recommendations made and affects the entire population at risk in her jurisdiction.

Scenario 3: After several years of briefings and lobbying by various community groups, a policy-maker supports legislation to increase funding for a health programme.

Scenario 4: A community action group re-interprets surveillance data to show how lack of public health services in their area magnifies a particular health problem. Their findings are released to the media.

The purpose of this chapter is to explore the multiple dimensions of use embedded in these scenarios. The seemingly simple question—"Did they use it?"—is not nearly so straightforward when considering the dimensions of use. How much was it used? By whom? Why? With what fidelity to intent was it used? When and how often was it used? How well? These questions are explored from a multi-disciplinary perspective, with examples drawn from the surveillance context. The preceding scenarios are re-visited at the end of the chapter, and recommendations to facilitate use of surveillance findings are made.

2. SURVEILLANCE ASSUMPTIONS AND CONTEXT

For too long we have believed in the better mousetrap theory as applied to public health: "If we produce more and better information, people will use it in policy and strategy development." Yet even well-developed surveillance systems, such as the U.S. Behavioral Risk Factor Surveillance System, have failed to meet the developers' expectations (Remington, 1988; Figgs et al., 2000). Contributing to lack of use are some problematic assumptions about surveillance and the nature of the context in which use occurs.

Surveillance is taken to mean a systematic and consistent approach to data collection on health status and related phenomena. Within the surveillance system, the maximum use of existing data is facilitated or constrained, in part, by the relevance and quality of the data (Figure 1). Relevant data are driven by needs, action oriented, timely, responsive, feasible, and adaptable. Quality data are scientifically rigorous, able to be integrated with other data sets, understandable, and credible. A preliminary intention in establishing a surveillance system to provide data that will be used to better health outcomes is assumed. Indeed, there would be no point in establishing or maintaining a surveillance

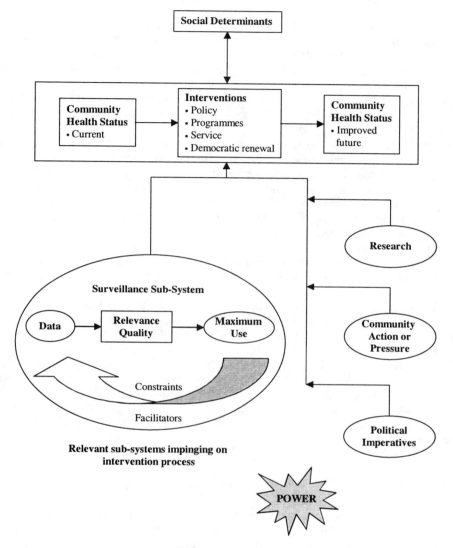

Figure 1. The broad surveillance context.

system not intended to produce a health benefit. In the short term, it may produce interim benefits such as publications, formation of networks, and employment, but even these are not sustainable unless they produce policies leading to health gains.

The surveillance system is only one of many influences on community health status. Interventions (e.g., policies and programmes) intend to positively intervene between current community health status and some level of improved future state of health. These interventions are influenced by social determinants of health (e.g., income distribution or education levels) and relevant sub-systems (e.g., research, political imperatives, or democratic renewal). Included among these sub-systems is surveillance. These sub-systems interact in ways that can facilitate or hinder the improvement of community health. The power differentials embedded in this context influence surveillance implementation and use in multiple ways, including participation in the planning of surveillance systems, access to data, and control over resources. For example, political pressure and funding to collect surveillance data on HIV/AIDS may steamroll community demands for information about toxic waste.

Failure to consider the surveillance context and how this may impinge on what information is collected and ultimately used may mean inappropriate use of the data and failure to achieve a desired or planned outcome. An assumption that a surveillance system is complete when sufficient quality information is collected may underlay the argument to ignore or minimise the role of context in surveillance. Or the assumption may extend to the use of information in the design of policy, services, and programmes. A related assumption is that a surveillance system is not responsible for implementing policy or interventions.

These assumptions are problematic. First, they are based on an activity focus (e.g., data collection or data analysis) rather than a system perspective (e.g., inter-action or lack of action among components). A surveillance system needs system-level thinking, along with quality activity. Second, these assumptions do not clarify who and what is included within the surveillance system. Is the system limited to public health professionals, or is the community a part of a surveillance system? Third, these assumptions have no specific plan for use. Assumed use is not planned use. Last, they do not recognise that surveillance has a secondary role in monitoring the effects of evidence-based interventions. At all stages of surveillance activity there are a number of influences that determine how and by whom the system is accessed and used. These influences may also determine the paradigm that is brought to bear on the issues under investigation. In effect, the quality of the evidence produced and used in, or from, a surveillance system will be determined by the impact of the surveillance context.

3. UNDERSTANDING THE DIMENSIONS OF USE

In light of the surveillance context and assumptions, the definition and dimensions of use are explored here. Use is defined as putting something into practise or operation, carrying into action or effect, employing or handling something for a certain end or purpose, or being able to use or needing to use something (Simpson and Weiner, 1989). Use involves action and purpose. It is about "intended use by intended users" (Patton, 1988, p. 14). Studies about use in other fields such as evaluation (Patton, 1997), sociology (Lindblom and Cohen, 1979), and public policy (Weiss, 1977) along with related concepts such as application (Ottoson, 1995) and diffusion (Rogers, 1995) are brought to bear here on the surveillance context. In addition, the experiences and recommendations of academics, government representatives, and practitioners at two international meetings on surveillance contributed to the ideas of this chapter.[†] The various dimensions of use to be explored are discussed in the following sections and summarised in Table 1.

[†] One meeting was "Analysis, Interpretation, and Use of Complex Social and Behavioral Surveillance Data: Looking Back in Order to Go Forward," held June 2000 in Savannah, Georgia. The second was "Capacity

Table 1. Dimensions of surveillance use

Dimension	Considerations
What is used	• Ongoing • System components • Varying focus (e.g., health indicator, behaviour) • Intended link to policy and practise • Multiple products • Quality characteristics • Relevance
The kinds of uses	• Primary and secondary • Incentives • Action or decision making • Intended or unintended • Underlying theories of change (e.g., radical versus incremental)
Who uses it	• Public health professionals or others • Stakeholders, users, definers • Roles (e.g., policy-maker, manager, frontline practitioner, community groups, media) • Number of people using data or findings
When it is used	• Immediately, eventually, never
How direct the derivation is	• Instrumental (short term) • Enlightenment (long term)
How much effect is needed before data are considered used	• Proportion of data collected that is used (all, some, or none)
How well it is used	• Standards (performance measures and indicators) • Relevance of data • Importance of information

3.1. What Is Used?

The characteristics of *what* is used shapes *how* it is used. Depending on the context, what is used could be a technology, a concept, data, a system, an innovation, or power. Technology use is more likely to be transferred intact than applied in variation like a concept (Ottoson, 1997). A system requires more holistic and complex use than a limited set of data. The use of power requires political strategy and tactics that a new technology may not. Understanding what surveillance is begins the understanding of surveillance use.

Building, Comparability, and Data Use in Behavioral Risk Factor Surveillance: Focus on Global Surveillance Issues," held September 2000 in Atlanta, Georgia. Both meetings were sponsored by the U.S. Centers for Disease Control and Prevention, National Center for Chronic Disease Prevention and Health Promotion.

Public health surveillance is the ongoing collection, analysis, interpretation, and dissemination of health data to describe and monitor health events, with the explicit provision that these activities be systematic, timely, and linked to public health practises such as planning, implementation, and evaluation of intervention and prevention programmes (Thacker and Berkelman, 1992; Thacker and Stroup, 1994). Surveillance is an ongoing process that might be likened to a 24-hour surveillance camera. Once the camera is focused, it picks up and records what is in its sight without prejudice. Second, surveillance involves decisions about which foci are included or excluded from the system. Who focuses the camera? Further, the "products" of surveillance vary over time, moving from raw data to interpreted results to applied actions. Last, a surveillance system is developed out of general scientific knowledge about the public's health, and its products are intended for application in specific practise settings.

A new generation of researchers is also concerned about focus. What gets included in the system? What is counted as evidence? Such questions are part of an eco-social framework of health and are concerned with more complete explanations of health problems than are provided in traditional risk factor surveys. They go beyond risk factor epidemiology and seek more comprehensive explanations of the societal dynamics of health and disease (Susser, 1985; Schwartz et al., 1999). This approach also considers the appropriateness of the research paradigm being used and is more likely to select the method appropriate to the research question. This is likely to involve mixed-method research approaches using both qualitative and quantitative skills in the design of the surveillance questions. The narrative of the qualitative method is less exclusive than the skills of the quantitative methods and more likely to involve communities and individuals in owning and using data.

In surveillance systems we are concerned not only about the extent and type of a disease or disorder, but also with service delivery and other initiatives that will modify the problems. It is important, therefore, to the epidemiologist, the sociologist, or other researcher involved in surveillance to build partnerships—not only among themselves but with policy implementers—that will lead to the use of data to achieve desired health outcomes.

These characteristics of surveillance affect its use. Concern about use of surveillance findings needs to be as ongoing as the surveillance process itself. It is too late to initiate thinking about use after data collection has begun. A surveillance system produces various kinds of products, from raw data to constructed recommendations. Each of these products might be designed, implemented, promoted, and used differently if end users were kept in mind from the beginning. To treat use in a surveillance system as a monolithic process is to miss the complexities of the system. Underlying the decisions about surveillance foci are issues of access. Are the intended users of surveillance findings involved in the up-front decisions about focus, or involved only after the fact to figure out what to do with what someone else designed? Form shapes function.

3.2. What Are the Kinds of Uses?

Surveillance data and findings can be used in different ways. Primary use includes provision of baseline measurements and monitoring of the status of different groups or disease trends. These are traditional public health uses. Secondary use for surveillance data and findings includes policy and programme development, community action, and

Table 2. Kinds of surveillance use

Kind of surveillance use	Examples
Warning	• Needs assessment • Environmental scanning • Strategic planning • Monitoring health status and needs of different groups
Guidance	• Healthy public policies • Health-friendly policies in other sectors • Improved interventions
Re-conceptualisation	• Development of knowledge • Research • Evaluation of policies and programmes
Mobilisation	• Increased public information and awareness • Education and training of professionals • Enhanced community capacity • Strengthening and empowering of communities • Advocacy

research. These differences are determined, in part, by who labels use as primary or secondary. The scientific community has more control over primary use than secondary use.

Policy-makers use information in the policy process: as warning, guidance, re-conceptualisation, and mobilisation (Weiss, 1990). Examples of these kinds of uses in surveillance are found in Table 2. Embedded in these examples are hints at the possible incentives for using surveillance data (e.g., problem solving versus mobilising community action). Probably most important is the recognition that users may have very different incentives that prompt use. These incentives need to be tapped if use is to be enhanced.

Use can involve decision making or action. Most persons would agree that taking an action, such as changing a policy or mobilising a workforce, counts as use. But can decision making without an observable action count as use? For example, are surveillance findings used if a programme manager proclaims to have made a decision to mobilise resources, but no action is taken to do that? If decision making alone counts as use, does decision making at some stages count as better use than at other stages (e.g., assessing needs, seeking a solution, or implementing a solution)?

Related to the kind of use is the reason surveillance data and findings are used. Of major interest is the extent to which data and findings are used for intended purposes and unintended purposes. For example, changing a programme's direction to fight an epidemic or monitoring vital health indicators might have been intended. Showing government inaction and rallying political support for more resources or change in leadership might have been unintended. Of course, the underlying question is, "Who labels use as intended and unintended, thereby giving it more or less credibility?"

The concepts of use and change are linked. If the purpose of surveillance data and findings is to create change, the espoused or practised theory of change needs to be understood (Shadish et al., 1991). Two common theories of change are the radical model and the incremental model. Is use of surveillance data and findings expected to create radical, complete, and observable change? Or is change understood as an incremental process and use will be tucked into small steps, over time? These different understandings of how change occurs affect how use of surveillance data and findings will be found and identified (e.g., immediate versus long term, or a grand impact versus a small embedded one). Function shapes form.

3.3. Who Uses It?

Group membership, role, and the number of people involved shape the use of surveillance data and findings.

Two related groups with an interest in surveillance data and findings are stakeholders and users. Either group might comprise representatives of various agencies and organisations (e.g., leaders or members, programme managers, professionals and administrators, policy-makers, researchers, academics, and the media). These representatives might be in the health sector or other sectors, and in public or private settings. Whether representatives of these various groups fall into the stakeholder or user category largely depends on the extent to which interest in surveillance data and findings is translated into use. Stakeholders include groups, partners, organisations, or institutions with interest in a health surveillance issue. This broad group could be affected at some level by surveillance findings. Users are a sub-set of stakeholders. They are the groups, partners, organisations, or institutions who can or do use surveillance information or findings.

A third group that could overlap with stakeholders and users is the definers of the system, particularly those who define data selection, collection, and analysis. By virtue of position or training, this group has the authority and credibility to establish the surveillance system. There are two central concerns about the "definers." The first concern is the scope of the surveillance system they establish. Does the system extend beyond data collection to needs analysis and use considerations for policy and practise? Is use part of the system established by the definers? The second concern is the extent to which the definers overlap with the users. Are those who establish the surveillance system the same or different from those who use surveillance data and findings? If these are two different groups, how is communication facilitated between them?

Historically, key people and organisations who could be involved in public health outcomes may have been excluded from the planning and development of surveys. This will inevitably result in less than optimum use or application of health data. Epidemiology, for example, has been accused of being more concerned with modeling relationships between risk factors than with their origins and implications for public health (Kreiger, 1994). A clearer focus on these latter two issues will logically involve a wider range of data users. Where surveillance systems can be freed from the political system, use by a range of community groups, organisations, and individuals may be more focused and applied. In Australia, the South Australian Health Omnibus is a user-funded surveillance system that employs a large representative population sample and conducts regular household health interviews (Wilson et al., 1992). The ability of a range of community health organisations to develop and purchase their own questions and analyses has led to important applications and health outcomes. Collaboration between these organisations has also produced data partnerships and enriched data use through unexpected cross-tabulation of data between the organisations.

The roles of actors within these groups also shape use of surveillance data and findings. Use is shaped by what data people in various roles need to perform their jobs, as well as the way in which they use data (Weiss, 1998). For example, front-line managers often put priority on data that shape the operations of the programme. What programme elements should be included or excluded? Programme managers are interested in data about best use of resources. Should resources be put into programme X or programme Y? Policy-makers may be involved in "go" or "no go" decisions about a programme and need data to inform or support their decision. People in these various positions use surveillance data or findings to make different decisions or take different actions, all of which occur in a complex political, economic, and organisational context that itself shapes use. The result is more likely a decision-making community in a political context than a sole actor (Smith and Chircop, 1989).

A last consideration is the number and location of people. Are surveillance data and findings used if one policy-maker in an agency of a thousand uses it? Are they used if five programme managers in a low-priority part of the country use it? The answers to these questions about scope and coverage may vary by type of surveillance, but are part of the consideration of what counts as use.

3.4. When Is It Used?

Whether something is used and used well depends, in part, on the timing of use. For example, if surveillance data are used within a week of detecting an epidemic to change public health practise, its use would be considered far more successful than if it were used 2 years after the fact. If the findings from a surveillance report are used within 3 years of the issuance of the report, is that successful use or not? When surveillance products are used may depend on several factors, including the nature of the product (e.g., raw data versus a finished report) and the urgency of the health problem (e.g., an epidemic versus chronic disease). Concern about use needs to be as ongoing as the surveillance system itself.

3.5. How Direct Is the Derivation?

Another use dimension is the fidelity of implemented use relative to intended use. Two different kinds of use have been identified in the evaluation literature: instrumental and enlightenment (U.S. Department of Health and Human Services, 2000). In the former, use is clearly linked to data and findings in a relatively short period of time. In the latter, use may occur over time and be informed by things other than the surveillance data and findings. For example, with instrumental use surveillance data might be used within a day or a week by a programme manager who can clearly identify the source of information for his or her decision or action. With enlightenment, use may come over many months or even years, and the user is unclear about which one of many different kinds or sources of information effected a decision or action. Instrumental use is comparatively easier to observe, measure, and get credit for. Enlightenment is much more difficult to evaluate, but common in the complexities of practise.

These two different understandings of use also shape the ways in which surveillance data and findings might be communicated. Instrumental use fits with a straight marketing approach, whereas enlightenment fits with more diffuse approaches to communication (e.g., policy debates, conferences, or hearings that include staff, commissions, media, interest groups, and scientists). Do both kinds of information processing count as use? Under which circumstances?

3.6. How Much Effect Is Needed before Data Are Considered Used?

The amount of surveillance data and findings engaged shapes use. How much of the surveillance data and findings need to be engaged or ignored—in decision making or action—before use is considered to have occurred or not? Is it use or non-use to have 1 data point out of 50 considered, to have 2 recommendations out of 25 brought forward, or 3 months of data out of 24 months analysed?

3.7. How Well Is It Used?

We have already mentioned the importance of data standards in improving the use of surveillance data, but more needs to be said. Data standards should include agreement on the performance measures or indicators that will populate surveillance systems, and some thought needs to be put into what will be relevant in assessing health status and measuring progress in public health. The U.S. Department of Health and Human Services (2000) has adopted 10 leading health indicators considered to fundamentally affect the health of individuals and communities. Although there are likely to be regional differences in health indicators or in their order of importance, it is still important to obtain fundamental agreement. This allows for two further developments. First, it allows comparisons across communities, regions, and countries and is likely to provide more accurate evaluation of public health initiatives. Second, it can lead to further work and agreement of question modules which reliably and validly measure the health indicators. Both of these developments are fundamental to improved data use through greater reliability, validity, and consistency. The first step to more widespread use by communities is to demonstrably improve data in surveillance systems.

4. IMPLICATIONS FOR USE

Determining whether surveillance data and findings are used is much more complex than the simple question posed by this chapter title. Use moves from the technical and scientific process of gathering data to the complex context of application in which political, sociological, psychological, and economic factors facilitate or hinder use. Recommendations to enhance the use of surveillance data and findings at different stages in the process are described in Table 3.

It can be argued that each of the scenarios presented at the beginning of this chapter counts as use. In each scenario the actors, motivations, objectives, strategies, and timing varied. A few of the scenarios could even be described as mis-use of data produced from surveillance; however, in a democracy this outcome is always a possibility. The point to be made is that use is highly inter-twined with access. In each scenario different groups were able to access the data for their own purposes. Restriction of access can occur at a variety of levels. First, approved users only may be a different list from those who would

Table 3. Approaches to enhancing use of surveillance data and findings, by stage of surveillance

Stage of surveillance	Approaches to enhancing use of surveillance data
Planning	• Mandate involvement of intended users in the design of a surveillance system • Respond to needs of different segments of users and stakeholders • Identify incentives for use • Clarify expectations from and limitations of surveillance, including data relevance and quality • Promote multiple ownership of surveillance data • Set objectives for the intended use of surveillance data and findings • Identify resources and responsibilities to support use
Implementation and analysis	• Make use as ongoing a focus as surveillance itself • Move beyond data collection to interpretation with user involvement
Communication	• Use intermediaries to translate data for stakeholders and users • Market data and findings appropriately to segments of users and stakeholders • Link surveillance data and findings to health problems and interventions • Develop a dissemination plan • Use best practises • Consider timeliness and policy and planning cycles
Capacity building	• Educate users and stakeholders about using the data and the dangers of mis-use • Develop guides for not only using surveillance data and findings, but setting up surveillance systems • Use education to turn interest in surveillance data and findings into use
Evaluation	• Assess whether and how surveillance data and findings are used • Gather users' suggestions for improving surveillance systems • Use evaluation of surveillance systems in planning new systems

like to have access. Second, use can be restricted because of the lack of partnerships, the lack of skills required to access the data, or the level at which data are made available.

Examples of working partnerships include the National Consultation for Health Surveillance in Canada (Mowat et al., 2000) and the National Information Infrastructure (NII) initiative in the United States (Lasker et al., 1995). The Canadian approach to health surveillance argues for better integration of systems, the development of common standards, skill for users, and improved applications of technology. The NII in the United States has identified facilitators of access, including effective collection, analysis, use, and communication of health and related information as well as improved technology skills and applications. Barriers to effective access and use of information in state and local public health agencies include lack of partnerships among public health, health care, research, and informatics groups and lack of development of uniform frameworks for data standards and data sharing that address privacy issues. The NII initiative identifies that timely and effective action is under-pinned by the collection, analysis, use, and communication of health information and describes these activities as the quintessential public health service (Lasker et al., 1995).

Five guiding principles for enhancing use were reached. (1) Shift concern about use of surveillance data from an afterthought to a forethought. This changes the use question from "Now that we have these data, how can we get people to use them?" to "If surveillance data were collected, who would use them and how?" (2) Involve potential users in decisions about the design, content, and interpretation of surveillance systems. Such involvement not only helps sharpen the relevance of data and findings, but encourages an ownership in the system that facilitates use. (3) Acknowledge that surveillance data are not the only influence on community health interventions. This is not to diminish the importance of good quality data, but to recognise them as one of many influences on decision making. (4) Acknowledge that surveillance data cannot be useful unless they are relevant and of acceptable quality. "Clearly officials believe that their case is strengthened when they have credible... findings to provide a rationale" (Weiss, 1990, p. 175). (5) Recognise that the value of surveillance data comes with their use, not their collection. These five principles can be used to evaluate the whole of a surveillance system.

A number of factors will facilitate or bar the recommendations offered. Facilitators include acceptable leadership, conviction about the importance of surveillance use and communication of that conviction to others, community capacity and better trained analytic staff (Mowat et al., 2000), and alliances between diverse users and stakeholders. These contextual facilitators complement good surveillance science. Barriers include lack of resources, lip service towards use and stakeholder involvement, failure to demonstrate efficiency and effectiveness, and presentation of findings mis-matched to intended users. If we are to achieve the mission of public health, we must increase the use of public health information by putting it in the hands of users who understand it and are able to apply it. This should occur by strategy rather than serendipity.

5. ACKNOWLEDGEMENT

We thank Prof. Jennie Popay, Salford University, England, for her advice on creating Figure 1.

6. REFERENCES

Figgs, L. W., Bloom, Y., Dugabety, K., et al., 2000, Uses of Behavioral Risk Factor Surveillance System data, 1993–1997, *Am J Public Health.* **90**:774–776.

Kreiger, N., 1994, Epidemiology and the web of causation: Has anyone seen the spider? *Soc Sci Med.* **39**:887–903.

Lasker, R. D., Humphreys, B. L., and Braithwaite, W. R., 1995, Making a Powerful Connection: The Health of the Public and National Information Infrastructure (February 6, 2002); http://nnlm.gov/fed/phs/powerful.html.

Lindblom, C. E., and Cohen, D. K., 1979, *Usable Knowledge: Social Science and Social Problem Solving*, Yale University Press, New Haven, CT.

Mowat, D., Goselin, P., Beddard, Y., et al., 2000, Improving Health Surveillance in Canada—What Are the Needs? (February 6, 2002); http://itch.uvic.ca/itch2000/papers/abstracts/ob-32a.htm.

Ottoson, J. M., 1995, Reclaiming the concept of application: from social to technological process and back again, *Adult Educ Q*. **46**:1–30.

Ottoson, J. M., 1997, Beyond transfer of training: using multiple lenses to assess community education programs, in: *New Directions for Adult and Continuing Education, No. 75*, A. D. Rose and M. A. Leahy, eds., Sage, Thousand Oaks, CA, pp. 87–96.

Patton, M. Q., 1988, The evaluator's responsibility for utilization, *Eval Pract*. **9**:5–24.

Patton, M. Q., 1997, *Utilization-Focused Evaluation: The New Century Text, Third Edition*, Sage, Thousand Oaks, CA.

Remington, P. L., 1988, Communicating epidemiologic information, in: *Applied Epidemiology: Theory to Practice*, R. C. Brownson and D. B. Pettiti, eds., Oxford University Press, New York, pp. 323–348.

Rogers, E. M., 1995, *Diffusion of Innovation, Fourth Edition*, Free Press, New York.

Schwartz, S., Susser, E., and Susser, M., 1999, A future for epidemiology? *Ann Rev Public Health*. **20**:15–33.

Shadish, W. R., Jr., Cook, T. D., and Leviton, L. C., 1991, *Foundations of Program Evaluation: Theories of Practice*, Sage, Newbury Park, CA.

Simpson, J. A., and Weiner, E. S. C., eds., 1989, *The Oxford English Dictionary, Second Edition*, Clarendon Press, Oxford, UK.

Smith, N. L., and Chircop, S., 1989, The Weiss-Patton debate: illumination of the fundamental concerns, *Eval Pract*. **10**:5–13.

Susser, M., 1985, Epidemiology in the United States after World War II: the evolution of technique, *Epidemiol Rev*. **7**:147–177.

Thacker, S. B., and Berkelman, R. L., 1992, History of public health surveillance, in: *Public Health Surveillance*, W. Haperin, E. L. Baker, and R. R. Monson, eds., Van Nostrand Reinhold, New York, pp. 1–15.

Thacker, S. B., and Stroup, D. F., 1994, Future directions for comprehensive public health surveillance and health information systems in the United States, *Am J Epidemiol*. **140**:383–397.

U.S. Department of Health and Human Services, 2000, *Healthy People 2010: Understanding and Improving Health, Second Edition*, U.S. Government Printing Office, Washington, DC.

Weiss, C. H., ed., 1977, *Using Social Research in Public Policy Making*, Lexington Books, Lexington, MA.

Weiss, C. H., 1990, Evaluation for decisions: Is anybody there? Does anybody care? in: *Debates on Evaluation*, M. C. Alkin, ed., Sage, Newbury Park, CA, pp. 171–184.

Weiss, C. H., 1998, *Evaluation, Second Edition*, Prentice-Hall, Upper Saddle River, NJ.

Wilson, D., Wakefield, M. A., and Taylor, A., 1992, The South Australian Health Omnibus Survey, *Health Promot J Aust*. **2**:47–49.

CHAPTER 11

HARMONISING LOCAL HEALTH SURVEY DATA
The EURALIM Experience

Alfredo Morabia, Mary E. Northridge, Sigrid Beer-Borst, and
Serge Hercberg for the EURALIM Study Group[*]

1. INTRODUCTION

Previous chapters of this book have stressed the growing interest in continuously monitoring and comparing distributions of health determinants across populations to better inform public health workers and guide needed actions. Several authors have pointed to the need for a worldwide collection of survey data. We deal in this chapter with what appears to be a major paradox of global surveillance projects to date: data are currently available from many independent and locally based health studies, but the results cannot be directly compared across populations because of methodological variability.

Our objective in this chapter is to demonstrate the importance and feasibility of a regional and eventually a global surveillance system to monitor the determinants of population health by pooling data from local surveys. We posit that the integration of existing systems will help ensure that surveillance data collected worldwide are more directly comparable across populations. This approach will also contribute to including those regions of the world that lack even the most basic surveillance infra-structure and resources (e.g., records of births and deaths). Its success depends on recognising and sharing expertise among all partners, the development of a core monitoring instrument, and co-ordinated efforts at fund-raising for central functions such as database maintenance.

To date, three main techniques have been used to compare data across national and international studies, namely (1) centralised, standardised studies based on a uniform protocol, (2) meta-analyses of published—and sometimes unpublished—results, and

[*] Alfredo Morabia, University Hospitals of Geneva, CH-1211 Geneva, Switzerland; Mary E. Northridge, Mailman School of Public Health of Columbia University, New York, New York 10032, USA; Sigrid Beer-Borst, Projects in Nutritional Sciences, CH-3098 Koeniz, Switzerland; Serge Hercberg, National Conservatory of Arts and Crafts, 75003 Paris, France. See Appendix for detailed list.

(3) harmonisation of data from independently conducted studies. The third approach is usually rejected out of hand because of methodological inconsistencies across surveys. Indeed, protocol differences are known to severely limit direct comparability of data, both in published tabulations used for most meta-analyses and in pooling efforts. But the potential advantages of harmonising data from local surveys are worth careful consideration because ongoing surveillance systems using concerted, centralised protocols are too costly and therefore unsustainable for most of the world's population.

We review here EURALIM, a collaborative European project designed to determine the practical and theoretical extent to which local survey data can be harmonised and potentially integrated into a global surveillance system of health determinants. More detailed accounts of the methods and results of EURALIM have been published (Morabia et al., 1998; Beer-Borst et al., 2000a, 2000b, 2000c; Morabia, 2000).

2. EURALIM

In 1995, the directors of the Division of Clinical Epidemiology in Geneva and the Institut Scientifique et Technique de la Nutrition et de l'Alimentation in Paris jointly launched a series of meetings with other interested European epidemiologists to discuss the development of a regional surveillance system to compare social and biological determinants of health across European populations. The result was a project entitled Europe Alimentation (EURALIM): Coordination and Evaluation of a European Information Campaign on Diet and Nutrition. The major aim of EURALIM was to determine the extent to which health survey data could be pooled and harmonised in a common database for comparisons across populations. EURALIM was jointly funded by the European Community and the Swiss Federal Office for Education and Science.

2.1. Objectives

The EURALIM team pursued three main objectives that were achieved in a series of steps between March 1997 and September 1998: (1) improve methods for comparing European data in health determinants that were collected in separate studies, (2) inform diverse audiences—including the general public, public health workers, and politicians—about contrasts in health determinants (e.g., by gender, age group, and social class) found within and across European populations, and (3) develop a technical document to assist public health researchers in the critical interpretation of survey data originating from various study designs and populations.

2.2. Study Design

EURALIM comprised seven independent European studies of high internal validity: SU.VI.MAX, France (Hercberg et al., 1998), Monitoring Project on Cardiovascular Disease Risk Factors, the Netherlands (Verschuren et al., 1993), Progetto ATENA, Naples, Italy (Panico et al., 1992), Progetto MATISS, Province of Latina, Italy (Giampaoli et al., 1997), Bus Santé 2000, Canton of Geneva, Switzerland (Morabia et al., 1997), Belfast MONICA Project, Greater Belfast area, Northern Ireland/United Kingdom (Evans et al.,

1995), and Catalonia Nutrition Survey, Province of Catalonia, Spain (Serra-Majem et al., 1996). EURALIM sites and their associated key personnel are provided in the Appendix.

Data from these seven local studies conducted using different designs and methods of data collection across sites were harmonised and compared. Database management and statistical analyses were performed centrally at the data co-ordination center in Geneva. An overview of the study plan for EURALIM is shown in Figure 1.

2.3. Harmonisation and Database Management

Study protocols, questionnaires, and variable lists from the participating sites served as the basis for the EURALIM team to jointly define new, common variables covering demographic, diet, health, and social factors. A EURALIM coding manual (EURALIM Study Group, unpublished, 1997) was prepared which defined the exact content of each variable, along with its prescribed length and order of assembly in the common database. Each of the independent research partners prepared its own EURALIM data set, performed detailed quality control checks, and transferred its data in ASCII text files to the data co-ordination centre (EURALIM Advisory Group, unpublished, 1997). Additional quality control checks were performed centrally to eliminate any remaining inconsistencies. Finally, the seven individual data files (comprising 227 common variables) were merged into a common EURALIM database.

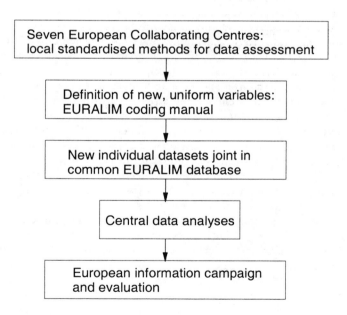

Figure 1. EURALIM study plan—harmonisation approach. [Reproduced from Beer-Borst, S., Morabia, A., Hercberg, S., et al., 2000, Obesity and other health determinants across Europe: the EURALIM project, *J Epidemiol Community Health.* 54:424–430 with permission from the BMJ Publishing Group.]

The resulting EURALIM database thus comprised data from seven population-based studies with somewhat different designs (Table 1). All final analyses were performed on a sub-sample of participants restricted to an age group represented in all seven studies (i.e., ages 40–59 years), for a total of 18,381 women and 12,908 men (Table 2).

A key task of the EURALIM team was to document inter-study differences in design and methods, such as sampling methods, population sizes, and age distributions. We illustrate this procedure using the dietary data to outline the component steps.

2.4. Harmonisation of Dietary Data

Dietary assessment methods varied substantially across sites. Salient aspects of the dietary assessment methods used by the participating studies are provided in Table 3. The Dutch study group considered their dietary assessment tool to be too different from the others to qualify for joint dietary comparison in scientific publications, so the Dutch tool was excluded from this assessment. The Catalonia survey used both a 24-hour dietary recall and a food frequency questionnaire (FFQ). Four of the remaining five groups assessed diet using FFQs. Only the two Italian studies used the same FFQ. The French study collected multiple 1-day records over 1 year (average for each participant, six records), which were subsequently re-coded as FFQs.

For the common database, fruits were defined as any type of fresh fruit (thus dried fruits, canned fruits, and fruit juices were excluded). Vegetables were defined to exclude potatoes and legumes. The resultant number and type of fresh fruits and vegetables listed varied considerably from questionnaire to questionnaire (Beer-Borst et al., 2000a). Because response categories also varied, conversion procedures were applied to obtain consistent information about the individual daily frequency of total fresh fruit and vegetable consumption. Definitions for low, medium, and high consumption of fruits (<1.5, 1.5–2, and >2 times/day) and vegetables (<2.5, 2.5–3, and >3 times/day) were based on U.S. dietary recommendations and guidelines (Wright et al., 1994). These guidelines consider only the frequency of fresh fruit and vegetable consumption reported for each day, without taking into account different serving sizes. As a result, individuals who consumed fresh fruits and vegetables at the recommended frequency (>2 and >3 times/day, respectively) were defined as "high" consumers (Wright et al., 1994; Krebs-Smith et al., 1995).

Required data to derive daily individual energy and nutrient intakes were obtained from the local dietary assessments. Composite measures were based on each survey's specific quantification method and national food composition database, but expressed in a common manner to allow for joint central analyses. For a crude assessment of diet composition, caloric density was calculated as the percentage of total energy intake derived from total carbohydrate, total fat, total protein, and alcohol intake. The percentage of energy derived from saturated fatty acids (not assessed in the Belfast MONICA project) and the measure of dietary fiber density were derived from total energy intake, including energy from alcohol.

Table 1. Characteristics and sampling methods of the participating EURALIM study populations

Population that study sample is representative of	Year(s) of survey	Urban and/or rural	Sexes and age (y) sampled	Sampling method	Response rate by sex
France	1995-1996	urban and rural	F, M: 35-65	random selection of a representative sample out of a large volunteer population (intervention study)	F: 86%; M: 81%
the Netherlands	1990-1992	mainly urban	F, M: 20-59	by gender, 5 year age strata	F: 62%; M: 57%
Naples (Italy)	1993-1996	urban	F: 30-69	Volunteer sample (95%) & random selection (5%)	Not applicable
Province of Latina (Italy)	1993-1996	rural	F, M: 20-84	random selection, stratified by sex, age	F: 72%; M: 67%
Geneva (Switzerland)	1993-1996	urban	F, M: 29-83	random selection by gender, 10 year age strata	F: 65%; M: 65%
Belfast (United Kingdom)	1991-1992	urban	F, M: 25-65	by gender, 10 year age strata	F: 47%; M: 49%
Catalonia (Spain)	1992	mainly urban	F, M: 25-75	multistage sample, stratified by region	F: 72%; M: 66%

[Reproduced from Beer-Borst, S., Morabia, A., Hercberg, S., 2000, Obesity and other health determinants across Europe: the EURALIM project, *J Epidemiol Community Health.* 54:424-430 with permission from the BMJ Publishing Group.]

Table 2. Number and percentage of 40-59 year old participants by EURALIM population

Population that study sample is representative of	Women		Men		Total
	number	*%*	*number*	*%*	
France	6 424	35.0	4 791	37.1	11 215
the Netherlands	5 664	30.8	5 144	39.8	10 808
Naples (Italy)	3 013	16.4	0	0.0	3 013
Province of Latina (Italy)	1 254	6.8	1 084	8.4	2 338
Geneva (Switzerland)	1 083	5.9	1 040	8.1	2 123
Belfast (United Kingdom)	538	2.9	550	4.3	1 088
Catalonia (Spain)	405	2.2	299	2.3	704
Total	18 381	100.0	12 908	100.0	31 289

[Reproduced from Beer-Borst, S., Morabia, A., Hercberg, S., 2000, Obesity and other health determinants across Europe: the EURALIM project, *J Epidemiol Community Health*. 54:424–430 with permission from the BMJ Publishing Group.]

Table 3. Dietary assessment methods employed in six participating EURALIM studies

Methods	Population study sample is representative of:					
	France	*Naples (Italy)*	*Province of Latina (Italy)*	*Geneva (Switzerland)*	*Belfast (UK)*	*Catalonia (Spain)*
Recall/Record	*1 day record*					*24 h recall*
n observations	1–12					2
Administration	Self-administered by Minitel					Face-to-face interview
Quantification	Photo book	N/A[a]	N/A[a]	N/A[a]	N/A[a]	Household measures
Season(s)	All year					Spring, winter
Day of the week	All days					All days
Food frequency questionnaire		*Semi-quantitative*	*Semi-quantitative*	*Semi-quantitative*	*Semi-quantitative and qualitative sections*	*Qualitative*
Reference period		12 months	12 months	1 month	1 week to 1 month	12 months
Administration		Face-to-face at research unit	Face-to-face at research unit	Self-administered at home	Self-administered at home	Face-to-face at home
Season(s)	CN/A[b]	All year	All year	All year	All year; none in July or August	Spring
Total number of items[c]		127	127	88	78	77
Number of vegetables[d]		19 (26)[f]	19 (26)[f]	9 (11)[f]	5 (9)[f]	8
Number of fruits[e]		17 (18)[f]	17 (18)[f]	5 (17)[f]	5 (6)[f]	5 (8)[f]

[a]N/A = not available; [b]CN/A = currently not available; [c]one question can consist of several items; [d]potatoes and legumes excluded; [e]considers total number of vegetable or fruit items listed within single questions. [f]dried fruits, canned fruits and fruit juices excluded;

[Reproduced from Beer-Borst, S., Hercberg, S., Morabia, A., et al., 2000, Dietary patterns in six European populations: results from EURALIM, a collaborative European data harmonization and information campaign, *Eur J Clin Nutr.* 54:253–262 with permission from the Nature Publishing Group.]

2.5. Comparison of Within-Population Contrasts

Despite harmonising and pooling of data from separate surveys into a common EURALIM database, problems inherent in comparing data from independent surveys remained. Regarding the dietary data just discussed, for example, variability across surveys was demonstrated in the type of assessment tool, reference period, number of food items listed, response categories provided, size of standard portions, method of interview, and seasons covered by the questionnaires. These differences were deemed insurmountable and precluded *direct* comparisons of most dietary items across sites.

As a result, the EURALIM team developed an approach that directly compared groups *within* populations and examined these contrasts *across* populations. We illustrate this approach here using body mass index (BMI) as an index of adiposity (BMI is defined as weight in kilograms divided by height in meters squared). Directly comparing BMIs across populations could be severely biased if the methods for assessing weight and height differed importantly among sites. The major methodological differences identified across surveys were the types of balances used and the manners and frequencies of their calibrations, the height measurement devices used, measurement precision, and clothing worn during measurements. The Swiss and Dutch body weight data were made more comparable to those obtained in the other surveys by subtracting 1 kg to account for the difference in assessing weight in full dress versus weight in undergarments only. Next, assume that the measurement error of height and weight was similar for men and women within the same population. This is a fairly reasonable assumption because the survey protocols were essentially similar across gender in all component surveys. If the BMI measure is mis-classified by a co-efficient δ which is similar for men and women, the resultant gender *ratio* of BMIs is unbiased:

$$\frac{\text{BMI measured in men}}{\text{BMI measured in women}} = \frac{\text{true BMI in men} \times \delta}{\text{true BMI in women} \times \delta} = \frac{\text{true BMI in men}}{\text{true BMI in women}}$$

The situation is somewhat different for gender *differences*, namely:

$$\text{BMI measured in men ! BMI measured in women}$$
$$= \text{true BMI of men} \times \delta \text{ ! true BMI of women} \times \delta$$
$$= (\text{true BMI of men ! true BMI of women}) \times \delta$$

While the *measured* difference may be biased, the *direction* of the difference is expected to remain the same.

Finally, if we compare genders at a given exposure level, such as the prevalence of obesity (defined as a BMI $\exists$ 30 kg/m^2), both the gender *ratio* and the gender *difference* will be biased. This is because a given δ of measurement error (say, 1 kg/m^2) will correspond to different areas under the BMI distributions in the compared groups (e.g., men and women) if the distribution curves are not identical. The magnitude of this phenomenon in six EURALIM populations (the Naples study did not include men) using the scenario of a 3% error in (under-) measuring body weight is illustrated in Table 4. For this example, it was assumed that the measurement error was similar for men and women. The nominal prevalence of obesity changed with the measurement error present, affecting

Table 4. Impact of a 3% measurement error for body weight on gender differences and ratios of obesity (BMI $\geq$ 30 kg/m²)

| Population that study sample is representative of | Error | Obesity | | Difference | Ratio |
		% in men	% in women	Men minus women	Men to women
France	0%	8	7	1	1.14
	3%	5	6	−1	0.83
the Netherlands	0%	12	14	−2	0.86
	3%	8	11	−3	0.73
Province of Latina	0%	20	37	−17	0.54
(Italy)	3%	14	30	−16	0.47
Geneva	0%	11	9	2	1.22
(Switzerland)	3%	8	7	1	1.14
Belfast	0%	15	16	−1	0.94
(United Kingdom)	3%	11	13	−2	0.85
Catalonia	0%	11	22	−11	0.50
(Spain)	3%	7	18	−11	0.39

[Reproduced from Beer-Borst, S., Morabia, A., Hercberg, S., 2000, Obesity and other health determinants across Europe: the EURALIM project, *J Epidemiol Community Health.* 54:424–430 with permission from the BMJ Publishing Group.]

direct comparisons across groups (e.g., between women from Latina and the Netherlands). Nonetheless, the impact of measurement error on the comparison of gender differences was minimal. Although the gender differences and ratios changed, the qualitative interpretation remained the same; that is, there was more obesity among women than men in southern Europe but similar levels of obesity among women and men in northern Europe. It is reasonable to expect that the qualitative relationship (i.e., whether men are more obese than women or vice versa) will not be affected if the two distributions have comparable variances.

Using these premises, the EURALIM team set out to generate *within*-population contrasts by gender, age group, and other known health determinants (e.g., education level and smoking status). These provided the basis for valid comparisons *across* populations. Two models of graphic presentation of these comparisons were developed, one for the general public and one for public health workers.

Results were targeted and disseminated to the general public via a European health promotion campaign. Data interpretation to the general public is modeled by Figure 2, which is part of the EURALIM brochure *Nutrition and the Heart: Healthy Living in Europe* (EURALIM Study Group, 1998a). A second, more detailed pamphlet was developed for public health workers. It discusses the major sources of variability among surveys, provides additional analyses, and explains the rationale for interpreting results on the distribution and determinants of health across populations (EURALIM Study Group, 1998b). An example of age-standardised gender differences in the prevalence of obesity and the associated 95% confidence intervals, as presented in the public health workers' pamphlet, is presented in Figure 3. Additional analyses stratified by age group (40–49 versus 50–59 years), educational level, and smoking status permitted further insights into the distribution and determinants of health within and across the considered populations.

2.5.1. Body Mass Index

The distributions (inter-quartile ranges) for men were usually shifted upward compared with the corresponding inter-quartile ranges for women (note that the median values were 1–2 kg/m^2 higher for men than for women), except for the populations from Catalonia and Latina (Figure 4). BMIs for women from Naples resembled those of women from Catalonia. Women from all populations showed greater variability in measured BMIs than did men (i.e., women's inter-quartile ranges, or P25–P75, were as much as 2 kg/m^2 larger). Additional analyses revealed that in all populations examined, being overweight (BMI = 25–30 kg/m^2) was significantly more prevalent in men than women. Few differences by gender for obesity (BMI ∃ 30 kg/m^2) were found in the populations of France, the Netherlands, Geneva, and Belfast. In Catalonia and Latina, however, more women than men were obese. These same results were also presented to the general public.

This North-South European gradient of gender differences in obesity may be a true reflection of varying social and economic conditions among the examined populations, as well as different kinds of occupational and leisure-time activities and dietary habits by gender. As demonstrated previously, differences in study design or in method of assessing body weight and height among studies are probably too small to meaningfully influence the gender contrasts found.

HOW TO READ THE GRAPHS

For most risk factors, the results are presented in two different ways:

> On the left side is shown the **typical value** of a population measured for a risk factor. Half the population will have values that fall within the range shown. These values are called **percentiles**.

> On the right side is shown the **percentage of women and men** that have risk factor values equal to or greater than defined critical values. These values are called **frequencies**. They are presented as **bar charts**.

Here is an example using blood cholesterol, measured in the population from the greater Belfast area.

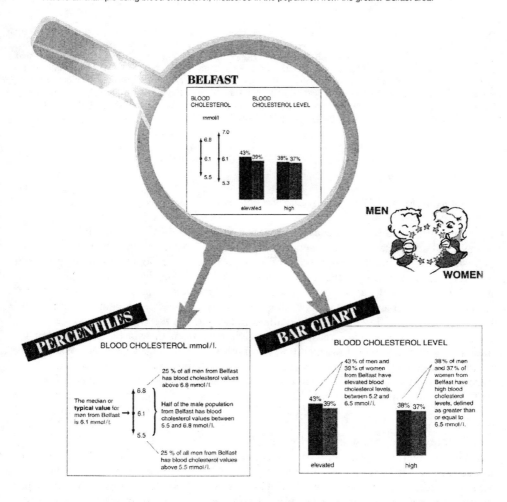

Figure 2. Explanation of percentiles and bar charts from the EURALIM brochure for the general public, "Nutrition and the Heart: Healthy Living in Europe." [Original is printed in color. For each set of bars, data for men are on the left and data for women are on the right. Reproduced from EURALIM Study Group, 1998, *Nutrition and the Heart: Healthy Living in Europe, First Edition*, European Communities, Geneva with permission from the European Communities.]

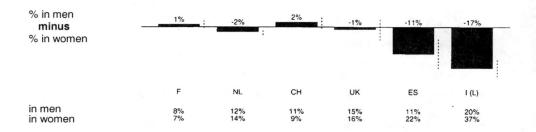

Figure 3. Supplement for public health professionals. Age standardised gender difference in the prevalence of obesity (BMI ∃ 30 kg/m^2) with their associated 95% CIs, 40–59 years. [Percentages and percentage point differences correspond to data in Table 4 for observed error. Dotted lines represent confidence intervals. Dotted lines that do not intersect the horizontal bar indicate statistical significance. F = France; NL = the Netherlands; CH = Canton of Geneva, Switzerland; UK = Greater Belfast area, Northern Ireland/United Kingdom; ES = Province of Catalonia, Spain; I (L) = Province of Latina, Italy. Reproduced from Beer-Borst, S., Morabia, A., Hercberg, S., et al., 2000, Obesity and other health determinants across Europe: the EURALIM project, *J Epidemiol Community Health.* 54:424–430 with permission from the BMJ Publishing Group.]

2.5.2. Consumption of Fresh Fruits and Vegetables

We investigated the frequency of fresh fruit and vegetable consumption across local surveys, without considering differences in portion size. Although the obtained *frequency* of fresh fruit or vegetable consumption might be higher in one population than another, it does not necessarily follow that the *quantity* of consumption (in grams per day) is also higher. The choice of cut-off points used for high, medium, and low frequency of consumption were influenced by the fact that the current U.S. recommendations and guidelines are considered high for most individuals in Europe and the United States.

The proportion of male and female participants (from the six populations that included both genders) with low, medium, and high fresh fruit and vegetable consumption are provided in Figures 5 and 6, respectively. Overall, more men than women were low consumers of fresh fruits and vegetables ($p < 0.01$ for all gender contrasts except for fresh fruits in the Catalonia population). Age-standardised gender differences in the prevalence of low consumption ranged between 7% and 18% for fresh fruits and between 5% and 15% for vegetables.

The prevalence of low fruit and vegetable consumption did not vary significantly by educational level, except in France and Belfast. In those populations, individuals with less education consumed fresh fruits and vegetables less frequently per day than did those with more education. Smokers in all populations consumed fresh fruits fewer times per day than did non-smokers (age-standardised differences ranged from 4% to 20%); differences in the frequency of vegetable consumption were less pronounced (age-standardised differences ranged from 1% to 9%).

OVERWEIGHT & OBESITY

Excessive body weight increases the risk of hypertension, unhealthy lipid profile, heart disease, diabetes, and some cancers. Overweight and obesity can be assessed using Quetelet's Body Mass Index (BMI) calculated as weight in kg divided by height in meters^2 (e.g., a woman weighing 70 kg and measuring 1.6 m, BMI = 70/(1.6 x 1.6) = 27 kg/m^2). **Overweight** is defined as a BMI in the range of 25 to 30 kg/m^2, and **obesity** as a BMI of equal to or greater than 30 kg/m^2. BMI values between 20 to 25 kg/m^2 indicate desirable body weight.

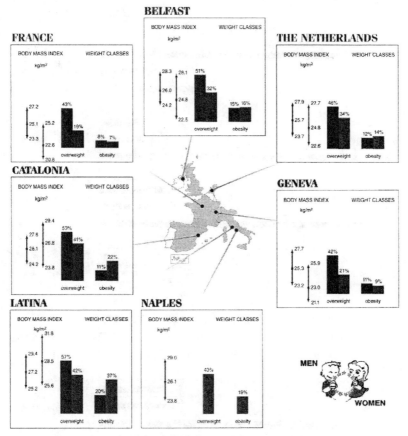

> In general men have higher Body Mass Indices than women. In the Province of Latina and in Catalonia however women have higher Body Mass Indices than men.
> More men compared with women are overweight, but in almost all populations more women than men are obese.
> Weight reduction in overweight and obese individuals can reduce the risk of heart disease. A diet with less calories and fat, as well as regular physical activity, will help a person to lose weight and to maintain the weight loss.

Figure 4. Brochure for the general public—Overweight and Obesity. [Original is printed in color. For each set of bars, data for men are on the left and data for women are on the right (the Naples chart shows data for women only). Reproduced from Beer-Borst, S., Morabia, A., Hercberg, S., et al., 2000, Obesity and other health determinants across Europe: the EURALIM project, *J Epidemiol Community Health*. 54:424–430 with permission from the BMJ Publishing Group.]

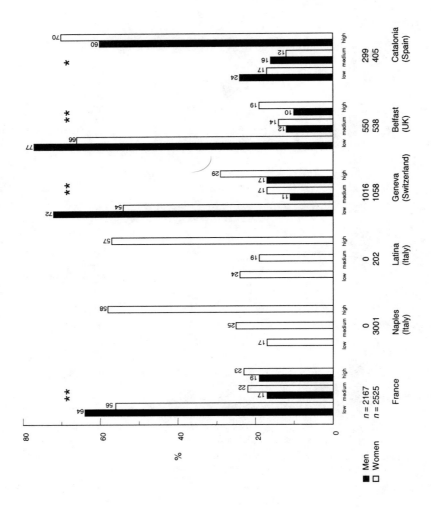

Figure 5. Age-standardized prevalence of low (<1.5 times/day), medium (1.5–2 times/day), and high (>2 times/day) fruit consumption in men and women aged 40–59 y, by EURALIM population. X^2 **$P < 0.01$, *$P < 0.05$ for gender differences. [Reproduced from Beer-Borst, S., Hercberg, S., Morabia, A., et al., 2000, Dietary patterns in six European populations: results from EURALIM, a collaborative European data harmonization and information campaign, *Eur J Clin Nutr*. 54:253–262 with permission from the Nature Publishing Group.]

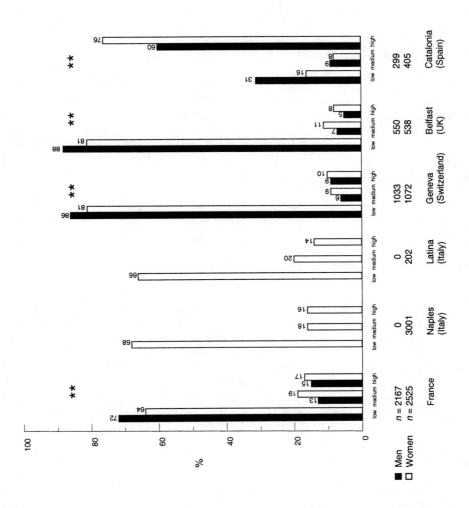

Figure 6. Age-standardized prevalence of low (<2.5 times/day), medium (2.5–3 times/day), and high (>3 times/day) vegetable consumption in men and women aged 40–59 y, by EURALIM population. X^2 **$P < 0.01$, *$P < 0.05$ for gender differences. [Reproduced from Beer-Borst, S., Hercberg, S., Morabia, A., et al., 2000, Dietary patterns in six European populations: results from EURALIM, a collaborative European data harmonization and information campaign, *Eur J Clin Nutr.* 54:253–262 with permission from the Nature Publishing Group.]

2.5.3. Energy and Nutrient Intakes

Overall, much less variability was observed across populations in nutrient intake than was observed for specific food items. The distributions of total energy intake (including energy from alcohol) in mega-joules per day for women and men separately, age-standardised for the six included populations, are presented in Figure 7. As expected, energy intake was higher for men than for women in the four populations in which required data were collected for both genders. No observed variability was found by gender for median caloric densities expressed as percent energy from carbohydrate, fat, protein, or alcohol (Beer-Borst et al., 2000a).

2.6. Information Campaign

"EURALIM Day" was held on May 19, 1998, in all seven participating centres, to kick off the information campaign which ultimately reached close to 1,500 public health workers across Europe. The general public brochure was subsequently distributed to more than 60,000 individuals through these 1,500 contacts. The information campaign was evaluated by participating public health workers in all seven collaborative centres by administering a common evaluation questionnaire. The response rates were low, which served as a reminder of how essential yet difficult it is to carefully evaluate large-scale public health campaigns (Beer-Borst et al., 2000c).

3. THE EURALIM EXPERIENCE

3.1. Co-ordination of Locally Based Surveys

The EURALIM team sought to determine the extent to which health survey data that had already been collected could be harmonised and pooled for comparisons across populations. Within a relatively short time frame and with limited resources, it was possible to identify a sub-set of common health determinants in all seven participating surveys. Locally run public health programmes often have the required features of successful surveillance systems; that is, they are population based, decision and action oriented, relevant, timely, readily accessible, and effectively communicated. Nonetheless, if such surveys are to become part of ongoing surveillance programmes to monitor the distribution of health determinants across time and place, certain modifications will be necessary to ensure better comparability.

3.2. Definition of New Uniform Variables

The development of a pooled database was a key step in EURALIM that allowed for joint, comparative analysis. Still, only a fraction of the examined variables were even remotely similar across all seven sites. Methods for assessing important factors such as physical activity, social class (e.g., education and occupation), and smoking habits varied considerably across studies. For certain factors (e.g., physical activity) it was not possible to define a common variable, as the methods used were so dissimilar. Since educational

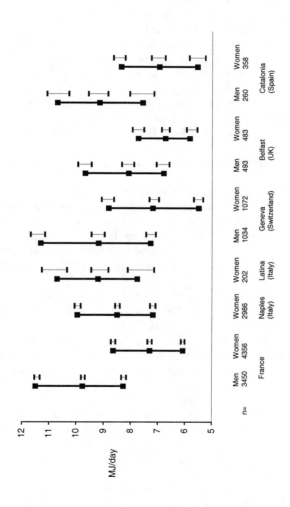

Figure 7. Age-standardized daily total energy intakes (MJ/day) by gender for six participating EURALIM populations, presented as 25th (P25), 50th (P50), and 75th (P75) percentiles with their associated 95% confidence intervals. [Reproduced from Beer-Borst, S., Hercberg, S., Morabia, A., et al., 2000, Dietary patterns in six European populations: results from EURALIM, a collaborative European data harmonization and information campaign, *Eur J Clin Nutr.* 54:253–262 with permission from the Nature Publishing Group.]

systems differ substantially across Europe, the best possible common cut-point was to set "high education" equal to "university or equivalent degree." Thus, the category "medium or low education" comprised a large, diverse spectrum of degrees. For smoking habits, it was possible to distinguish "never," "former," and "current" smokers across sites, but not to provide any common information on duration or intensity of smoking.

3.3. Age Standardisation

Age is an important determinant of most chronic diseases; therefore, age standardisation is a crucial step in comparisons of health determinants across populations. Several situations were encountered in EURALIM that future projects may also encounter. For example, the over-representation of the youngest age group in the Catalan population was due to reliance on what turned out to be incorrect census information. The inclusion of volunteers was in part responsible for the unequal age distributions in the samples from France and Naples. Very real differences in age distributions across populations are expected when, for example, poor and developed countries are compared. Age standardisation is therefore essential in any global surveillance system of health determinants (statistical methods are provided in Beer-Borst et al., 2000b).

3.4. Contrasts by Gender, Age Group, and Social Class

As discussed in Section 2.5, measurement error tends to be cancelled out or is usually negligible if the biases are essentially similar among the groups being compared. For example, if weight is over-estimated for both men and women in a given survey, the gender *ratio* of median BMIs will be unbiased. The gender *difference* of median BMIs will be slightly biased unless the gender difference is null. The situation becomes more complicated when the prevalence of a given condition (e.g., obesity) is compared by gender.

The central contribution of EURALIM that may be important in future comparisons of health determinants across populations is this: comparing the nominal prevalence of health determinants across populations is likely less valid than comparing contrasts by gender, age group, or social class. For example, in Latina obesity was more prevalent among women than men, but the reverse situation was found in France, the Netherlands, and Belfast. This observation may indicate that social and therefore potentially modifiable health determinants play important roles in the observed differences. Similar contrasts can be computed and compared for smokers versus non-smokers, upper versus lower social class, and various age groups. A disadvantage of ratio comparisons versus difference comparisons is that the former give no idea of the magnitude of the affected populations. Thus, differences among populations may be more useful for public health planning and preferred in standardised statistical reports (or presented along with ratio estimates).

The biological variables and physiologic measures investigated in EURALIM often had asymmetric distributions, thus limiting the mean as a measure of central tendency. Atypical individuals with outlying characteristics are also known to influence the usual estimates of means and variances. Accordingly, three percentiles were used to summarise the distributions of health determinants: the median or 50th percentile as a measure of central tendency, and the 25th and the 75th percentiles as measures of variability. The latter percentiles were preferred over the 5th and 95th percentiles because they can be more precisely estimated given the usually limited sample sizes of most local health surveys (Morabia et al., 1997).

✶ 3.5. Realistic Public Health Objectives

The EURALIM experience suggests that differences in the distributions of health determinants within and across populations are not fixed biologically, but may be largely culturally or socially determined. For example, the excess prevalence of hyper-cholesterolemia in men compared with women aged 40–49 years observed in Belfast (50% ! 44% = 6%, $p < 0.05$) and in Catalonia (47% ! 38% = 9%, $p < 0.05$) are likely modifiable since they were not observed in Geneva (37% ! 42% = !5%, $p > 0.05$) or in the Netherlands (44% ! 41% = 3%, $p > 0.05$). Thus, it may be reasonable to set the most favourable situations found among groups as attainable targets for the rest of the population, with the goal of eliminating disparities in health within and across populations.

4. STRATEGIES FOR GLOBAL SURVEILLANCE OF HEALTH DETERMINANTS

Two extreme strategies are outlined here to help delimit the boundaries for constructing a global surveillance system of health determinants. The first strategy uses a central-ised, standardised approach. Participating centres follow specific protocols to measure selected variables, and blood samples are shipped to and analysed in central laboratories. An advantage of this model is that the data collected across populations around the world are, in principle, directly comparable. Drawbacks of this approach are that it requires a heavily centralised organization, is prohibitively expensive, and cannot be implemented in populations lacking strong public health infra-structures. A model for this approach is the MONICA project (Tunstall-Pedoe, 1988), which has provided valuable and extensive information on determinants of cardiovascular disease across Europe and other select-ed countries. However, MONICA was conceived as an etiologic investigation into the causes of cardiovascular disease and therefore embodies methodological constraints that need not encumber global surveillance systems.

A second strategy towards developing a global surveillance system of health de-terminants would be to forego any a priori attempts at standardising protocols across locations. The EURALIM project is an example of this approach, in which central statistical analyses on major determinants of cardiovascular health were conducted after joint consideration of methodological issues by the original investigators of locally con-ducted surveys. Advantages of this alternative strategy include its relatively low cost and rapid time frame for reporting results. Nonetheless, serious obstacles prevent direct com-parison of data across populations due to the large variability in the methods employed for measuring key variables such as physical activity, social class, and smoking habits.

The EURALIM experience led to the conclusion that pooling and harmonising data from independently conducted surveys is not a suitable strategy for creating a global surveillance system of health determinants. The MONICA experience highlighted the challenges in creating a fully centralised and standardised system at the regional level of Europe, where the available resources are vastly greater than in most other countries.

From a financial viewpoint, it is clear that no international agency will be able to continuously fund a centralised global project of the magnitude of MONICA. This is a serious obstacle, as the vast majority of the countries of Asia, Africa, South America, and Eastern Europe have limited resources to devote to public health. Further, public health agencies and researchers around the world are likely to strongly resist complying with a centrally run system that over-rides local needs and considerations. In addition, conditions for surveillance vary dramatically across populations (e.g., no reliable and comprehensive telephone coverage exists for most of the globe).

A recent debate about the possible creation of a European centre for disease control (Stephenson, 1999) revealed a strong sentiment towards internet-driven centralisation as opposed to physical centralisation, which has bearing on this debate as well. Furthermore, it is not at all clear that full standardisation is the optimum way to go. The constraints of following a rigid protocol may impinge on high participation rates and desired flexibility to better adapt to each population's priorities and needs. Extensive standardisation may impose excessive delays in releasing collected information in a timely manner to the public and prohibit inclusion of those locales with little public health infra-structure or experience in surveillance techniques.

A workable system undoubtedly lies somewhere between the MONICA and EURA-LIM extremes. Neither a fully centralised nor a fully decentralised global surveillance system of health determinants are realistic options. The EURALIM team instead proposed an intermediate solution based on a short monitoring instrument (SMI) that would be common to all locales and added to ongoing surveillance instruments worldwide. The detailed characteristics of the SMI still need to be worked out, and input from *all* areas of the globe—thus far largely confined to Europe, North America, and Australia—is essential. The important features of the SMI are that it be short, easily administered, and of global relevance. As a start, monitoring for major determinants of cardiovascular disease may satisfy the criterion of global relevance since, within 20 years, coronary heart disease will become the major cause of premature death worldwide. The SMI is envisioned as a one- or two-page document, combining key social determinants of health (e.g., age, gender, race, ethnicity, social class, immigration status, occupation, and geographic location) with self-reported health information (e.g., smoking, diet, and physical activity) and perhaps selected clinical measures (e.g., weight, height, blood pressure, and total blood cholesterol). Clearly, the exact content of the proposed SMI remains to be worked out—collaboratively.

The developed SMI and essential protocols would then need to be translated and validated in each population in which they are used. A centralised database accessible through the internet may be the most efficient method for combining the collected data. This method would allow for public availability via the World Wide Web soon after the data have been entered. A collaborative but relatively sparse scientific and administrative team would be needed to routinely check the eligibility of the candidate data and to continuously maintain the integrity of the database. Continuous surveillance of the distribution and determinants of health across populations may allow for more careful assessment of the impact of health and other policies on the world's health, and to help us monitor progress towards health for all populations.

5. ACKNOWLEDGEMENT

EURALIM was supported by the European Community (DG V) project 96CVVF3-446-0 and the Swiss Federal Office for Education and Science OFES 96.0089.

6. REFERENCES

Beer-Borst, S., Hercberg, S., Morabia, A., et al., 2000a, Dietary patterns in six European populations: results from EURALIM, a collaborative European data harmonization and information campaign, *Eur J Clin Nutr.* **54**:253–262.

Beer-Borst, S., Morabia, A., Hercberg, S., et al., 2000b, Obesity and other health determinants across Europe: the EURALIM project, *J Epidemiol Community Health.* **54**:424–430.

Beer-Borst, S., Morabia, A., Hercberg, S., et al., 2000c, Public health professionals evaluate EURALIM, a European information campaign on diet and nutrition, *Rev Esp Nutr Comunitaria.* **6**:123–131.

EURALIM Study Group, 1998a, *Nutrition and the Heart: Healthy Living in Europe, First Edition*, European Communities, Geneva.

EURALIM Study Group, 1998b, *Nutrition and the Heart: Healthy Living in Europe. Supplement for Public Health Professionals: Additional Analyses and Rationale for Interpretation, First Edition*, European Communities, Geneva.

Evans, A. E., Ruidavets, J. B., McCrum, E. E., et al., 1995, Autres pays, autres coeurs? Dietary patterns, risk factors and ischemic heart disease in Belfast and Toulouse, *QJM.* **88**:469–477.

Giampaoli, S., Poce, A., Sciarra, F., et al., 1997, Change in cardiovascular risk factors during a 10-year community intervention program, *Acta Cardiol.* **52**:411–422.

Hercberg, S., Preziosi, P., Briancon, S., et al., 1998, A primary prevention trial using nutritional doses of antioxidant vitamins and minerals in cardiovascular diseases and cancers in a general population: the SU.VI.MAX study. Design, methods, and participant characteristics, *Control Clin Trials.* **19**:336–351.

Krebs-Smith, S. M., Cook, A., Subar, A. F., et al., 1995, U.S. adults' fruit and vegetable intakes, 1989 to 1991: a revised baseline for the healthy people 2000 objective, *Am J Public Health.* **85**:1623–1629.

Morabia, A., 2000, Worldwide surveillance of risk factors to promote global health, *Am J Public Health.* **90**:22–24.

Morabia, A., Bernstein, M., Heritier, S., et al., 1997, Community-based surveillance of cardiovascular risk factors in Geneva: methods, resulting distributions, and comparisons with other populations, *Prev Med.* **26**:311–319.

Morabia, A., Beer-Borst, S., Hercberg, S., 1998, Locally based surveys, unite! The EURALIM example. EURALIM Study Group, European Information Campaign on Diet and Nutrition, *Am J Public Health.* **88**:1153–1155.

Panico, S., Dello Iacovo, R., Celentano, E., et al., 1992, Progetto ATENA, a study on the etiology of major chronic diseases in women: design, rationale and objectives, *Eur J Epidemiol.* **8**:601–608.

Serra-Majem, L., Ribas Barba, L., García Closas, R., et al., 1996, *Avaluació de l'Estat Nutricional de la Població Catalana (1992–93): Avaluació dels Hàbits Alimentaris, el Consum d'Aliments, Energia i Nutrients, i de l'Estat Nutricional Mitjançant Indicadors Bioquímics i Antropomètrics, First Edition*, Generalitat de Catalunya, Departament de Sanitat i Seguretet Social, Barcelona.

Stephenson, J., 1999, Creation of a "European CDC" debated, *JAMA.* **281**:1477–1478.

Tunstall-Pedoe, H., for the WHO MONICA Project Principal Investigators, 1988, The World Health Organization MONICA Project (monitoring trends and determinants in cardiovascular disease): a major international collaboration, *J Clin Epidemiol.* **41**:105–114.

Verschuren, W. M. M., van Leer, E. M., Blockstra, A., et al., 1993, Cardiovascular disease risk factors in the Netherlands, *Neth J Cardiol.* **4**:205–210.

Wright, J. D., Ervin, B., Briefel, R. R., eds., 1994, *Consensus Workshop on Dietary Assessment: Nutrition Monitoring and Tracking the Year 2000 Objectives*, U.S. Department of Health and Human Services, Hyattsville, MD.

7. APPENDIX: EURALIM SITES AND KEY PERSONNEL

EURALIM Collaborating Centres

France
Institut Scientifique et Technique de la Nutrition et de l'Alimentation, Paris
Principal investigator: P. Galan
Key personnel: S. Hercberg and P. Preziosi

Italy
Department of Clinical and Experimental Medicine, Federico II University of Naples
Principal investigator: S. Panico
Key personnel: R. Galasso (Regional Hospital of Oncology, Rionero in Vulture) and E. Celentano
    (Tumour Institute, Naples)

Laboratory of Epidemiology and Biostatistics, National Institute of Public Health, Rome
Principal investigator: S. Giampaoli
Key personnel: F. Pannozzo, C. Lo Noce, and M. F. Vescio

Northern Ireland/United Kingdom
Department of Epidemiology and Public Health, Queen's University of Belfast
Principal investigator: A. Evans
Key personnel: J. Yarnell, E. McCrum, and J. Weston

Spain
Community Nutrition Research Group, University of Barcelona, and Department of Clinical Sciences,
    University of Las Palmas de Gran Canaria
Principal investigator: L. Serra-Majem
Key personnel: L. Ribas and J.M. Ramon

Switzerland
Division of Clinical Epidemiology, University Hospitals of Geneva
Principal investigator: M. S. Bernstein
Key personnel: A. Morabia, S. Héritier, and S. Beer-Borst

The Netherlands
National Institute of Public Health and the Environment, Bilthoven
Principal investigator: W. M. M. Verschuren
Key personnel: J. C. Seidell, S. Houterman, and P. C. W. van den Hoogen

EURALIM Data Co-ordinating Centre, Geneva
Division of Clinical Epidemiology, University Hospitals Geneva
Responsible officer: A. Morabia
Key personnel: S. Beer-Borst and S. Billard (database management) and O. Vitek (biostatistics)

Associated EURALIM Collaborating Centre
Harlem Health Promotion Center, Mailman School of Public Health of Columbia University, New York
Principal investigator: M. E. Northridge
Key personnel: C. Leu

EURALIM Steering Committee
Project co-ordinator: S. Hercberg (Paris)
Project director: A. Morabia (Geneva)
Project manager (associate): S. Beer-Borst (Geneva)

EURALIM Advisory Group
Biostatistics: S. Héritier (Geneva)
Database management: P. Preziosi (Paris)

CHAPTER 12

ANALYSIS, INTERPRETATION, AND USE OF COMPLEX SOCIAL AND BEHAVIORAL SURVEILLANCE DATA

Looking Back in Order to Go Forward

David V. McQueen and Linda Gauger Elsner[*]

1. INTRODUCTION

During the past 20 years the international public health community has increasingly recognised the importance of understanding chronic diseases and the risk factors associated with them. Although a plethora of social and behavioural data has been accumulated by economically advanced countries during these years, much of the information is neither fully analysed nor used. For example, most analyses have been limited to descriptive statistical reports. While these types of reports are valuable and useful, they clearly do not represent all possibilities for analysis, interpretation, and use of data.

Participants at the September 1999 conference "Global Issues and Perspectives in Monitoring Behaviors in Populations: Surveillance of Risk Factors in Health and Illness," held in Atlanta, Georgia, concluded that new analytic approaches are needed to allow public health officials to appropriately understand and solve many current health problems. Further, in light of the sophistication of current computer technology and the development of advanced statistical models, the participants agreed that now is the optimum time to begin using more complex analytic approaches. To foster the development of such approaches, two follow-up meetings were held to address the needs versus demands of surveillance activities in developed and developing countries, respectively.

The first meeting, "Analysis, Interpretation, and Use of Complex Social and Behavioral Surveillance Data: Looking Back in Order to Go Forward," was held in Savannah, Georgia, in June 2000. It brought together data analysts (e.g., statisticians), interpreters of data (e.g., epidemiologists, theorists, social scientists), users of data (e.g., policy-makers, programme planners), and representatives of other groups who have a vested interest in the surveillance dialogue (e.g., Ministries of Health, federal agencies, scientific journal editors, the World Bank, the World Health Organization and its regional offices) from

[*] Centers for Disease Control and Prevention, Atlanta, Georgia 30341-3717, USA.

developed countries. The meeting's structure and dynamics contributed to some unexpected but valuable messages for countries that have not yet developed surveillance systems, as well as obvious points of importance to countries with advanced behavioural monitoring systems. This chapter details the Savannah meeting, the major purpose of which was to identify messages and recommendations for developing countries that had not yet established surveillance systems. These messages and recommendations were presented at the second follow-up meeting, "Capacity Building, Comparability, and Data Use in Behavioral Risk Factor Surveillance: Focus on Global Surveillance Issues," which was held in Atlanta in September 2000.

2. FRAMEWORK AND GOALS OF THE MEETING

The Savannah meeting was by invitation. Participants were invited for their experience with data analysis, interpretation, or use. The meeting included fewer than 50 people from 13 economically advanced countries and had an open format designed to force the participants to think through the issues and learn from each other. The meeting opened with a half-day plenary session, which introduced participants to the purpose and format of the meeting and established questions to be discussed over the next several days.

After the plenary session, each participant met in one of three assigned working groups and deliberated for the next day and a half. The Analysis Group shared new approaches for analysing data, the Interpretation Group learned about new techniques and spoke with statisticians about the best ways to present data to users, and the Data Use Group discussed the types of information that were most useful to them for planning and evaluating programmes. Each group spent the greatest portion of their time listening to informal presentations and discussing relevant issues.

On the third and final day of the meeting, all meeting participants re-convened for an assembly wherein each working group described their findings and all meeting participants discussed those issues. In this chapter, the assembly debates are summarised under the relevant working group section. After the debates a closing session was held, during which the meeting participants developed "single over-riding communication objectives" to be used at the September 2000 meeting.

3. PLENARY SESSION

The opening plenary session set the stage for group discussions by establishing the vast differences in how data are collected, analysed, and used in developed versus developing countries. In many official reports for developing countries, footnotes might indicate that the data came from surveys in only certain geo-political sections or one city, yet the data are presented as being representative of the entire country. On the other hand, the problem in the United States and most other Western countries is generally the opposite: enormous stores of data are available—some collected systematically and some not—yet most analyses are relatively primitive, very few studies try to interpret the data in depth, and much of the data are never used. Over the past decade modern surveillance systems have tried to address these issues, but they are still a long way from being resolved.

Specific sets of questions that had arisen during the September 1999 conference were proposed as starting points for each working group, and during the opening plenary session more questions were added, especially for the Data Use Group. These questions are listed under each working group section. The groups could change the questions or discard them altogether. What looked like a small task at the outset was actually a much larger undertaking, but ample time was allowed for contemplation and discussion.

Many data systems relevant to the factors that affect population health are generated *outside* of the public health field. When researchers focus only on data collected in the public health domain, they miss the mark because the real issue is integrating data sets on the environment, economy, labor market, income levels, and other areas. This lack of integration applies especially to developing countries that cannot always afford to duplicate with multiple health surveys. This issue was applicable for all of the working groups to consider. Furthermore, the working groups would have to think about the definitions of "surveillance" and "multiple surveys." If surveillance is defined as a continuous collection of data with time as a key variable, very few true surveillance systems around the world exist. Also, many systematic surveys and other data systems may need to be connected with surveillance systems (e.g., surveys related to the environment, transportation, housing), depending on the desired outcome. This issue is especially relevant for developing countries that might need to build on currently available information, but integration of systems is problematic even in Western countries.

Meeting participants discussed the need to consider not only behaviour but also the changing burden of disease—the epidemiologic transition that has occurred in almost all of the world's countries. Except in a few sub-Saharan African countries, chronic diseases are now the primary causes of disability, mortality, and morbidity. Because of this, there is a real concern with the determinants of those chronic diseases, and most researchers believe they should look at behavioural risk factors first. For example, many discussions focus on global surveillance for tobacco use, but broader discussions are needed about related issues pertaining to the environment, social determinants, and context of all the variables and whether these mean the same things in developing countries as in developed ones.

Indicators (e.g., heart disease, suicide, homicide) often appear to be independent in data analysis, but they are all likely inter-related in some way. Although it is not yet clear whether this inter-relationship could actually be formulated through advanced analysis, it is misleading to look at only one or two indicators. The ways in which factors are related may be quite subtle, however. Money invested in lung cancer prevention might also help prevent heart attacks, but it would be a non-reciprocal relationship: putting money into heart attack prevention would not necessarily prevent lung cancer. These relationships are not necessarily intuitive and investigators would have to look at the effect of one indicator on the rest of them in an interactive way, which would be extremely complicated. Translating research findings from the West to the developing world is even more difficult because completely different indicators are used. Even if one could develop indicators applicable across many countries, fully comprehending the interactions among the indicators in the varied cultural contexts would be difficult.

The opening discussion revealed the incredible diversity of issues that arise when even straightforward questions are posed. Of particular interest was the issue of surveillance as evidence and knowledge, and what these might be in different contexts. This issue may apply more to the developing world than to industrialised countries. Many people working in health promotion and public health believe that the basic surveillance strategy (i.e., highly measured, highly analytic scientific approach) is not leading to any understanding of the basic problems that populations face. To some extent, this problem may be related to the analysis, interpretation, and use of data. Knowledge is more than just data; therefore, surveillance ultimately must tap other dimensions beyond its database and include other types of knowledge.

Because they probably could not fully develop specific recommendations for codes of practice and best practice in the given time frame, the meeting participants instead tried to develop suggestions for minimal data sets. Even this task was difficult because the whole concept of variables of interest, of what *should* be included in surveillance systems, is a highly Western-derived and -based system. The participants needed to get beyond this ethno-centric approach to develop messages for surveillance system planners in other countries.

4. WORKING GROUPS

4.1. Analysis Group

4.1.1. Questions

A specific set of questions that had arisen during the September 1999 conference was proposed as a starting point for the Analysis Group. These were as follows:

- Which statistical models and analytic techniques do you most often use?
- How did you decide which set(s) of data to use?
- How did you decide which analytic methods to use? Do you think there were more appropriate techniques to use? If so, why were the more appropriate methods not used?
- How can we increase our knowledge base of analytic techniques?
- How can public health researchers and practitioners make the transition from using descriptive statistics to using more sophisticated analytic techniques?

4.1.2. Report

The Analysis Group reported that only one of several presentations to the group had specifically addressed the assigned questions, but a great deal of the discussion was indirectly related to them. The working group discussed models and analytic techniques, and various members of the group described procedures they were currently using. Discussion topics included logistic regression, regression techniques, time-series analysis, neural network analysis, non-linear dynamics, the nature of surveillance systems and data sets, change point analyses, and correspondence analyses.

The subject of "black boxes" and methods came up repeatedly. The group realised that analysis itself is a highly technical endeavor with many complications, and they discussed at length the extent to which, for people who are not analysts or statisticians, the analysis used for surveillance remains a black box, or an unknown entity, out of which something comes. This topic arose as a particularly important issue because many policy-makers and others making decisions based on data think they understand surveillance, or think they know what surveillance *should* do. This is the reason analysts continue to produce rather simple analyses. This concept caused questioning among the working group about why analytic techniques that have been around for at least a century or so continue to be used, and why possibly more appropriate techniques that have been developed in recent years (e.g., neural network analyses, non-linear analyses, change point analyses, correspondence analyses) have not entered into the accepted practice of public health analysis. Many of these cutting-edge analytic procedures are routinely used in fields outside of public health. The public health community continues to grind out gray literature of cross-tabulations and other reports, however.

The Analysis Group discussed whether analysis is for exploration or confirmation (i.e., whether the researchers are looking at data to explore new ideas and pull information that is not readily apparent out of the data, or they are just analysing data to confirm what is already known or suspected). Most data sets are probably used for confirmation— they are analysed to answer questions and expectations about patterns built in by others.

Regarding linear and non-linear analyses, much of the discussion kept coming back to *who* asks the questions and how that drives the type of analysis that is used. A great deal of debate centred on surveillance systems and what they measure, the kinds of variables and indicators they have, and the difference between "surveys" and "surveillance." The latter is an issue because most surveillance systems are built on a survey structure, but a survey is but a piece of a surveillance approach. The working group did not question this issue, but did discuss data acquisition and the fundamental structure of surveillance systems.

This group also discussed the role of measurement and its relationship to analysis. Analysis is highly affected by measurement issues, and most of the variables in surveillance systems have complicated underpinnings in terms of measurement. Some of the variables are purely dichotomous and quite simple, some are more like indicators, and some are really conceptual ideas put into numeric form. This complexity has many implications and, of course, almost all systems use a mixture of types of measures.

The Analysis Group also talked about surveillance systems in terms of combining with other systems, synthetic data, and synthetic estimates. If a surveillance system were designed to be as simple as possible and to collect a data stream that is stable over time, and if it were composed of basic fundamental components that changed so little that the system could monitor trends over time, how could researchers then develop a richness to that data that would allow more exploratory analyses and, therefore, more explanations? One approach might be to link those surveillance data to other data collection efforts and other indicators that are in some way "out there" synthetically. Yet even in countries with advanced and numerous surveillance systems, there are many difficulties and challenges in linking systems from different groups or agencies. For example, efforts have been made to link data on health services payment with data on risk factor surveillance. At first glance it seems an easy task, until the question arises of how and why data are acquired. The data acquisition issue made it very difficult to create synthetic data. In one agency data were collected to learn how medical bills were paid and how much particular procedures cost, not to answer epidemiologically inspired questions; these were essentially accounting data, so linking to surveillance or research data proved problematic.

The Analysis Group considered what researchers and surveillance practitioners should be doing today to conduct surveillance. The working group participants broadly discussed whether they should focus on methods, questions, interventions, policy making, or other areas. This discussion was followed by reflections on surveillance in general and early thoughts on recommendations that could be made. One issue that required attention was *who* is running surveillance systems *where*, particularly in the developing world. There was some debate about where such systems are based—in universities, a nation's central government, or global organisations. Typically, universities conduct surveys rather than surveillance, and using universities as a base for running surveillance systems is limited because such systems often are tied to individual professors or to projects with finite funding that might not be renewed. On the other hand, university staff have the necessary research and analytic skills that government personnel may not. Government agencies might be good at data acquisition (e.g., obtaining money to fund data collection efforts and putting together huge amounts of data), but universities are full of theoretical and social statisticians who can actually put the data to greater use if they have access to it. These are important questions for both the developed and developing worlds because people who help develop surveillance systems have to consider the skills each country's public health system will need to surveil and to analyse data, and where those skills should be placed (e.g., analysis may need to be done by universities, not by government agencies).

Ethics, which at first glance does not appear to have anything to do with analysis, generated an interesting and powerful discussion. This topic arose because many countries have national ethics committees or institutional review boards (e.g., the National Bioethics Advisory Commission in the United States) that look at ethical issues regarding data collection. Sometimes, to protect the subjects being interviewed or surveilled, the committee or board introduces conditions that lower the response rate of surveys or set limits on who can participate. Such restrictions may have a profound effect on surveillance and data analysis. A lower response rate is one thing, but putting conditions on who may respond can eliminate a lot of people. Also, fully informing subjects about the research (to meet requirements for "full informed consent") sometimes changes the way people interpret survey questions. Data analysis takes into account the quality and characteristics of the data, so efforts to protect subjects may result in unexpected findings.

The Analysis Group then confronted various approaches to analysis, the collection and analysis of continuously collected data, and how trends are identified. The working group debated the need to have (1) analytic techniques that look at data over time to best show trends, (2) many data points, and (3) a minimal gap between data collection points to provide truly continuous data. Having these advantages would give researchers many options for looking at various things. The working group also talked about using surveillance data to carry out impact analyses of public health phenomena—either those that occur naturally or purposive interventions. They discussed change point analysis, for example, with regard to how a continuous data stream could be examined to see where change *really* occurred temporally. The group agreed on the importance of examining surveillance data over a long period.

When data collected at many points over a period of time are plotted, the resulting charts usually show data points that appear "all over the chart." To data interpreters, these erratic and apparently unstable variable lines may be disconcerting and challenging. However, in a sense all analysis involves data reduction, which means removing much of the variance from a very complex data stream so the data can be more easily understood. Many methods exist for doing that, such as regression analyses, logistic approaches, and change point analyses. The Analysis Group extensively discussed truncating data and presenting them as reality to end users, and how people make decisions based on that "reality." Presenting such a model of reality is acceptable because it is all most people can deal with.

The working group went on to talk in depth about using surveillance data for evaluation and impact analysis. For example, if researchers have data collected over a long time, they can look at such things as how long an intervention really lasted or what the real dynamics of that intervention were. Only with surveillance-type data collected over time can they actually look at the dynamics, form, and shape of any intervention. The group discussed, for example, why cardiovascular heart disease community projects are often seen as failures and considered whether the approaches and models used to analyse such large-scale public health interventions may be inadequate. The group also discussed the underlying model in many analyses of surveillance and other types of data— the randomised, controlled clinical trial—and the inadequacy of that design for highly dynamic and non-linear data.

Neural networks and non-linear systems are increasingly common in the physical sciences, but their use in analysing surveillance-type data has been rare, even though they represent a potentially powerful analytic approach to complex data. Such approaches have arisen out of recent concerns about complex or seemingly chaotic data (especially when viewed over time), as with the U.S. Behavioral Risk Factor Surveillance System. Some surveillance efforts also include data of very mixed value, consistency, and reliability that were collected in very different ways. The neural network approach is not concerned with the nature and quality of the data, but fits the data into clusters and patterns that reveal a lot about each other and their relationships. This approach also examines the probability of members of the clusters moving from one cluster to another. Thus, neural network analysis is a potentially important approach for looking at global data when researchers want to know, for example, how Country X compares with Country Y.

4.1.3. Assembly Discussion

Some meeting participants in the assembly session questioned whether including qualitative data in a surveillance context is appropriate; others argued that many surveillance data *are* qualitative, perhaps not in the sense of in-depth personal interviews, but in their evaluation. When subjects are asked how they feel about their health and how many days they felt good in terms of their physical movement in the last month, that is a form of collecting qualitative data, and it is certainly included in surveillance systems already. Many of the analytic approaches currently being used appropriately recognise the distinction between qualitative and quantitative data, whereas historically analyses often treated qualitative data as if they were parametric.

The issue of social, institutional, and time costs was raised. In many developing countries, community and other public health workers spend much time conducting surveys on nutrition, respiratory diseases, diarrhoea, and other topics (e.g., the National Nutrition Survey). In Mexico, for example, at one point some community workers spent 2 days a week conducting different kinds of surveys rather than operating programmes. Such costs are also an issue for teachers who have to conduct surveys during school.

A related issue is returning the data. Ministries of Health may not have the capacity to analyse and interpret surveillance data, but certainly they are expected to apply the findings. Often the data are not returned to the people who carry out programmes in a way that can be used. Also, some surveys that might be helpful are never conducted because they are closely tied to illegal pursuits (e.g., drug use) and respondents are not likely to reveal their participation in such activities.

A fundamental problem with most surveys and surveillance systems, particularly ones conducted by governments, is getting the data used. One difficulty that interferes with the timely use of data is that some people believe that data have to be perfect— "the perfect gets in the way of the good." The mission of public health agencies is to improve people's health, not to produce perfect data. The meeting participants agreed that "good enough" data should be collected and analysed correctly, then must be returned to the people who are in a position to make public health decisions. Advances in technology and computer processing could look at data in a very timely fashion, but as long as people keep using current methods, they will continue to worry about having perfect cells. This perfectionism creates a major problem for end users.

Linking databases may be useful, but it is only tangentially an issue of analysis and more an issue of data acquisition and collection. Even so, such links are relevant in terms of people working in their own categorical areas and surveillance systems. A possible direction for the analytic agendae might be the development of, and attention to, methods that help bring together data from other sources to enhance the information already collected independently by each system. Such links would not cause changes in any particular surveillance system but would allow integration into other kinds of information.

Multi-level modeling and other valid statistical approaches to analysing complex data were explored. Although some analytic techniques are capable of comparing data collected from parallel sources and in different places, often it is difficult to get two or three groups together to plan a strategy for merging the pieces that might be related, even among congenial groups in the same agency. In most large countries, Ministries of Economy, Education, Labor, Interior, and Fisheries; Departments of Agriculture and Transportation; and other government agencies likely have economic data sets relevant to public health and could be linked, and the technology to link them is probably available. Easy mechanisms for linking the information (e.g., between agencies or institutions) generally do not exist, however. Universities often encounter this same problem.

Contextual analyses are very much en vogue in epidemiology. In a recent study examining income and equality, data from the U.S. Behavioral Risk Factor Surveillance System were easily used because they included state and county codes. These codes allowed researchers to run a multi-level model to look at inequalities between states, which many epidemiologists want to be able to do more easily. This simple analysis received a lot of recognition, so something more meaningful would likely be exceptionally well received. The entire assembly acknowledged that as more journal editors and publishers accept reports on these kinds of analyses, recognising that these are valid approaches to use, the situation will improve. But data collection agencies still need to think about how to integrate different data sets.

The "level" issue often goes back to the expectations of the data user. If users expect cross-tabulations as the output, they will be sorely disappointed because of the fundamental rules for statistical sampling. For example, if an accepted sampling strategy requires surveying 1,500 persons to make estimates for the United States, the same sampling strategy would require 1,500 to make estimates for the state of Georgia and 1,500 for a neighbourhood in Georgia. This requirement is problematic because millions of interviews cannot be conducted to allow every neighbourhood to be represented. Various data analysis solutions may be used, but when estimates from other kinds of analysis are used, programme planners and policy-makers are not satisfied. Instead, they want the same kind of local data that the state has. Perhaps the surveillance community needs to re-educate the end users of data systems about what analysis is and what can realistically be expected. Large surveillance systems simply cannot provide local data because they are not designed to do so, but they could provide local data if the view of what analysis is can be changed.

4.2. Interpretation Group

4.2.1. Questions

A specific set of questions that had arisen during the September 1999 conference was proposed as a starting point for the Interpretation Group. These were as follows:

- What is the relationship between theory and analysis?
- Why do we continuously make inferences without proper analysis?
- How do we know when to stop collecting data (how much data are enough)?
- How can we increase the sophistication of interpretation?

The working group debated these questions and altered them as they deemed appropriate (see Section 4.2.2.). Further, during the opening plenary session, the following topics were added:

- The increasing sophistication of analysis and the problem of making inferences without proper analysis. (This topic was also assigned to the Data Use Group.)
- How to treat the data and what types of theory are applicable.

4.2.2. Report

The Interpretation Group stayed very close to the original questions in its delibera-tions. After struggling in the beginning, the group was able to clarify the given issues and questions and to develop a first set of recommendations. Several factors affected the group's discussions. First, strong egos in the room encouraged and started dialogues, but sometimes dominated the discussions. Second, for participants whose native language was not English, the open discussion format posed difficulties. Some members had prob-lems following the native speakers, especially those who spoke quickly or whose mean-ing was unclear. Third, the U.S. Behavioral Risk Factor Surveillance System anchored this working group, which was helpful because the group could draw on the experience of the people representing that system, but it also tended to limit thinking about the use-fulness of other approaches to surveillance. The Interpretation Group constantly referred to the U.S. Behavioral Risk Factor Surveillance System, either implicitly or explicitly, even during discussions of general issues related to surveys, not surveillance systems.

Much of this working group's difficulties arose because it was asked to address spe-cific questions about interpretation, even though some general issues related to surveil-lance were not clear. The group attempted to address specific questions against a rather unspecific background. Why is surveillance needed? Should it provide information only on what is going on in a population, or should it be more explanatory and help answer questions about why things happen as well (e.g., why certain behaviour patterns occur and, even more complicated, how to change those behaviour patterns)? The Interpretation

Group did not actually try to answer these questions because they were outside the realm of these discussions, but they were overarching themes throughout the deliberations.

The role of theory in surveillance is another complex topic the Interpretation Group studied. The working group discussed what was meant by "theory" but decided not to try to define it. However, the group agreed what theory meant in the context of surveillance and considered whether the focus should be on existing surveillance systems, those that are planned, or some "ideal" system. This, too, was a permanently open question that contributed to the group's difficulty in answering more specific questions.

The Interpretation Group decided that the first question assigned to it, "What is the relationship between theory and analysis?", is more suited to a discussion on analysis than on interpretation. Therefore, the question was rephrased as "How does interpretation relate to theory?" The answers were general because a relationship can be specified by claiming that theory guides interpretation either implicitly or explicitly, although most of the time it is only implicitly. Some thinking or ideology lies behind every variable chosen, so there is always some theoretical consideration. The working group also considered the "ideal" relationship—that interpretation of data builds theory—which does occur on occasion. If they focused on evaluation and judgement, the working group could declare that evaluation reflects theory and principles of epidemiologic, social, and behavioural research and that judgement reflects theories of causation of disease (or determinants of health problems) and theories of policy development.

The Interpretation Group dismissed the second question assigned to it, "Why do we continuously make inferences without proper analysis?" and rewrote it as "What properties of surveillance data affect the value as evidence contributing to either causal explanation or development of health policy?" Sub-questions were added: "How frequently do we need to collect data?" and "How specific do we need to be in terms of sub-groups and target groups?" The answers depend on whether the goal of the surveillance is description, explanation, or evaluation; on the level of analysis; and on other factors. The resulting discussion reflected the view that a number of properties of surveillance data are relevant to interpretation, and in acknowledgement the working group chose to focus exclusively on the questions "How much data are enough?" and "How long should data be collected?" [These two questions derive from the third assigned question, "How do we know when to stop collecting data (how much data are enough)?"]

What properties of surveillance data, then, affect their value as evidence contributing to causal explanation or development of health policy? The following items are appropriate properties to consider, especially in the evaluation of the data: (1) study design (the appropriateness of the design to the question at hand, and the rigour of the plan with respect to the sampling and the design of observation or data collection), (2) conduct (the reliability of the data as actually collected, and the representativeness of actual data with respect to true underlying variation in the phenomenon measured over time, between places or populations, or by personal attribute), and (3) analysis (the appropriateness of the analysis to the question, design, and actual data as collected). In many cases people can obtain money for collecting information, but no money may be available for analysing it. The working group considered how to decide when to stop collecting data. The possible criteria include statistical power, resources and funding, and policy development. Perhaps data collection should end when there is nothing new revealed through the surveillance, but perhaps ongoing surveillance systems must be in place to reveal the unexpected.

Assigned question 4, "How can we increase the sophistication of interpretation?", was incorporated into a new question, "How can quality of interpretation be enhanced?" The following sub-items were added: (1) identify and illustrate relevant considerations about evidence for health policy, then disseminate, debate, and seek general concurrence, (2) articulate clearly the question(s) at issue, (3) apply the considerations to the evidence in the context of the specific question(s), and (4) recognise and evaluate the contributions of additional evidence, interests, and influences in relation to those from surveillance data. The first sub-item is a general task, and the remaining sub-items are approaches to specific issues.

In exploring the question "How can quality of interpretation be enhanced?", the Interpretation Group referred to two products of surveillance: causal inference and policy development. The literature contains extensive reports on causal inference, but not as many on policy development. Therefore, guidance is lacking for interpreting the results of surveillance or other data specifically as evidence contributing to development of health policy. In this area, then, is room for two broad types of activity. The first is to identify and illustrate relevant considerations about evidence for health policy, then to disseminate, debate, and seek general concurrence about those considerations. The word "consideration" was borrowed from a paper by A.B. Hill. What he proposed were criteria for judging causality based not on epidemiologic associations, but on considerations about the evidence that, more or less fulfilled, would add greater or lesser credence to the interpretation that an association reflects cause and effect rather than chance or other interpretations. The second activity was conceived as a three-step process that could improve the quality of interpretation: (1) articulate clearly the question at issue, (2) apply whatever considerations are adopted to the evidence in the context of the specific question at hand, and (3) recognise and evaluate the contributions of additional evidence from other sources, interests, and influences in relation to those from surveillance data.

In the context of social and behavioural surveillance data, interpretation encompasses two distinct functions: evaluation of the data, and judgements about the data. The Interpretation Group considered first the evaluation of the data with regard to their validity, generality, strengths, and limitations. For example, data might be considered quite reliable as a basis for inference and have acceptable breadth of coverage of the population, but be relatively recent. To incorporate more or less current concepts or constructs or to be of longer or shorter duration, and therefore evaluate the data as a part of interpretation, the working group had to address these aspects. Second, judgement about the implications of the data as evidence should be considered. One might consider a number of the uses of surveillance data, for example, to distinguish between surveillance data as evidence for causation of health problems or as evidence for development of health policy. In the view of this working group, interpretation means evaluation of the data and judgement about their implications for these kinds of applications.

After reflecting on their debates, the Interpretation Group suggested the following statements as a starting point for discussions at the September 2000 meeting for developing countries:

- Base interpretation on international comparison, not data per se. Also base interpretation on situations and experiences related to surveillance systems, especially previous experiences (before surveillance was implemented), experiences at the beginning of implementation, and—most of all—experiences with pitfalls that could be avoided if surveillance were undertaken in a different manner.

- Invest as much in interpretation as in data collection to avoid one of the motivators behind the Savannah meeting: a history of collecting a great deal of data at high cost but rarely interpreting or analysing those data. This advice reinforces the point that data analysis and interpretation are as important, and should be as great an effort, as data collection.
- Ensure interpretation (like surveillance) is an ongoing and long-term process.
- When interpreting data, establish local priorities derived from local analysis for different groups.
- Carefully interpret data collected at multiple points in time. Mistakes have been made when policies were developed based on data that did not actually reflect a trend because they were collected over too short a time period.
- Establish or take into account some broad ethical guidelines for interpretation.

4.2.3. Assembly Discussion

An inquiry was made about who the Interpretation Group believed should interpret data and at what point interpretation should occur. Should interpretation occur during the reporting, in the data system, or in the feedback loop? Is interpretation a scientific, political, or social process? The Interpretation Group reported that they discussed these issues and concluded that interpretation had to be inter-disciplinary and involve experts from different perspectives. "Experts" could include lay people because quite often, when it comes to individual health, the individual is the expert. But no matter who provides input, politicians and others will always try to interpret the results to their own advantage. Therefore, the working group decided to leave this issue to the Data Use Group but pointed out there is too little emphasis on interpretation: unless surveillance systems invest in the provision of sound interpretation, data use will not increase. A suggestion was made to form groups of interpretation experts with different backgrounds.

Strict interpretation of data does not help on two other questions: "What might be going on, or what might be the causes?" and "What do we need to do as a result of what these data, even minimal data, say?" During internal agency reviews and clearance, conjecture about causes is the first thing to be cut out of reports because such conclusions do not come from the data and because papers that include them would not be accepted by journal editors. Epidemiology is a science and it should be based on good principles, statistics, and design. Somewhere along the line, however, people will have to take a risk and say, "And this might be what is going on, which needs further validation or further study." Public health practitioners who are trying diligently to deliver programmes and make differences in a community need to know what the experts recommend based on the data.

Surveillance data alone cannot provide the basis for recommending action. But surveillance data along with additional survey data, which provide more context, could provide the basis for recommendations as well as reports relevant to applied practice. For example, if the question is whether an association reflects cause and effect, the writer can point to a number of widely recognised considerations to justify his or her speculation. There is room for development of a similar set of considerations or rationale to strengthen speculations about the practical meaning of the data for policy change or other actions.

Such considerations may help increase the acceptability and credibility of these aspects of interpretation in surveillance reports.

"Interpretation" does not mean just the causality; it could also mean the translation of the data and information towards policy and intervention development or public health practice. More data are collected than are interpreted or described, and a lot of useful data are under-used. A risk for developing countries is that data collection could become an end rather than a first step towards taking action. This happens everywhere—collected data are never interpreted and never put to use—and has gone on for decades. Having the data collected and interpreted by the same agency might improve the feedback loop and increase the likelihood that only data that would be interpreted and used are collected. When collected by one agency for interpretation by others, data may not be passed on by the surveillance staff or the interpreters may not know why the data were collected and therefore may not interpret them correctly. The use of interpreted data for the development of policies or interventions is still more art than science, and using interpreted data for such activities will depend on prior research and on local circumstances, culture, and people. Broad interpretation beyond the area in which the data have been collected may not be sensible because so much depends on local situations. An expert in one country may not do a good job of interpreting local data from another country. Therefore, using local expertise is essential.

The scientific community has to maintain credibility and take risks cautiously. Yet surveillance provides a data stream precisely for taking public health action, and it implies different kinds of interpretation and analysis at different stages. For example, different levels of interpretation are needed for infectious disease data (to allow for rapid assessment and action) and for chronic disease and behavioural data. The very basis for public health practice is looking at available data, interpreting what they mean, then making recommendations to people seeking the public health community's assistance in addressing the issue. Recommendations should be based on theory, previous public health experiences, and perhaps other data. To say that the scientific community's surveillance role ends with a written interpretation but no recommendations undermines the credibility of public health surveillance systems.

Researchers rarely have all the information they need to make a decision. At times, they have to make an educated guess based on the available data. The assembly considered such guessing to be an integration of scientific and practical approaches. Sometimes the recommendations will be wrong, but data interpreters must take risks because their success (in terms of increasing the use of data to improve the public health) and ultimately their ability to maintain funding may depend on how well they meet the needs of people who want consultation or information. If recommendations are not provided, people will look for them elsewhere.

Finally, the assembly addressed the problem of declining response rates. This decline is clearly evident in developed countries, and the literature indicates that response rates in developing countries are even worse. Interpretation obviously begins with the analysis of good data. Response rates certainly affect data interpretation and use. This issue would be covered in the September 2000 meeting with representatives of developing countries.

4.3. Data Use Group

4.3.1. Questions

A specific set of questions that had arisen during the September 1999 conference was proposed as a starting point for the Data Use Group. These were as follows:

- Who really uses the data to set policy (politicians, political staffers, advocates, programme planners, the media)?
- Are the data useful the way we usually present them now (i.e., descriptive statistics such as cross-tabulations)?
- Are descriptive statistics satisfactory? If not, what can analysts do to improve the usefulness of the data? If so, is using more sophisticated techniques a waste of time?
- How do some areas become "hot topics" (e.g., social capital, community planning)?
- Are decisions based on evidence or do other factors, such as political will or economics, have a stronger influence on policy decisions?
- How do we know when to stop collecting data (how much is enough)?

During the opening plenary session, the following ideas were added to the Data Use Group's list:

- How good or how perfect and pristine the data must be to be used, and for what purposes they should be used.
- Guidance and advice that can be given to developing countries about beginning surveillance when their sophistication and resources vary so widely.
- The increasing sophistication of analysis and the problem of making inferences without proper analysis. (This topic was also assigned to the Interpretation Group.)

4.3.2. Report

The Data Use Group discussed the original questions assigned to them and ultimately decided they were unconnected, too specific, and did not get to the heart of the matter. They believed the greater issues to be data applications and outcomes, not simply "data use." After a great deal of debate, the working group decided the most important question they could ask was, "Are we really concerned only about data use and applications, or are we concerned about the information and intelligence that can be generated from data?" An additional question was, "How can we maximise the use of the data?" The surveillance community's relationship with others associated with the data also appears to be overlooked. Surveillance is not a one-way process. Other people are involved, and their needs must be acknowledged and considered as well when planning surveillance systems. Other critical questions the group asked included, "How do we use data to make a difference?", "If other people (e.g., stakeholders) are involved, how do we involve them in our processes?", and "Do we all agree that the basic reason for generating information in the first place is to promote health, and should we focus on that outcome as part of our thinking in terms of the use of data?" Instead of planning to use data in isolation, perhaps the focus should be on stakeholders, outcomes, and the important end users of the data.

These deliberations led to a gestalt for the Data Use Group that energised their thinking and established a platform for the rest of their considerations. The working group agreed their fundamental task was to improve the use of information gathered in surveillance systems and concluded the key factor in doing so would be enhancing the relevance and quality of surveillance information for stakeholders (i.e., provide or use information that meets an important public health-related need). The working group also discussed the definitions of stakeholders and users, whether there are differences between stakeholders and users, and if so, what those differences are. Stakeholders were defined as the individuals, groups, partners, organisations, or institutions with interest in health surveillance. Users were defined as the groups, partners, organisations, or institutions who use the information product; users are a subset of stakeholders. These definitions were important in distinguishing between the models the Data Use Group developed.

Following the gestalt, relevance became the key issue. In their report at assembly, the working group discussed relevance and explained the basic model that relevance was part of, explained how everything fit into the prototype surveillance framework the group developed, and discussed why it is important to focus on the most important uses of data—and from that, on the users of data. The following sections detail these discussions.

4.3.2a. Relevance. Rather than answering the specific questions they had been given, the Data Use Group stepped back and developed a framework for answering these and other questions that might be generated. The working group viewed surveillance as a subsystem within a wider system designed to intervene between a population's current health status and its future improved health status. The group examined the notion that certain social determinants affect the relationship between current and future health status. More specifically, they were looking for interventions, policies, and programmes that focused on health, including movements towards democratic renewal and people's greater involvement in the process of shaping health. Surveillance is only one of the sub-systems that inform those interventions, policies, and programmes; therefore, the working group focused on that wider system. To illustrate why, one of their assigned questions was, "How do some areas become 'hot topics' (e.g., social capital, community planning)?" These hot topics could badly skew the work of surveillance systems by several possible mechanisms: the interaction between the different sub-systems or between the managers and producers of the surveillance systems, the researchers who wanted to use the data or were trying to shape the data that were collected, the communities (e.g., some U.S. communities exerted pressure to collect more information about toxic waste, which changed some of the surveillance systems), and politicians or others exerting political pressure. Essentially, those mechanisms exist at different levels of power in society. Depending on where one is in the surveillance sub-system, power from different parts of the other sub-systems would be more or less apparent. For example, at the level of national and global organisations, political pressure to do certain things could subsume community pressures.

In summary, some of the questions the working group was asked to address could be re-framed. The working group was able to answer questions more systematically by looking at them within the kind of framework they had developed. A more detailed discussion of the surveillance sub-system follows.

4.3.2b. The Surveillance Framework. This segment focuses on the relationships between data users (e.g., researchers, educators, policy-makers, advocacy groups). The Data Use Group examined how different people use the information, how they apply the information they already have in their research and evaluation, and how these activities affect health. One of the problems was the idea of presenting data to the users. The assigned question "Are the data useful the way we usually present them now (i.e., descriptive statistics such as cross-tabulations)?" implies that data are presented, users apply them, and the data application makes a difference. Starting with the idea of *presenting* data seems too simplistic, however, so the working group added the processes of *obtaining* information and *applying* it to the data system and described the whole as a "surveillance loop" that users should be part of from the beginning.

Looking back to the broader framework, including social determinants and their context as well as community and population health, the working group examined the relationship between these factors and tried to show how it determines the need for information of some sort. The group suggested that information needs to come out of the loop between context (e.g., structures, economics, politics, culture) and community and population health. They examined such things as why some people or groups (e.g., researchers, advocacy, public groups, interveners, public health practitioners, and front-line workers) would suddenly become data users, and what the need for information was to begin with.

Additionally, the possibility of partnerships between users and people who develop the data was discussed. People in charge of developing surveillance systems usually consider what is possible, feasible, and politically acceptable regarding data collection, but often overlook users' needs. The Data Use Group discussed the possibility of an "information data partnership" becoming part of the surveillance system process. It is important to know what the users intend to do with the data (e.g., use them to answer a research question, evaluate a programme, educate the public, increase awareness) when the information or data system is being shaped, and equally important for the users and developers to determine together what should be included in the system.

Although many databases already exist, the working group considered how the user–developer partnership might be involved in collecting new data that might be needed. One element of any data system is the kind of data that are collected (e.g., quantitative, qualitative, other). Relevance is embedded in all aspects of a system, but the issue of data quality should also be part of the data collection system. Then the working group deliberated about the kinds of products that come out of the system:

- Are they cross-tabulations, raw data, or information?
- Do they contain analysis?
- What do the products look like?
- Are the producers of the data just handing over the data?
- Is it information?
- What format is it in?
- How is it made relevant?
- How are people going to be able to use the data?

The working group explored how to move the data back to the users, whoever they might be. At this point the group considered including communications strategies, dissemination plans, diffusion approaches, and even capacity building in the surveillance system to help people *use* the data. If at the beginning of the collection process some of the stakeholders do not consider themselves potential users of the data, surveillance system planners should think about how to help the stakeholders discover ways the data might be useful. This is another way that surveillance can be made more relevant.

Finally, the Data Use Group discussed the ways users translate ideas and products from the surveillance system into practice; that is, how users apply them in their own context for research, evaluation, education, policy making, and other activities. The working group also considered what actually constitutes "use." Must the data be used within 1 week or within 5 years? How much of the data product has to be used? If someone untangled a minor variable and it was distorted in some way and that was used to make a point, did that count as use?

4.3.2c. Focusing on Uses and Users. A group member shared the story of a presentation he made in northern Canada using data indicating that the Inuit were less healthy than the non-native people of the region. The Inuits listened patiently, but at the end of the presentation an Inuit elder said, "But what did you ask about their spiritual health?" That was an important lesson because it revealed that the researchers had not talked to the users before the researchers audaciously informed the Inuit how healthy they were by someone else's measures. Belatedly discovering the importance of spiritual health to this population demonstrated that researchers should not talk *to* or *at* users at the end of a process; instead, they should find out what "health" means to the users before measures are developed.

Surveillance data are of no value whatsoever unless or until they are used. Silos full of data are available and millions and billions of dollars are spent on collecting data, but much less is spent on actually turning them into useful information (e.g., reports, fact sheets, workshops, seminars, web sites). One of the major aspects of data use—and one that receives less attention than it deserves—concerns the ways in which surveillance data can contribute to the broader public health effort. Many people talk about the difficulty of getting funding for surveillance, but the answer to getting money is to show the value of what would be received in return. Much of the value of using surveillance data comes from turning the data into information products that enhance public health and well-being and promote equity and social justice throughout the population.

The Data Use Group discussed other uses of surveillance data, especially how the data could be turned into products that would be used with *other* things to contribute to increased public information and awareness, better education and training of professionals, or enhanced community capacity. Surveillance information could help improve prevention, care, treatment, and support programmes and contribute to better evaluation of policies and programmes, particularly state-wide interventions. Surveillance data already are often used for advocacy (e.g., tobacco use) and have been used successfully to develop public policies that promote good health and health-friendly policies in other sectors (e.g., transportation, education, private industry). These numerous and widely varied private sector policies (e.g., regulations regarding smoking in the workplace or on airplanes) substantially affect public health as well.

In their considerations of uses and users of data, the Data Use Group focused largely on the use of surveillance information in what they called "empowerment of intermediaries"—the vast numbers of people and the inter-relationships between them in the field. Surveillance contributes to a broad spectrum of public health efforts and is imperative in many dimensions. Because surveillance does not stand alone but is part of a massive effort to improve the overall public health and well-being, the working group defined uses and users together in functional terms. "Users" are people who work to increase public information and awareness as part of any major national health strategy (e.g., cardiovascular health, HIV/AIDS, breast cancer prevention), especially in those components for educating and training health professionals. Users who have other objectives are excluded from this definition, because a national surveillance programme is not concerned with them other than to ensure that if and when they use information, they use it responsibly; however, this involves a different set of criteria.

4.3.2d. Maximising Data Use. The Data Use Group considered two key dimensions related to maximising data use: relevance and quality. To maximise data use, data relevance and data quality must be maximised as well. Relevance comes out of a close dialogue between users and stakeholders. The notion of who the users and stakeholders might be is not simplistic, nor are the relationships simple between the producers of information, people who analyse and interpret it, and people who use it. These relationships are based on relative power and control. Data are most relevant if they are needs oriented (e.g., provide relevance, meet a need, promote public interest or understanding, recognise diversity and differences in populations and communities, are informed by policy analysis) or action oriented (e.g., make a difference, lead to action, provide a clear link to applications).

High-quality data support feasible activities, are timely and responsive, and are presented in a way that is understandable and believable by the potential users. Other dimensions are the quality inherent in analysis, interpretation, and the collection process. Yet another aspect is the added value from integrating or linking data sources, in that the more progress surveillance programmes make in linking the data they collect, the better quality the data will be. This aspect depends, though, on the methods used. Surveillance programme staff can maximise their chance of having outputs that are needs oriented, action oriented, timely, responsive, understandable, and believable if they have a close relationship with users and stakeholders and if the process includes a feedback loop. The quality assurance process will be undermined if surveillance programmes do not receive feedback from the people who use the data.

4.3.3. Assembly Discussion

There are clear examples of applications of surveillance for knowledge development and research. For administrative reasons, however, people carrying out surveillance must be sensitive to the distinction between surveillance and research. Some surveillance workers view themselves, and are viewed by others, as researchers; their ability to generate support and enthusiasm for, interest in, and relevance of surveillance in *their* settings might be constrained if they cannot define their activities as research. Furthermore, their surveillance activities may be undertaken for research. With that in mind, the assembly considered whether the distinction is necessary and, if necessary in some settings, whether it is universal or a position that may be regarded as circumstantial or adaptable to different circumstances. The Data Use Group acknowledged that, in certain places, this dichotomy had been discussed and debated for years. The debate about defining surveillance as research is frequently idiosyncratic to a particular bureaucracy, and how and why surveillance is defined is primarily a function of administrative needs (e.g., to determine whether a formal human subjects review is required). To reflect that research can be an application of surveillance data, for the Savannah meeting the working group opted to allow flexibility in the new framework.

The framework developed by the Data Use Group focused not only on users and stakeholders, but also on "stockholders" (i.e., those in the business world). Because in most of the developing world monumental external debt accounts for more than 50% of national expenditures and 90% of health expenditures go towards staff salaries, surveillance planners must consider how they can deal with research and other issues that probably will not be funded. The World Bank is limited to interacting with only governments, and the Pan American Health Organization and the World Health Organization respond only to requests from governments (not to individual organisations such as universities or non-governmental organisations). Thus, should governments take the initiative in seeking their own pattern of financial aid or support, or explore other funding mechanisms for meeting very basic and standard needs such as surveillance of behavioural risk factors?

More dis-aggregated data and more data useful at the community level are needed for decision making, policy development, programme planning, and other activities. This need had been discussed at length in the working group session when the Data Use Group talked about capacity building—not just in terms of users, but also because more people at the local level want to have the knowledge, skills, and competencies to produce their own data and to have data dis-aggregated enough by local areas (e.g., school, community, neighbourhood) to be useful to them.

Many technical advisors to the World Bank and their client countries take the approach that collecting *some* data is an important first step. The surveillance does not have to be fancy, perfect, or expensive. This concept is beginning to take hold at the World Bank, as some money is now being used for surveillance, household surveys, and early steps towards behavioural risk factor surveillance. The bank wants to assist in building infra-structure and capacity, but it is also concerned with how countries plan to sustain what is built with loan money, and plans for sustaining programmes must be included in proposals. If a proposal for surveillance called for only 1 year of data collection, it would likely not be supported; the bank is more interested in how surveillance fits into a long-term strategy and sustainable system.

By using the framework the Data Use Group created, countries could more easily explain how surveillance would be related to the interests of different stakeholders and users. Partnerships are also an important way for countries to secure investments in surveillance or health, with local community groups as well as international organisations.

The assembly discussion then touched on the relationship between different priorities and different users. Meeting participants noted the huge difference between data and information. The process that links data to information is analysis plus interpretation, and both must be embedded in the surveillance system. A surveillance system should not be simply a way of producing data; furthermore, it may not be efficient, necessary, or ethical to give data to everyone who wants to use it. It may be more appropriate to specify levels of access in surveillance systems in which many people provide data and many people have access, but in different ways—some to raw data, some to data plus information, and so on.

Sometimes different interpretations of the same data are viewed as errors when they simply reflect different world views. Resolving those interpretations should not involve deciding who is right and who is wrong; instead, the different political perspectives or experiences should be considered. Thus, some meeting participants argued that data should be freely available and that everyone involved should have an open discussion about errors and differences in interpretation.

During the individual working group sessions, the Data Use Group had discussed not only how the products might differ by the kind of user, but also what the strategy for tailoring products might be. The words that kept arising in the working group discussions were "sell" or "market" the product, but group members tried to think of other types of strategies for diffusing or disseminating data. Therefore, they considered the need to tailor strategies for returning data as well as what the products should be for different users.

Some assembly participants contended that the intended use, not the data themselves, should be the driving force behind surveillance. If a surveillance system can achieve its intended uses, it is sufficient.

The Data Use Group's proposed framework listed 13 possible categories of data users. Assembly participants suggested that the use of surveillance systems could be improved by sub-dividing the list of possible users under two types of surveillance—burden and intervention. An assembly participant likened surveillance as burden to a video camera that runs 24 hours a day in a business establishment with the intent of catching thieves. Surveillance as intervention is more complicated. For example, a smoke detector plus a water sprinkler is a more intelligent system that, aside from describing what is going on, is linked to an action (intervention) triggered by the smoke (findings from surveillance).

The question of the user and access to data is an interesting one, but most surveillance systems produce raw data that are absolutely meaningless in and of themselves. The question then is, "*Who* filters the data to get them to *where*?" It is critical to determine which people should be close to the data and how close those people should be. The logic model proposed by the Data Use Group must account for the many analysts between the raw data and the people who look at a finished analysis and interpret it. Such a logic model presents a challenge for research to flesh out what is really involved in each of its components. The model should not show how a surveillance system *does* work, but how the system *should* work. Therefore, it may be appropriate to see how a case study would fit, or not fit, in the framework. Such case studies could show whether the framework works or how it should be altered; this aspect of surveillance had been left out of the proposal. On the other hand, developing countries are not necessarily looking for a prescription of what should be in a framework, but instead are looking to countries that have built surveillance systems over time to learn how it was done, what the connections were, and other processes. The Data Use Group had been extremely sensitive about the use of the word "Model," moving from big "M" to little "m" to "framework." The name is not as important as the idea of putting together the pieces somehow. The framework was created from a use perspective and focused on how to improve use, not just increase use of surveillance data. It could be used not only for interrogating systems, but also for asking different kinds of questions about surveillance so planners of surveillance systems can look more broadly at what it takes for use to occur. The Data Use Group did discuss case studies and concluded it would be a good topic for a larger group discussion.

People who carry out surveillance have not really been held accountable for surveillance expenditures. Every other aspect of the health system needs to show the impact of funding expenditures on public health; however, there is virtually no evaluation of surveillance whatsoever in terms of impacts and outcomes of the value for money spent. Generally, evaluation ends with the product (e.g., publication in a peer-reviewed journal) and does not examine impacts and effects. This is an area in dire need of research and development, especially if funding for such systems is to be sustained. Although there are some examples of evaluations that examined the impact of strategies for data dissemination and utilisation, these were accomplished by going directly to users and specifically assessing the list of desired impacts. Evaluation is important because, ultimately, the future of surveillance systems will be determined by whether other people need them.

An inquiry was made as to whether, during its discussions of social and behavioural surveillance (how, when, and how extensively to implement it), the Data Use Group presumed that vital registration surveillance of events in the population already existed and whether alternative strategies are possible for initiating surveillance in countries where little or no surveillance is taking place. Effective implementation of behavioural surveillance might be an incremental step towards establishing credibility and marshaling resources to support local surveillance with intensive surveillance of vital events in a sentinel area, and perhaps will be done later or even never on a nation-wide basis. The assembly agreed this topic should be discussed further at the September 2000 meeting.

Regarding existing and new data, potential data users should be consulted on the front end. Buy-in might be better, thereby increasing response rates. And because consultations are time-consuming and expensive, seed money needs to be considered.

5. CLOSING SESSION AND DEVELOPMENT OF RECOMMENDATIONS

The closing session of the Savannah meeting was spent discussing, both within and between the working groups, future directions for surveillance of risk factors in chronic disease and public health and the "single over-riding communications objectives" the meeting participants wanted to put forward at the September 2000 meeting "Capacity Building, Comparability, and Data Use in Behavioral Risk Factor Surveillance: Focus on Global Surveillance Issues" in Atlanta. Two types of recommendations could be made:

- General recommendations about the analysis, interpretation, and use of data. Thinking globally or generally, meeting participants as a whole could consider what their over-riding general messages should be.
- Specific or process recommendations about how to continue this work, not only for the Savannah meeting participants, but for other people who want to do the same. Future processes, for example, might include networking or forming targeted working groups to look at specific problems.

The meeting participants considered whether the recommendations should be presented as formal consensus recommendations or informally as the results of their deliberations that might be helpful at the September 2000 meeting. Some attendees suggested that although several salient issues need a great deal of emphasis, input should be solicited from representatives of developing countries before any formal recommendations are presented. A suggestion was put out that only process-oriented recommendations be made, because many participants did not feel comfortable offering general recommendations about surveillance. Further, because the September 2000 meeting would be about capacity building for the developing world, that meeting did not seem to be the right forum in which to deliver strict recommendations. Therefore, the meeting participants decided against making formal, prescriptive recommendations and opted instead to flesh out process recommendations. They also agreed to create this chapter describing their deliberations and emphasising the benefits and importance of surveillance to public health. The following recommendations were proposed in the closing session:

- The costs-to-benefits ratio of surveillance work should be emphasised with regard to the effect of surveillance on populations around the world. Surveillance data can be severely compromised by constraints imposed by ethics boards due to the boards' lack of understanding about surveillance activities.
- An analysis network should be established. [This could be paralleled in other areas as well (e.g., data interpretation and data use).] Such a network could have several components, such as a co-ordination, data collection, and information dissemination centre (at the Centers for Disease Control and Prevention or some other institution); a core of experts who would meet over time to more fully develop recommendations for and ideas about analysis; an expert advisory panel or networking group; and a network web site.
- Publications (e.g., executive summaries) should be translated into various languages to allow greater accessibility for international public health audiences.
- A specific networking strategy should be developed to help raise awareness of the benefits of surveillance activities, generate greater demand for them, and guide funding for surveillance programmes by international organisations (e.g., Pan American Health Organization, World Health Organization, World Bank). Presentations could be made to potential funders attending the September 2000 surveillance meeting, the Pan American Health Organization's Directive Council Meeting, and other meetings as they arise.
- Stakeholders should be included at the outset of any surveillance endeavor, rather than be treated as end users to whom a product will be sold.
- To increase international understanding of surveillance issues and to foster the development of surveillance and interpretation activities, influential organisations such as the Centers for Disease Control and Prevention, Pan American Health Organization, World Health Organization, and World Bank should facilitate interaction between some of the less powerful groups involved in data interpretation.
- Surveillance should always be conducted in the context of local situations. There is no need to rush to using sophisticated analysis and interpretation techniques. Analysis and interpretation should be conducted at a level that will be understood and used by local policy-makers and surveillance users.
- Members of the Data Use Group should continue to work together (via e-mail, conference calls, or other means) to flesh out the framework it had developed.

6. CONCLUSION

The June 2000 Savannah meeting "Analysis, Interpretation, and Use of Complex Social and Behavioral Surveillance Data: Looking Back in Order to Go Forward" was different, difficult, and complicated. Although the meeting format was a challenge for people who were used to participating in more structured gatherings, each of the working groups coalesced in its own way. Mostly "left-brain" people were assigned to the Analysis Group, and they were highly focused. The Interpretation Group was constructed with a slightly different rationale, and group members immediately started to de-construct all of the questions they were given, then re-arrange and re-interpret everything; after all, that is what interpretation is about. The Data Use Group included more "right-brain" people and they immediately bonded, assembled, widened everything, became less focused, and moved towards creating models. Each group grappled with similar questions that came out of various meetings, and even though they were not expected to answer all these questions, the working groups succeeded in sharply defining these areas related to surveillance.

The interpretation of data is one of the most difficult aspects of surveillance, as it is dependent on the type and quality of analyses and on the skills of the interpreter. It is probably the most challenging area of surveillance work because it is neither easily taught nor easily understood. Many standardised texts exist on how to properly collect data, and there are many volumes on analytic techniques. The ideas on how to interpret data and make data useful are more uncertain; one has to rely on experience and years of practice to understand the data. This depth of knowledge was reflected in the discussions in Savannah.

CHAPTER 13

MEGA COUNTRY HEALTH PROMOTION NETWORK SURVEILLANCE INITIATIVE

Strengthening the Capacity of the World's Most Populous Countries to Monitor Non-Communicable Disease Behavioural Risk Factors

Kathy A. Douglas, Gonghuan Yang, David V. McQueen, and Pekka Puska[*]

1. INTRODUCTION

Eleven countries in the world have a population at or exceeding 100 million: Bangladesh, Brazil, China, India, Indonesia, Japan, Mexico, Nigeria, Pakistan, Russia, and the United States. Together, these diverse countries represent over 60% of the world's population. In 1998, in response to critical trans-national health issues and the transition of global disease burden from communicable to non-communicable diseases (NCDs) (Murray and Lopez, 1996), the World Health Organization (WHO) formed a network among these countries to combine efforts towards improving world health. This network, called the Mega Country Health Promotion Network, was born out of recognition that these highly populated countries have the potential to impact world health by working together to strengthen infra-structure for tackling common global health issues.

The Mega Country Health Promotion Network provides a platform for representatives from the 11 countries to work together to strengthen the capacity within each of these countries for collecting NCD behavioural risk factor data in a systematic and sustainable manner. The Network also provides these countries with a strategic, collaborative approach for responding to global initiatives, such as the WHO 53rd World Health Assembly resolution on Prevention and Control of Noncommunicable Diseases (WHO, 2000) and the WHO stepwise approach to NCD risk factor surveillance (STEPS) (WHO, 2001). Additionally, the Network works closely with partners such as the U.S. Centers for Disease Control and Prevention (CDC) and the National Public Health Institute of

---
[*] Kathy A. Douglas and Pekka Puska, World Health Organization, CH-1211 Geneva, Switzerland; Gonghuan Yang, Chinese Academy of Medical Science, 100005 Beijing, People's Republic of China; David V. McQueen, Centers for Disease Control and Prevention, Atlanta, Georgia 30341-3717, USA.

Finland, who have long-standing experience conducting behavioural multi-risk factor surveillance systems such as the Behavioral Risk Factor Surveillance System (CDC, 1997, 2000a), the Youth Risk Behavioral Surveillance System (CDC, 2000b, 2001a), the FINBALT Health Monitor (Prättälä et al., 1999), and the Countrywide Integrated Non-communicable Disease Initiative Health Monitor (WHO Regional Office for Europe, 1996, 2001), which was launched in 2001.

The mission of the Mega Country Health Promotion Network is threefold: (1) strengthen the capacity of the Mega countries for global and national health promotion, (2) enhance the health of the populations in these 11 countries, and (3) support the health of the world's population beyond the Mega countries (WHO, 1999). To achieve this mission, goals were established to facilitate the development of health promotion strategies, share successful health promotion policies and programmes, increase inter-sectoral collaboration, and provide training to increase each country's capacity for health promotion. A specific surveillance goal is to improve the evidence base for NCD prevention and health promotion by strengthening the Mega countries' abilities to monitor behavioural risk factors.

The link between NCDs and risk behaviours is well documented and provides the rationale for establishing public health programmes and policies directed towards changing the prevalence of NCD risk behaviours in populations (Harris et al., 1997; CDC, 1999; International Union for Health Promotion and Education, 2000; Teutsch and Churchill, 2000). Although systematic collection of information valuable in controlling communicable diseases is common in the Mega countries, systematic collection of data pertinent to controlling NCDs—particularly behaviourally related factors—is virtually non-existent in most of these countries. By 1998, as the global patterns of disease continued to shift from communicable diseases to NCDs (WHO, 1996), the value of collecting NCD behavioural risk factor data became apparent and created the impetus for developing the surveillance component of the Mega Country Health Promotion Network.

2. EXPERIENCES CONDUCTING CONTINUOUS BEHAVIOURAL RISK FACTOR SURVEILLANCE SYSTEMS IN THE UNITED STATES AND CHINA

When the behavioural risk factor surveillance component of the Mega Country Health Promotion Network began, two Mega countries—the United States and China—had already implemented continuous surveillance systems. Their experiences are being considered during the development of similar systems in other Mega countries.

2.1. U.S. Behavioral Risk Factor Surveillance System

Since 1984, CDC has continuously monitored health risk behaviours associated with chronic diseases, injuries, and preventable infectious diseases. This monitoring system, called the Behavioral Risk Factor Surveillance System (BRFSS), provides cross-sectional data on health risk behaviours, preventive practises, and health conditions and covers a wide range of topics, including health status, access to health care, tobacco use, alcohol consumption, physical activity, fruit and vegetable consumption, awareness of hypertension, awareness of high cholesterol, disability, immunisation, asthma, diabetes, arthritis, prostate cancer screening, colorectal cancer screening, and human immuno-deficiency virus (CDC, 1997, 1998a). (See Chapter 5 for more information about the BRFSS.)

Through a monthly series of telephone interviews conducted among representative samples of the general population, all U.S. states and territories collect standardised data on behaviours that place adults (persons aged 18 years or older) at risk for chronic disease, injury, and infectious disease (CDC, 2000c). The BRFSS identifies demographic differences and trends in health risk behaviours, provides useful public health data for guiding the development of disease prevention and health promotion programmes and policies, and measures progress towards state and national health objectives. Because it is continuous, the BRFSS can integrate emergent and critical health issues into the system as they arise (CDC, 1997, 1998b).

The BRFSS did not start out as a national surveillance system. In the early 1980s, CDC and several states worked together to develop the system. By 1984 15 states participated in the BRFSS, and by 1990 the number of participating states had increased to 45. Today the system is used by all states, the District of Columbia, and three U.S. territories (CDC, 1998b).

2.2. China's Adaptation of the BRFSS

In 1995, when the China surveillance system was being planned, CDC had more than 10 years of experience implementing the BRFSS. The World Bank, the China Ministry of Health, and the Chinese Academy of Preventive Medicine asked CDC for technical consultation on modifying the BRFSS for application in China as a part of a World Bank disease prevention project (No. P003589) (World Bank, 1995). The BRFSS questionnaire was modified to better reflect behaviours closely linked to the leading causes of mortality and morbidity in China, and the methodology was changed from telephone-based interview to household-based, face-to-face interview.

In September 1995 a pilot test of the modified questionnaire and methodology was conducted in Shanghai, and in January 1996 the adapted BRFSS was implemented among representative samples from seven municipalities (Beijing, Chengdu, Liuzhou, Luoyang, Shanghai, Tianjin, and Weihai). The survey was initially conducted for 3 weeks of each month in the seven municipalities, but this frequency of data collection was found to be too demanding to maintain. In January 1998 the data collection period was changed to 3 weeks each quarter, with the annual sample size maintained. Since that time, data have been collected for a 3-week period each quarter.

2.3. Comparison of U.S. and China Surveillance Systems

Because the China surveillance system was based on the U.S. BRFSS, obviously the two surveillance systems are quite similar. Yet the BRFSS was modified to be appropriately responsive to the contextual and health needs of China. For example, China and the United States differ on how their health services are organised, how their communities are structured, and the key risk factors associated with the leading causes of NCD mortality and morbidity. Another important difference is the prevalence of telephone use in households. Especially at the time when the surveillance system was first established in China, the rate of telephone use was too low to support a telephone-based surveillance system. It is this difference in data collection methodology that constitutes the largest difference between the two continuous behavioural risk factor surveillance systems. Descriptions of the U.S. and China surveillance systems—including the questionnaires used, sampling plans, data collection, data management, data analysis and reporting, management of the surveillance systems, and quality assurance procedures—are summarised in Table 1.

2.4. Lessons Learned

The application of a modified version of the U.S. BRFSS in China has revealed a number of strengths about this surveillance system. First of all, this system maintains its scientific under-pinnings yet is adaptable enough to be useful in diverse contexts. A rigid, over-prescriptive surveillance approach that does not offer this kind of flexibility would certainly fail when applied to other settings because it would not be truly responsive to a country's specific surveillance needs. Therefore, an effective surveillance system is one that carefully balances science with the need to remain flexible for use in a wide range of contexts.

Second, this surveillance system effectively balances the different data collection needs at both the national and local levels. It does this by incorporating a standardised sub-set of questions into the questionnaire for comparison across locations, while ensuring that enough room remains on the questionnaire to add locally developed questions for addressing health problems of particular relevance to each participating location. Using common core questions for data comparison plus additional questions of local relevance provides valuable information to decision-makers at both the national and local levels.

Another strength is that this behavioural risk factor surveillance system uses an effective partnership model. Both China and the United States use a national agency to provide central over-sight and management to the data collection efforts, yet the participating states or municipalities have a voice in how the system is maintained and expanded over time. At the national level, a central, co-ordinating agency helps ensure that questions included in the questionnaire address the priority national health issues and that data are collected and analysed consistently across participating locations. At the local level, co-ordinators integrate questions into the questionnaire that are of high priority to that location, and they oversee the implementation of their local system to ensure quality control of the interviews and data collection process. Thus, participants at national and local levels collaborate to reap the benefits of the information produced through their systematic efforts.

Finally, this surveillance system builds capacity in several important ways. First, by empowering local professionals to maintain ownership of the local data, participation in the surveillance system allows these professionals to increase the capacity of their data collection skills and efforts to address priority health problems within the local context. Second, although the number of participating locations may be small when the surveillance system is first implemented, the capacity of the system is increased towards a national data collection system as other locations see the value of collecting this type of data and want to participate. Third, as the surveillance system provides information on trends and patterns of key risk factors across a number of important NCD health problems, the capacity to target specific problems in need of further research through point-in-time surveys can be identified.

Table 1. Summary of United States and China behavioural risk factor surveillance systems

	United States	China
	Questionnaire	
Sections	The questionnaire consists of three main sections: • core questionnaire, which consists of fixed, rotating, and emerging questions (topics included in the core questionnaire may shift from year to year), • optional modules, which states may decide to use, and • state-added questions that are a priority to each state.	The questionnaire consists of two main sections: • core questionnaire, which consists of 12 modules (listed below), and • municipality-added questions that are a priority to each municipality.
Topics	Topics vary from year to year. In the 2000 core questionnaire, topics included: • demographics, • health status, • access to health care, • tobacco use, • exercise, • fruit and vegetable consumption, • weight control, • care giving, • asthma, • diabetes, • women's health, and • human immuno-deficiency virus/acquired immuno-deficiency syndrome (HIV/AIDS).	Core topics are: • demographics, • health status, • health services, • tobacco use, • alcohol use, • hypertension awareness, • cholesterol awareness, • breast and cervical cancer screening, • injury control, • physical activity, • dietary behaviour, and • sexually transmitted infections, including HIV infection.

Table 1. (continued)

	United States	China
	Sampling Plan	
Sampling Design	Probability sampling, in which all households with telephones have an equal chance for inclusion in the state survey.	Probability sampling, in which all households within the municipality have an equal chance for inclusion in the municipality survey.
Sampling Frame	Although various sampling designs may be used, all states now use dis-proportionate stratified sampling in which: • lists of state telephone numbers are randomly generated, • telephone numbers are randomly selected from the lists, and • households are contacted and an adult aged 18 years or older within the household is randomly selected to participate in the survey.	Each municipality uses a three-stage cluster random sampling procedure in which: • neighborhoods are randomly selected from a census list of all municipal neighborhoods, • households are randomly selected from the neighborhoods, and • households are contacted and a family member aged 15 years or older within the household is randomly selected to participate in the survey.
Sample Size	During the first 5 years of the China surveillance system (1996–2000), the U.S. BRFSS was implemented in 50 states, the District of Columbia, and Puerto Rico. In 1996, the number of completed questionnaires in each state ranged from 1,096 to 4,482 (national sample size, 120,354). In 2000, the number of completed questionnaires in each state ranged from 1,716 to 8,149 (national sample size, 184,450).	During the first 5 years of data collection (1996–2000), the China BRFSS was implemented in seven municipalities (Beijing, Chengdu, Liuzhou, Luoyang, Shanghai, Tianjin, and Weihai). The sample size was doubled in 1996, during the start-up period of the surveillance system, to collect data from 400 adults each month in each municipality. For the second year of data collection (1997), 200 adults were surveyed each month in each municipality. Because the monthly schedule of data collection became too labour-intensive to maintain, beginning in 1998 data were collected from 600 adults each quarter in each municipality (sample size, 2,400 per year in each municipality).

Table 1. (continued)

	United States	China
Data Collection		
Methodology	Most states collect data using computer-assisted telephone interviewing (CATI). CATI is based on an inter-active computer programme that aids the interviewer in following correct questionnaire skip patterns and checks for valid data entry.	The seven municipalities collect data using household-based face-to-face interviews. Genders are matched between the interviewer and respondent to handle sensitive questions.
Frequency	In most states, telephone interviews are conducted during a 2-week period each month. Within each 2-week period, interviews are conducted 7 days a week during the daytime and evening.	From January 1996 through December 1997, municipalities collected data for 3 weeks each month. Since January 1998, interviews are conducted for 3 weeks every quarter. Within each 3-week period, interviews are conducted 7 days a week during the daytime and evening.
Data Management		
Questionnaire Review	The questionnaire is reviewed each year and decisions are made regarding which topics to include in the core and optional modules. The final questionnaire is programmed into the computer by the Centers for Disease Control and Prevention (CDC) to facilitate analysis.	The questionnaire is reviewed each year to ensure the questions continue to solicit accurate responses. The questionnaire is programmed into the computer by the Chinese Academy of Preventive Medicine (CAPM) to facilitate analysis.
Data Aggregation	As monthly data from states are received at CDC, the data are combined for each state across the months during a 1-year period.	As quarterly data from municipalities are received at CAPM, the data are combined for each participating municipality across the quarters during a 1-year period.

Table 1. (continued)

	United States	China
Data Analysis and Reporting		
Data Preparation	Data: • are adjusted for multiple sampling levels, • are edited for response errors and inconsistencies, • are weighted to reduce bias, and • provide representative prevalence estimates.	Data: • are adjusted for multiple sampling levels, • are edited for response errors and inconsistencies, • are weighted to reduce bias, and • provide representative prevalence estimates.
Analysis Software	Data are analysed using SAS and SUDAAN software.	Data are analysed using SAS and SUDAAN software.
Reports	Monthly quality control reports to ensure accurate data are produced by CDC and disseminated to states. CDC also prepares and disseminates state reports and annual summary prevalence reports to states.	Municipal reports and annual summary prevalence reports are prepared by CAPM and disseminated to the participating municipalities, Ministry of Health officials, and World Bank officials.
Surveillance System Management		
Managing Agency	Oversight and management of the surveillance system is housed at CDC, under the U.S. Department of Health and Human Services.	Oversight and management of the surveillance system is housed at CAPM, under the China Ministry of Health.
Central-Level Tasks	CDC maintains central-level responsibility by: • co-ordinating development of the annual questionnaire, • preparing documents that support the questionnaire and surveillance system process, • providing telephone samples, • editing monthly raw data from states, • weighting the data, • producing reports, and • providing quality assurance for system adherence at the state level.	CAPM maintains central-level responsibility by: • programming the questionnaire, • preparing documents that support the questionnaire and surveillance system process, • helping the municipalities generate samples, • editing quarterly raw data from municipalities, • weighting the data, • producing reports, and • providing quality assurance for system adherence at the municipal level.

Table 1. (continued)

	United States	China
	Surveillance System Management (continued)	
Local-Level Tasks	Surveillance co-ordinators maintain state-level responsibility by: • recruiting interviewers, • recruiting supervisors to ensure consistency in interview delivery, • managing the interviewing process in conjunction with telephone bank operations, • conducting the initial editing procedures on state data, • analysing the state data, • producing state reports, and • providing input into the future direction of the U.S. Behavioral Risk Factor Surveillance System	Surveillance co-ordinators maintain municipal-level responsibility by: • recruiting interviewers, • recruiting supervisors to ensure consistency in interview delivery, • managing the logistics of the household-based interviewing process, • analysing the municipal data, • producing municipal reports, and • providing input into the future direction of the China behavioural risk factor surveillance system.
	Quality Assurance	
Protocol Requirements	Systematic, unobtrusive electronic monitoring is a routine and integral part of monthly survey procedures for all interviewers.	Monitoring with tape recorders is a routine and integral part of quarterly survey procedures for all interviewers.
Interview Verification	A 5% random sample of completed interviews is called back each month to verify that interviews were properly conducted and that the responses were correctly coded. These verification callbacks require less than 10 minutes to complete.	A supervisor or the municipal co-ordinator reviews at least one interview per interviewer during each annual interview period. Feedback is given to the interviewer to improve performance.

2.5. Issues for Further Consideration

The application of a behavioural risk factor surveillance system in both the United States and China has highlighted several issues that need further consideration as other countries prepare to collect systematic NCD behavioural risk factor data. These issues pertain to methodology, response rates, and using surveillance data to evaluate and support interventions.

2.5.1. Methodology

The surveillance methodologies initially used in the United States and China reflected appropriate choices for implementing the surveillance systems in these countries at the time (Frey, 1983; Fowler, 1988), and the advantages of each method within its cultural context outweighed the disadvantages. Even so, problems arose. Early in the implementation of the modified BRFSS in China, it became clear that using a household-based, face-to-face methodology to collect the required number of interviews was not tenable within 2 weeks each month, the time frame used by most states in the United States to conduct telephone-based interviews. Although the data collection period of 3 weeks per month was attempted in China, it was soon apparent it would be impossible to maintain this pace over a long period of time. Continuous household-based, face-to-face interviews are much more labour-intensive than telephone interviews, especially when follow-up interview attempts are factored in to obtain completed interviews with the selected respondents. Yet the household-based, face-to-face interview is at present the most practical approach to population-based data collection for many countries, and the frequency of data collection must be carefully considered to strike a balance between costs and generating sufficient data for trend analysis.

A problem also exists with the telephone-based method used in the United States. Because of changes in telephone technology, the explosion of companies using telephones to sell products and services, and the influx of mobile telephone use during the past few years, telephone habits have shifted dramatically in the United States. Future U.S. surveillance efforts might be hampered by these changes, including the use of answering machines and devices to display the caller's telephone number ("caller ID"), which relieves individuals from feeling compelled to answer the telephone, especially if the number identified is not recognised. Even in households not equipped with the latest telephone technological advancements, household members may simply refuse to answer their telephone to avoid telemarketers. Further, the proliferation of mobile telephones now means that a person can be reached while in a car, in a work environment, or in other settings inappropriate for conducting the interview. Moreover, because the BRFSS is based on the premise that the telephone is tied to respondents in households, the proliferation of mobile telephones creates a whole new set of challenges for sampling design. State-based sampling procedures will become even further complicated because eventually people may be able to take their telephone number with them when they move across states.

Maintaining telephones as a viable interview method will require exploring ways to keep up with, and adequately address, these shifting patterns in telephone use. While difficulties in telephone and face-to-face interview methodologies are a normal part of data collection challenges, as more countries develop and expand surveillance systems, technology advancements within the context of each country will need to be carefully considered.

2.5.2. Response Rates

In the United States, the percentage of persons who participate in and complete the surveillance interview has decreased, from 84.1% in 1991 to 61.7% in 2000 (CDC, 1998c, 2000d, 2001b) (Figure 1). The trend is likely due, in great part, to the telephone technology advancements and shifting use patterns just described. In contrast, the response rates for the seven participating municipalities in China were stable the first 5 years of implementation, ranging from 77.5% in 1996 to 81.8% in 2000 (Chinese Academy of Preventive Medicine, 1997–2001).

The ability to maintain adequate response rates in the future may be affected by the complex and inter-related societal issues that contribute to busy lives and the competing demands people are increasingly experiencing around the world. Issues that may affect future surveillance participation rates include (1) improvements in and increased access to the computer internet, where information is exchanged around the world at ever-increasing rates, influencing local norms and perceptions about whether to participate in interviews, (2) increased urbanisation (where lifestyles are affected by urban sprawl and by transportation design, mode, and availability) and work demands (including the

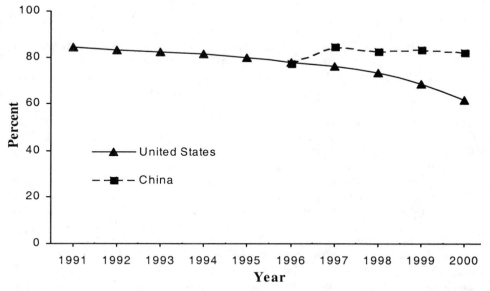

Figure 1. Estimated response rates for the United States and China behavioural risk factor surveillance systems. U.S. estimates are based on median upper bound response rates of the participating states (CDC, 1998c, 2000d, and 2001b), and China estimates are based on averages of the seven participating municipalities (Chinese Academy of Preventive Medicine, 1997–2001).

competition for limited positions or resources) that contribute to an overall decrease in "free time" that participants are available and willing to use to participate in interviews, (3) housing quality factors (where lifestyles are affected by safety and crowding) that make it difficult to gain access to questionnaire respondents or conduct confidential interviews (United Nations Research Institute for Social Development, 1995), and (4) increased solicitation of individuals to take part in all kinds of surveys, especially for commercial marketing, which may encourage persons to ignore any requests for interviews, including those for behavioural risk factor surveillance. As the world continues to move at a faster and faster pace, steps will need to be taken to help ensure adequate participation in important surveillance activities.

2.5.3. Using Surveillance Data to Evaluate and Support Interventions

Traditionally, surveillance data have not been used to their full potential in evaluating the effectiveness of health interventions, perhaps because the work of staff involved with surveillance activities is typically different from, and not well connected to, the work of staff who design, implement, and evaluate interventions. Indeed, in many countries survey research and intervention planning are considered completely different functions. Combined with under-staffing and budgetary restrictions, it may not be possible to include a staff person with evaluation expertise on the surveillance team. And with attention focused primarily on keeping up with the various tasks essential to maintaining an effective surveillance system, little or no time may be available to forge a better link with intervention planning and evaluation.

The lack of integration between surveillance and intervention programmatic areas accentuates the problems associated with the timing of data collection. For example, if the surveillance data are not produced during a time period useful for intervention planning, the value of such data may be questioned. But without data to target the development of programmes or evaluate the impact of such programmes on health trends, intervention planners often cannot demonstrate programme progress or effectiveness. Conducting continuous surveillance systems can help alleviate this problem by offering timely data. The chief stumbling block remains the lack of integrated public health programmes that strategically incorporate surveillance data as a part of the ongoing planning, implementation, and evaluation procedures. This issue is part of a broader problem of public health infra-structure.

Despite this lack of integration, the United States and China have effectively used surveillance data to evaluate some interventions. In the late 1980s, for example, U.S. health officials were concerned that women aged 40 years or older were not getting mammograms to screen for breast cancer (CDC, 1998b). The 1987 BRFSS results verified this concern, showing that only 44% of women this age had received a mammogram to screen for breast cancer that year. Public health departments throughout the United States used this information to justify developing educational programmes to inform women about the need for mammograms. By 1995, 82% of women surveyed had received mammograms to screen for cancer, demonstrating that the educational programmes had worked.

In China, various intervention strategies used to increase rates of blood pressure measurement among people aged 35 years or older were compared among the seven municipalities collecting behavioural risk factor data (Yang, in press). Because some doctors did not consistently assess blood pressure as a part of their routine medical work when they first saw a patient, one strategy was to introduce a municipal regulation requiring all doctors to do so. Other interventions included developing community-based health education programmes on the benefits of getting blood pressure checked to avoid diseases related to hypertension, such as stroke. The surveillance data revealed that the number of persons aged 35 years or older who had their blood pressure tested increased significantly in the municipality that had all intervention strategies in place.

Much of the focus to date has been on using behavioural risk factor surveillance data to target the development of programmes and policies; using such data to evaluate intervention effectiveness needs to be encouraged. Creating better links between surveillance data and intervention planning and evaluation will gain importance as surveillance experts strive for ways to communicate their data more effectively. Making such data readily available and publicising results in a way easily understood by target audiences will be powerful tools in health interventions.

3. MEGA COUNTRY HEALTH PROMOTION NETWORK SURVEILLANCE GOALS

The purpose of the Mega country surveillance initiative is to enable the most heavily populated countries in the world to strengthen their capacities to conduct behavioural risk factor surveillance by using integrated, systematic approaches that will support the sustainability of NCD data collection over time. As the Mega countries work towards national data collection, they can benefit from the U.S. and China experiences in continuous surveillance as well as from surveillance experiences of countries involved in other WHO initiatives, such as the Countrywide Integrated Noncommunicable Disease Initiative programme. Through the application of systematic surveillance approaches that move beyond the implementation of single point-in-time surveys, the Mega countries will be in a position to more effectively address the critical NCD health needs of their populations. By responding to their own national NCD data collection needs, these countries also will be able to significantly contribute to global data collection efforts.

3.1. Moving from Surveys to Surveillance

The characteristics of risk factor surveys differ from those of risk factor surveillance (Table 2). While both surveys and surveillance provide important information for addressing the NCD prevention agenda, they represent different strategies and should not be confused. Characteristics associated with surveillance include providing public health information on factors that compromise health, collecting this information across a range of critical health problems so that trends and patterns can be examined over time, and examining these health trends and patterns in the general population so that programmes and policies can be developed to help people live healthier lives. Collecting information systematically over time requires dedicated infra-structure for this activity. With infra-structure in place, procedures and processes can be clearly defined to ensure that scientific integrity is maintained in the system over time, opportunities for making improvements to the system can be acted upon, and risk factors associated with emerging health problems can be easily incorporated into the system to be addressed

Table 2. Survey and surveillance characteristics

Surveys	Surveillance
Research driven	Public health driven
Theory based	Atheoretical; helps develop theory
Goes into depth within (categorical) health issues	Looks at broad trends and patterns across multiple health issues
Single point in time	Continuous (time is a variable)
Results point to the way things were	Results point to the way things are changing
Static design: new surveys are developed to address emerging health issues	Dynamic design: emerging health issues are integrated into the system fairly quickly
Inefficient: re-starting and re-training are required; does not generate capacity building	Efficient: ongoing system generates efficiencies with start-up, training, and capacity building

in a timely manner. Surveillance is a dynamic tool for collecting critical and current health information.

Surveys, on the other hand, often involve single data collection periods for examining risk factors in one or more health topic areas. Historically, health surveys were developed as research tools to help explain relationships among risk factors. Because of their depth, surveys provide very good detailed information about these relationships. However, they are often unable to include questions across a broad range of health topics typically included in surveillance systems. Because surveys are conducted at a single point in time, the findings reflect relationships among risk factors only at the point in time when data were collected. Surveys also are static; they are terminated when data have been collected and results have been disseminated. Consequently, efficiencies are lost with regard to staffing, establishing systematic procedures for data collection, integrating procedural improvements, and building capacity for long-term data collection.

While both surveys and surveillance are useful tools, surveillance provides a snapshot of how risk factors occur over time, illuminating the trends and patterns of critical health behaviours as they occur. A surveillance system also offers the possibility of incorporating point-in-time surveys into the ongoing data collection approach.

3.2. Addressing Critical Population-Based NCD Health Needs

Most of the Mega countries do not have surveillance systems in place to collect NCD behavioural risk factor data on their adult populations. With current realities and constraints, some countries have indicated it would be less expensive and easier to conduct surveillance among adults by using a settings-based approach (e.g., data collection at work sites) rather than a population-based approach. Both approaches are viable, but the trade-off regarding population coverage or generalisability and expense is clear: a population-based approach is more expensive than a settings-based approach, but it is also more equitable and useful because data are collected to reflect the larger, general population rather than a specific or unique sub-group.

Because many countries currently collect blood sample information in hospital or clinic settings, a common recommendation made by medical researchers is to incorporate NCD risk factors into the hospital-based data collection system. The information obtained from this approach can certainly be used, particularly in a treatment and curative sense, but it does not offer a means to provide extensive or timely information for the broader public health NCD prevention agenda. Rather, this approach focuses primarily on collecting morbidity indicators among those individuals who have access to health care at the point when treatment is being sought. It is only through collecting data among adults in the broader community that useful information on preventable risk factors can be obtained for individuals across all economic levels, including those who cannot afford health care.

Population-based surveillance among adults in the broader community requires a commitment of time, resources, and effort. The information yielded, however, will be better able to address the public health needs of the entire population. Further, incorporating the collection of multiple risk factors across a number of important NCD health problems in the same surveillance questionnaire, rather than developing separate questionnaires to address each specific health problem, is an efficient way to gather NCD health information, especially in countries where little NCD risk factor information is yet available. Using a multi-risk factor, population-based approach is a very good way to demonstrate "evidence" of need across a number of health problems relatively quickly so that disease prevention and health promotion programmes and policies can be developed.

3.3. Contributing to Global NCD Data Collection

WHO developed STEPS as a framework for global NCD surveillance (WHO, 2001). STEPS, described in Chapter 3, recommends that countries collect data on those risk factors that contribute most to the global NCD burden. This approach incorporates three dimensions: one for different types of risk factor assessment (self-report behavioural risk factor measures, physical measures, and blood samples), one for the types of questions asked on each topic contained in the framework (core, expanded, and optional questions), and one for the NCD health topics included in the framework (self-report behavioural risk factor topics included in the framework: tobacco and alcohol use, physical inactivity, and nutrition; physical measures included in the framework: blood pressure, height, weight, and waist circumference; and blood samples included in the framework: blood glucose and cholesterol). The surveillance component of the Mega Country Health Promotion Network supports the collection of core questions contained in the STEPS framework.

4. SURVEILLANCE CHALLENGES IN THE MEGA COUNTRIES

Mega countries will have to overcome a number of challenges to implement effective behavioural risk factor surveillance systems. First of all, Mega countries have large, and sometimes complicated and cumbersome, bureaucracies to negotiate in order to implement national initiatives and reach their populations. Although most Mega countries will begin their behavioural risk factor surveillance systems in limited, geographically defined areas, the long-term goal is to build towards nationwide coverage. The U.S.

BRFSS provides an example of how one surveillance system expanded over time, beginning as state-based point-in-time surveys, shifting approximately 3 years later to a surveillance system in which a small number of states participated, then over the course of the next 10 years expanding the yearly cycle of data collection to more and more states until all states and territories participate in the system today. Beginning with only a limited number of participating locations can help ensure that data are analysed and communicated effectively, which in turn helps to demonstrate the value of the information collected, generate additional resources, and motivate other locations to participate in the surveillance system.

Second, adequate surveillance infra-structure must be built up, then maintained. Many of the Mega countries currently face a large disease burden from both NCDs and communicable diseases, without a national health budget to address both arenas adequately. In the midst of the sometimes intense competition for resources, establishing a long-term surveillance infra-structure to address NCD risk factors might seem unattainable and would likely need to be developed in stages, as described in Section 3.3. Combining this "staged" approach for building infra-structure with other strategies, such as working with partners from the communicable disease arena and learning to communicate information more effectively with various groups of data users, may translate into increased funding and support to maintain and expand the surveillance system over time. For example, questions concerning risks associated with communicable disease control, such as vaccinations or sexually transmitted infections (including human immunodeficiency virus), can be incorporated into a questionnaire to help provide valuable prevention information and link the communicable and NCD health arenas together. Further, working more closely with communication specialists or public relations professionals can help transform surveillance results from scientific statements into meaningful information that comes alive for decision-makers, politicians, citizens, and others who respond in different ways to the data.

Another challenge concerns balancing local, national, regional, and global data collection needs. As the Mega countries move forward to develop and expand surveillance systems to address their own national priorities, they also will contribute to global data collection efforts, such as the WHO STEPS approach (WHO, 2001), which necessitates more equivalence and consistency across countries and across time. Issues that affect the consistency of global data collection efforts include the standardisation of measures and respondent age groups and the time frame for data collection. As critical NCD determinants take on increasingly global features, nations will increasingly overlap in the type of information needed and the need for data at the global level will intensify. Although international collaboration helps individual countries strengthen their own surveillance efforts and offers the possibility of comparing results globally, the collection of comparable data among nations ultimately rests on convincing individual countries that such data relate highly to national public health interests.

5. CONCLUSION

Surveillance is an essential under-pinning for NCD prevention and health promotion efforts. It is "the tool that provides the necessary data to define the disease burden, identify populations at highest risk, determine the prevalence of health risks, and guide and evaluate disease prevention efforts" (CDC, 2000a, p. 1) at national and local levels. Behavioural risk factor surveillance is essential in NCD prevention because practical prevention and health promotion work are based on a few behaviours that greatly impact disease risks and quality of life. And because behaviours can be modified, "promoting positive health behavior choices, through education and through community policies and practices, is essential to reducing" (CDC, 1999, p. vii) the overall NCD burden. Therefore, behavioural surveillance should be considered a cornerstone of effective NCD programme and policy planning.

Focusing on health risk behaviours provides a concrete and common pathway for the 11 Mega countries to work together towards strengthening their own NCD prevention and health promotion programmes as well as contributing to world health. This is a long-term commitment to building capacity within the most populated countries of the world to establish and maintain population-based surveillance of NCD risk factors. Data collected from these surveillance systems can then be used to develop and implement targeted NCD prevention and health promotion policies and programmes within each of these countries. Because of the projected burden due to NCDs, mental health disability, and injury by the year 2020 (Murray and Lopez, 1996), capacity must be built now to provide these essential data for controlling the NCD epidemic. Working together, the Mega countries can share information and learn from each other's surveillance experiences to effectively address this great need.

6. REFERENCES

Centers for Disease Control and Prevention, 1997, *Health Risks in America: Gaining Insight from the Behavioral Risk Factor Surveillance System, Revised Edition*, CDC, Atlanta.

Centers for Disease Control and Prevention, 1998a, *Behavioral Risk Factor Surveillance System User's Guide*, CDC, Atlanta (October 3, 2001); http://www.cdc.gov/nccdphp/brfss/pdf/userguide.pdf.

Centers for Disease Control and Prevention, 1998b, *BRFSS Overview*, CDC, Atlanta (October 3, 2001); http://www.cdc.gov/nccdphp/brfss.

Centers for Disease Control and Prevention, 1998c, *1995 BRFSS Summary Quality Control Report, Revised*, CDC, Atlanta.

Centers for Disease Control and Prevention, 1999, *Chronic Diseases and Their Risk Factors: The Nation's Leading Causes of Death*, CDC, Atlanta (October 3, 2001); http://www.cdc.gov/nccdphp/statbook/statbook.htm.

Centers for Disease Control and Prevention, 2000a, *Tracking Major Health Risks in America: The Behavioral Risk Factor Surveillance System At-A-Glance*, CDC, Atlanta (October 3, 2001); http://www.cdc.gov/nccdphp/brfss/at-a-gl-2000.htm.

Centers for Disease Control and Prevention, 2000b, Youth Risk Behavior Surveillance—United States, 1999, *Morb Mortal Wkly Rep CDC Surv Summ.* 49(SS-5):1–96.

Centers for Disease Control and Prevention, 2000c, *1999 BRFSS Summary Prevalence Report*, CDC, Atlanta (October 3, 2001); http://www.cdc.gov/nccdphp/brfss/pdf/99prvrpt.pdf.

Centers for Disease Control and Prevention, 2000d, *1999 BRFSS Summary Quality Control Report*, CDC, Atlanta.

Centers for Disease Control and Prevention, 2001a, *Assessing Health Risk Behaviors Among Young People: Youth Risk Behavior Surveillance System At-A-Glance*, CDC, Atlanta (October 3, 2001); http://www.cdc.gov/nccdphp/dash/yrbs/yrbsaag.htm.

Centers for Disease Control and Prevention, 2001b, *2000 BRFSS Summary Data Quality Report, Revised*, CDC, Atlanta.

Chinese Academy of Preventive Medicine, 1997–2001, *Behavioral Risk Factor Surveillance System Annual Reports*, CAPM, Beijing.

Fowler, F. J. Jr., 1988, *Survey Research Methods*, Sage Publications, Newbury Park, CA.

Frey, J. H., 1983, *Survey Research by Telephone*, Sage Publications, Beverly Hills, CA.

Harris, J. R., McQueen, D. V., and Koplan, J. P., 1997, Chronic disease control, in: *Principles of Public Health Practice*, D. Scutchfield and C. W. Keck, eds., Delmar Publishers, Albany, NY, pp. 216–224.

International Union for Health Promotion and Education, 2000, *The Evidence of Health Promotion Effectiveness: Shaping Public Health in a New Europe*, the Union, Brussels.

Murray, C. J., and Lopez, A. D., eds., 1996, *Global Burden of Disease and Injury Series, Volume 1: The Global Burden of Disease. A Comprehensive Assessment of Mortality and Disability from Diseases, Injuries, and Risk Factors in 1990 and Projected to 2020*, World Health Organization, Geneva.

Prättälä, R., Helasoja, V., Kasmel, A., et al., 1999, *FINBALT Health Monitor: Feasibility of a Collaborative System for Monitoring Health Behaviour in Finland and the Baltic Countries*, National Public Health Institute, Helsinki (October 1999); http://www.ktl.fi/eteo/finbalt/index.html.

Teutsch, S. M., and Churchill, R. E., eds., 2000, *Principles and Practice of Public Health Surveillance, Second Edition*, Oxford University Press, New York.

United Nations Research Institute for Social Development, 1995, *States of Disarray: The Social Effects of Globalization. A UNRISD Report for the World Summit for Social Development*, UNRISD, Geneva.

World Bank, 1995, *Staff Appraisal Report: China Disease Prevention Project*, World Bank, Washington, DC (Report No. 14912-CHA).

World Health Organization, 1996, *Noncommunicable Diseases: WHO Experts Warn Against Inadequate Prevention, Particularly in Developing Countries*, WHO, Geneva (WHO Fact Sheet No. 106).

World Health Organization, 1999, *WHO Mega Country Health Promotion Network: The Most Populous Countries Working Together for a Healthier World*, WHO, Geneva.

World Health Organization, 2000, *Global Strategy for the Prevention and Control of Noncommunicable Diseases. Report by the Director-General*, Fifty-third World Health Assembly, WHO, Geneva (Provisional Agenda Item 2.11; A53/14).

World Health Organization, 2001, *Summary: Surveillance of Risk Factors for Noncommunicable Diseases: The WHO STEPwise Approach*, WHO, Geneva.

World Health Organization Regional Office for Europe, 1996, *Countrywide Integrated Noncommunicable Diseases Intervention (CINDI) Programme: Protocol and Guidelines*, WHO, Copenhagen.

World Health Organization Regional Office for Europe, 2001, *CINDI Health Monitor: Proposal for Practical Guidelines*, National Public Health Institute, Helsinki.

Yang, G., in press, Application of BRFS data in World Bank Project, *Chin Prev Control Chron Non-Commun Dis*.

CHAPTER 14

EPIDEMIOLOGICAL SURVEILLANCE SYSTEM IN LATIN AMERICA AND THE CARIBBEAN
Perspectives, Challenges, and Solutions

Ligia de Salazar[*]

1. INTRODUCTION

Summarising the experience of epidemiological surveillance in Latin America and the Caribbean in a brief chapter is not an easy task, given the diversity of countries that make up the region, the scarcity of literature addressing how surveillance systems operate, and the unknown effectiveness or impact of surveillance on controlling or eradicating risks and harmful factors under surveillance. Despite the challenge of discussing this topic, it is necessary to undertake it because of the growing importance of and need for surveillance in Latin America.

This chapter has two purposes: first, to point out the strengths and the more salient limitations of efforts deployed in the region to implement epidemiological surveillance systems; second, to propose some short- and medium-term answers to help create a culture that re-inforces the collection, processing, and use of data to improve health conditions and quality of life.

Most efforts to implement epidemiological surveillance systems in many Latin American countries are intended to help control communicable diseases rather than to address behavioural risk factors. Nevertheless, behavioural risk factors lead to chronic diseases, which have become endemic in Latin American cities because of worsening life conditions, rapid urbanisation, and dramatic changes in the states' role in Latin America.

Cities grow rapidly in developing countries, and this rapid urbanisation puts pressure on the physical environment that creates specific health threats for the city's inhabitants. In many economically deprived cities, the street has replaced the family as the source of housing and security for children and young people. These young people are exposed to a wide variety of health and behavioural problems: malnourishment, infectious diseases,

---

[*] Public Health Technology Assessment Center, University of Valle, Cali, Colombia.

accidents, substance dependence, prostitution, and—more recently—inter-personal violence (Ferguson, 1993). Ferguson argues that street children's access to services is more
limited than that of other urban residents because of poverty, inadequate documentation,
social stigma, lack of insurance, and inability to pay. Also, young street dwellers usually
consider health and social services as hostile, threatening, and useless. Health workers,
already overloaded, have been reluctant to face the complexity of the problems facing
these young people, whom they consider to be transitory and marginal.

Solutions to these problems are not immediately foreseeable, especially given current
social security systems, a consequence of ongoing state reforms in the region. Yet there
are possibilities for solutions, such as implementing a community-based epidemiological
surveillance system that is considered not only a process, but also a culture. In such a
system, the community does more than just collect data; it also assumes responsibility for data processing, analysis, interpretation, and use. In this manner, the community
is equally responsible for both implementing the system and finding solutions to detected problems.

Having such a community-based system does not absolve government institutions
of responsibility, nor does it conflict with national and local systems in which the community assumes a leading role. On the contrary, these systems are complementary—
although they respond to different logic, they are not diametrically opposed because both
build capacity and help develop local and national infra-structure for safeguarding the
public health.

The first part of this chapter addresses epidemiological surveillance in Latin America
in general, including its challenges and limitations. One of the main difficulties in documenting the surveillance processes in the region is a lack of published material. A few
references were found on local and national vertical programs; these references described
results, but did not include critical analysis of structural components and infra-structure
related to epidemiological surveillance initiatives within countries and the region.

The second part of this chapter points out some alternatives for overcoming constraints, paying special attention to the community-based surveillance system. Finally, a
practical example is presented to show the application of one of these systems (a school-
based behavioural risk factor surveillance system) that covers children and adolescents.

2. EPIDEMIOLOGICAL SURVEILLANCE IN LATIN AMERICA
AND THE CARIBBEAN

2.1. Background

Latin America and the Caribbean is a region with territorial, demographic, and particular socio-cultural characteristics that vary between and within countries. However,
these nations face a common challenge: economic and social development, in the context
of globalisation and state structural adjustment programs.

In most countries of Latin America and the Caribbean, growing poverty and unequal
distribution of income, resources, and opportunities are unavoidable realities. The governments try to apply social and economic policies simultaneously but, in practise, economic policy has been prioritised at the expense of social policy.

It is important to acknowledge how, beginning in 1978, ministries of health used the Health Decennial Plan for the Americas to execute policies and common goals that were strengthened by the Primary Health Care Strategy, the engine of health sector development. As a result of this strategy, programmes were successfully implemented to increase health care coverage, improve community and rural health, increase the population's access to basic health services, and improve environmental sanitation, nutrition, and other aspects of public health. Starting in 1983, when the foreign debt crisis exploded, the infra-structure and operative capacity of health services progressively deteriorated due to resource deficits. At the same time, health risks related to the growth of poverty increased among the population. In terms of disease and death, the health disparities between less privileged social groups and those that managed wealth became more visible.

The Pan American Health Organization (PAHO) recognises that social inequities are the greatest contributor to health problems in the Americas (Málaga and Castro, 2001). However, it is not possible to obtain information on the role national epidemiological surveillance systems have played in identifying the consequences of these inequities or the interventions used to close the gap. Several authors (Málaga and Castro, 2001; Ferguson, 1993; Organización Panamericana de Salud/Organización Mundial de Salud [OPS/OMS], 2000a) maintain that the association between a population's life conditions and health is demonstrated by the wide differences in the structure of health services and rates of diseases and death. They cited examples from Argentina, Colombia, Mexico, Peru, and Venezuela to illustrate this association.

In industrialised nations, the evolution of epidemiological surveillance has spanned more than a century and has passed through three very defined stages. In the first stage, the infectious diseases that accompany poverty, malnourishment, and inadequate environmental and personal hygiene were addressed step by step through improvements in housing and sanitation, better availability of drinkable water, and vaccinations. In the second stage, degenerative disease—such as cardiovascular disease, stroke, and cancer—began to replace infections as the main cause of mortality. The third stage reflects a growing concern with health problems caused by exposure to environmental contaminants and changing social conditions that may contribute to more widespread violence, drug dependence, excessive use of alcohol, and accidents.

In developing countries, these same three surveillance stages are occurring simultaneously. For this reason, the health picture in Latin America and the Caribbean has become a true epidemiological mosaic. Despite the recognition that is given to epidemiological surveillance, the same level of effort has not necessarily gone into translating the documentation of facts into policy and social management initiatives in Latin America and the Caribbean countries.

2.2. Limitations and Challenges

When reviewing epidemiological surveillance programs and statistical information from the Latin American and Caribbean region, one can appreciate the unequal development of national surveillance systems among the different countries. This can also be seen as an example of the inequities between the various health systems' infra-structures (OPS/OMS, 2000b).

A 1996 PAHO survey on health information infra-structure in 24 countries of the region (OPS/OMS, 1996) revealed the existence of serious problems and obstacles related to data gathering, use and dissemination of information, and human resource training. The survey also revealed substantial differences between Latin American and Caribbean countries in technological infra-structure, investment, and deployment of information systems. If, in addition to quantity, we assess the quality of information (as measured by validity of the data, opportunity in the notification, and utility and use of information to change situations that threaten the population's health), the picture becomes even more disproportionate.

Another element that causes concern is the weak or non-existent relationship between local and national surveillance systems. Can they be complementary, without losing their own identities and freedom to act according to the situation particular to each territory and group under study? How well do these systems perform in terms of moving from notification to action? Is there evidence that surveillance systems have contributed to better health and quality of life?

In general, the epidemiological surveillance systems in the Latin American region have restrictions that have kept them from re-orienting and energising the processes of change. Therefore, most of them have been unable to introduce interventions that would improve the population's health or modify health determinants.

PAHO and the World Health Organization (WHO) recognise that the most serious problem for information systems is data capture and precision (OPS/OMS, 1996). They also point out that the main obstacles system operators face have to do with quality of the data source, compilation of data, and timely registration of data. In general, almost all countries compile, register, and store health data systematically, based on guidelines and standards defined at national level (Table 1).

Table 1. Degree of development in four basic activities of information management in 24 Latin American and Caribbean countries

Activity	None (%)	Low (%)	Moderate (%)	High (%)
Systematic data collection according to national guidelines	4.2	20.6	62.5	12.5
Information related to epidemiological surveillance	0.0	12.5	75.0	12.5
Use of information for:				
Evaluation of services processes	12.5	54.2	29.2	4.2
Clinical decision making	25.0	50.0	25.0	0.0
Service management support	4.2	58.3	33.3	4.2
Dissemination of information via:				
Electronic networks	20.8	37.5	29.2	12.5
Meetings	8.3	37.5	37.5	16.7
Internet access	37.5	33.3	16.7	12.5
Information bulletins	12.5	29.2	50.0	8.3

Adapted with permission from OPS/OMS (1996), as cited by López-Acuña and Rodríguez 1996.

3. A COMMUNITY-BASED INFORMATION AND EPIDEMIOLOGICAL SURVEILLANCE SYSTEM: AN ANSWER TO THE OBSTACLES IN DEVELOPING COUNTRIES

3.1. Rationale

The ongoing socio-economic deterioration in Latin American and Caribbean countries may continue placing obstacles in the way of implementing epidemiological surveillance systems in the region. Even so, we are compelled to think of innovative ways to strengthen surveillance systems and to transform findings into social policies, educational campaigns, and permanent advocacy to respond to the problems of poor health determinants.

One innovation being tried in several countries is a locally or community-based epidemiological surveillance system. Such a system uses smaller units—such as the home, school, workplace, neighborhood, or *comuna*—as referents. The use of small units has both advantages and disadvantages.

Tognoni (1997) describes the following advantages of the community-based epidemiological surveillance system: participatory development of knowledge, participative management of interventions, sensitisation of participants to the surveillance, development of a pedagogic process, empowerment of the community, improvement of management processes, and development of a permanent source of information upon which to base public health actions. The following are also advantages of such epidemiological surveillance systems: they are centred on risks and problems in the community, providing motivation to act upon them; they allow the permanent creation of capacity and local infra-structure that are compatible with culture and resources in each setting; they specifically address the particular needs of the population; they generate conditions to introduce measures that improve the quality of registration; they facilitate intervention and follow-up because the smaller units can be used as indicators of what is going on in the larger population; and they facilitate collection, processing, analysis, and interpretation of data, dissemination of information, and the development of cohesive groups to act upon the identified obstacles and overcome them.

Among the limitations of using smaller units are the high percentages of illiteracy and functional illiteracy in most rural communities, the population's lack of education, and the lack of importance given by decision-makers to what is happening in them. Data gathered are not necessarily of institutional interest; consequently, there is a lack of institutional support to respond to the problems encountered. All these problems can be solved by building links between community and institutional systems; sensitising policy-makers and health managers about the importance of community systems; widely publicising achievements, especially when solutions are found through active community participation; and documenting processes that successfully point out the achievements and challenges.

3.1.1. Possibilities and Challenges of Epidemiological Surveillance in the Context of De-Centralisation

The political and administrative de-centralisation of territories in Colombia and several other Latin American countries was the result of a search for efficiency and cost containment in the 1980s. It is believed to be the central instrument for socio-economic development in the region. De-centralisation not only offers opportunities of growth and local development, but also demands changes in the political, administrative, and fiscal structure of the territorial units and in the relationships between the state and civil society. Therefore, the relationships between municipal development entities should be reconsidered in the new political context.

De-centralisation requires certain basic local conditions to become a real instrument of local development rather than a catalyst of under-development and poverty. It therefore requires the enactment of concrete regulations, such as those to transfer power and responsibility to territories; to establish leadership; to build technical, administrative, and financial capacity; to ensure social commitment among development partners; to set up effective systems of information, surveillance, and public communications; and to open up areas of negotiation and agreement.

Although the financial models are important and critical factors in shaping the power relationships between players in the surveillance system, finances are not the only influential factor. Other aspects of internal and external relationships within the environment should be considered. Little has been done to promote the development of local capacity and leadership that foster more balanced power relationships and legitimise the participation of communities in activities to improve their health and well-being. By means of active participation of the community, a surveillance instrument can be designed to assess the population's health and describe their current risk factors for chronic diseases.

In Colombia, for example, the Center for the Development and Assessment of Public Health Technology (CEDETES) has worked to create participatory systems, such as a community-based information and epidemiological surveillance system. These systems have sought to permanently guide community efforts in generating effective answers and addressing the inherent challenges of health and disease processes, most notably in the school population. Focusing on the future, this work started with recognition of a critical situation and tried to build health care strategies around it. In this way, the community response transcends a particular problem and occurs within an overall structure that facilitates and promotes a permanent cycle of activities (i.e., surveillance to action).

Endeavors to address child and adolescent health have been implemented worldwide and have been especially supported by WHO and its regional offices. Recently schools have been recognised as a development area. PAHO/WHO pointed out the need to expand health and wellness activities used in other sectors to the school setting, thereby providing an opportunity for human development, peace, and equity (OPS/OMS, 2000c).

According to Levinger (1994), an approach to child and adolescent health that takes into account the culture of the educational centers (e.g., the schools) offers the opportunity for young people to acquire techniques, knowledge, attitudes, and habits that promote personal, community, and national development. For these programmes to achieve their goals, they should be designed by those directly involved in young people's education and be supported by methodologies and technologies designed in conformance with the expectations and language of the school community.

3.1.2. Epidemiological Surveillance and Healthy Schools

In Colombia, the CEDETES proposal for behavioural risk factor monitoring and epidemiological surveillance for the school population strives to make the school a catalyst for strengthening local capacity and improving quality of life. This is developed through de-centralisation, in which each municipality assumes responsibility for its population's health.

The first step is to use small group settings or physical structures, such as schools, to build support for health-promoting behaviours in the rest of the community. Because the schools "belong" to local communities and reflect the area's interests, they are in a position to bring the community together and foster the development of collaborations around a common purpose, such as promoting health and quality of life among the school-age and adolescent populations and the community as a whole (De Salazar, 1996).

The next steps in developing and implementing a risk factor and health determinant surveillance and monitoring system in a school-age population are to consolidate and strengthen decision-making capacity and the population's action towards health and to bring together strategic alliances among key sectors to fulfill this purpose.

3.2. Information and Epidemiological Surveillance System for School-Age and Adolescent Populations (SIVEA)

3.2.1. The School-Age and Adolescent Populations: A Challenge for Public Health

Around the world, there are more than 1,000,000,000 adolescents between 10 and 19 years of age (Singh and Wulf, 1990). In 1996, the Latin American and Caribbean region had a population of 51 million young people between 15 and 19 years of age, and that number was projected to grow to 52 million in 2000. Currently, adolescents represent more than a fifth of the region's total population.

Latin America has two thirds of the adolescent population of the entire American continent. Population analysis shows that the median age in most Latin American countries is below 20 (Maddaleno and Suárez, 1995). It is calculated that in Latin America there are 50 million young people under the age of 15.

Health problems or specific conditions such as violence, hunger, and drug use hinder academic performance and prevent children and adolescents from taking advantage of available resources or effectively dealing with the life conditions they often experience (e.g., poverty, social exclusion). The boy or girl who cannot adapt to the school system because of such problems has a high probability of dropping out. This is a time when children are most at risk of beginning a dangerous cycle that includes greater marginalisation and the further development of anti-social behaviours—such as aggressiveness, drug use, and violence—and other problems.

Traditionally, programmes directed to children, girls, and adolescent populations have focused on health institutions and curative care. Other sectors and resources that contribute substantially to young people's development have been overlooked, even though they are a part of the population's daily life and culture.

The morbidity and mortality rates among children 6 to 18 years of age have been much lower than those of younger children. In general, morbidity and mortality in this age group are associated with accidents in almost all the countries of the American region. The tendency to practise risky health behaviours explains the high mortality and morbidity due to violent causes in adolescents (Florenzano, 1993).

Other studies in Latin America have pointed out that common problems among the region's young people—extreme economic deprivation, family history of behavioural risk taking, and the lack of a protective environment—underlie most cases of substance abuse, delinquency, pregnancy, and dropping out of school (Maddaleno et al., 1995). Mortality in adolescents is mainly the result of external causes—accidents, homicide, and suicide. A 1997 analysis of mortality rates in the region showed that the leading causes of death in children aged 10 to 14 years were accidents, violence, malignant tumors, and infectious diseases. For the adolescent population between 15 and 19 years of age, the main causes of death were accidents, homicides, suicide, malignant tumors, heart disease, and pregnancy complications (both during childbirth and immediately post-partum) (PAHO, 1998).

According to the Colombia Ministry of Health, the main reasons young people seek medical care, are hospitalized, or die are accidents and violence (30%) and infectious diseases (16%). Problems with teeth and gums are among the most frequent reasons for seeking medical care, but the most common reason continues to be accidents and violence (Colombia Ministry of Health, 1998). In these cases, young people are both the victims and the perpetrators of violence that results in death or injury.

According to data from the Colombian Institute of Family Well-Being (1992), every year between 50,000 and 100,000 children are mistreated or abused. Also, a study on underage offenders in Colombia showed that 30% were less than 15 years of age, and more than 15% of those were younger than 12 (Fundación para la Educación Superior, 1994).

Information compiled by the Ministry of Health concerning child labour in Colombia showed that in 1992, more than two million people 9 to 17 years of age were employed (Colombia Ministry of Health, 2002). In low socio-economic groups, almost 90% of children and young people in that age group were employed. Further, the proportion of young people who attended school was much smaller among workers: urban children aged 12 to 13 years who worked, 50% attended school; among non-workers the same age, 95% attended school.

The situation of these young people appears more dramatic when we examine the number of hours they work. Colombian children and adolescents work an average of 40 hours per week; the length of the work week increases with age and varies by location and by sex. Despite the number of hours they work, on average children earn less than half the legal minimum wage. Likewise, social security coverage for these young people is significantly low, due mainly to the high proportion of children and adolescents working informally. Only 13% of the urban young people and 8% of those living in the countryside have access to social security.

Because children and adolescents are among the region's most vulnerable and underserved populations, there is less opportunity to detect their risks and morbidity rates. However, these young people can become health "sentinels" in the school, in their own homes, and in the community as a whole.

By means of different techniques and methods, SIVEA collects, analyses, interprets, delivers, and uses socio-demographic data and information on the young people's extracurricular activities, sanitation and housing conditions, family composition and resources, academic performance, and health status (De Salazar, 1999). This information is then used to improve young people's health conditions and quality of life (Figure 1).

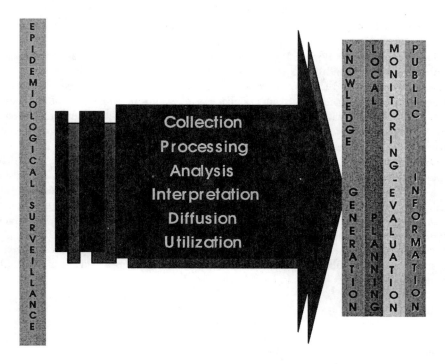

Figure 1. Information and epidemiological surveillance system for school-age and adolescent populations. SIVEA: methods and results.

3.2.2. Infra-Structure of SIVEA

The rationale for use of a school-based information and surveillance system is founded in a series of premises put forward by authors such as De Salazar and co-workers (1993, 1994), Kirby (1990), and Levinger (1984). Premises come from authors' experiences with similar initiatives and from recent studies on the topic. SIVEA was the result of seven years of work, in which 795 students and teachers at four schools were actively involved. Although this document discusses one example of epidemiological surveillance in a school population in Colombia, it is worth acknowledging that several Latin American countries are also implementing school-based information and surveillance systems.

SIVEA is a set of elements and inter-related resources. Its infra-structure takes into account local resources and particularly those from the school, especially its physical and human resources—students, teachers, and parents. Likewise, SIVEA takes advantage of resources that come from private institutions, such as non-government organisations, and from a number of public agencies in the health, justice, government, transit, and leisure sectors. It also receives support from a wide variety of community organisations that collaborate with the school. The university is one of those resources that also benefits from the surveillance system in terms of getting input and support for its academic programs and research.

4. CONCLUSION

The lack of behavioural risk factor surveillance compounded by rapid urbanisation, deteriorating health conditions, and growing rates of chronic diseases in many cities of the Latin American and Caribbean region have under-scored the growing importance of and need for surveillance in this part of the world. Solutions to these problems are not immediately on the horizon, although recent efforts to implement community-based epidemiological surveillance systems show great promise for finding ways to overcome the region's many health problems and surveillance limitations.

One example of such a system is SIVEA, a school-based surveillance system that attempts to fill in gaps in the majority of the region's epidemiological surveillance systems, which exclude information on behavioural risk factors. Although the system is school based, it is grounded in the society at large by using different entities and people in the epidemiological surveillance cycle and in the practical development of initiatives to address the identified health risks of the population. This system has clearly demonstrated that the school has an important role in the development process of children and young people and is a favourable venue for studying the local conditions and generating collective and inter-sectoral solutions to local health problems.

5. REFERENCES

Colombia Ministry of Health, 1998, *Escuelas Saludables. Lineamientos Generales de Escuelas. Documento Preliminar*, Santafé de Bogotá, Colombia.

Colombia Ministry of Health, 2002, Erradicación del Trabajo Infantil (January 28, 2003); http://www.minsalud. gov.co/NewSite/MseContent/images/news/DocNewsNo9418.htm.

Colombian Institute of Family Well-Being, 1992, Statistics (March 15, 2002); http://www.icbf.gov.co/ingles/ estadisticas.asp.

De Salazar, L., 1993, School health information system: a key element for health education. Outline on "How health education strategy will be conducted in Colombia," Tanzania. Unpublished mimeograph.

De Salazar, L., 1996, *Hacia una Escuela Saludable: Avances de una Estrategia Asociativa para el Abordaje de la Población en Edad Escolar y Adolescente*, Proyecto UNI-Cali, Universidad del Valle, Cali, Colombia.

De Salazar, L., 1999, *Escuelas Promotoras de Salud: Resultado de Alianzas Estratégicas entre la Academia, el Gobierno Municipal y la Comunidad*, Centro para el Desarrollo y Evaluación de Tecnología en Salud Pública, CEDETES, Universidad del Valle, Cali, Colombia.

De Salazar, L., Scott, M., et al., 1994, Improving health of school age children: a project in association with the Partnership for Child Development, Montreal. Unpublished conceptual document.

Ferguson, B. J., 1993, Youth at the threshold of the 21st century: the demographic situation, *J Adolesc Health.* **14**:638–644, 703–710.

Florenzano, R., 1993, Factores de riesgo y la juventud: el rol de la familia y la comunidad. *J Adolesc Health.* **14**:683–689.

Fundación para la Educación Superior, 1994, *Tres Estudios Inéditos sobre los Menores Infractores en Colombia*, la Fundación, Santafé de Bogotá, Colombia.

Kirby, D., 1990, Comprehensive school health and the larger community: issues and possible scenario, *J School Health.* **60**:170–177.

Levinger, B., 1984, School feeding programmes: myth and potential, *Prospects.* **24**:369–376.

Levinger, B., 1994, *La Nutrición, la Salud y la Educación para Todos*, Education Development Center, Programa de las Naciones Unidas para la Infancia, New York.

Maddaleno, M., Munist, M., Serrano, C., et. al., 1995, *La Salud del Adolescente y del Joven*, Organización Panamericana de la Salud/Organización Mundial de la Salud, Washington, DC (Publicación Científica No. 552).

Maddaleno, M., and Suárez, E., 1995, Situación social de los adolescentes y jóvenes en América Latina, in: *La Salud del Adolescente y del Joven*, M. Maddaleno, M. Munist, C. Serrano, et al., eds., Organización Panamericana de la Salud/Organización Mundial de la Salud, Washington, DC, pp. 70–84 (Publicación Científica No. 552).
Málaga, H., and Castro, M., 2001, *Cómo Empoderar a Los Excluidos en el Nivel Local. Promoción de la Salud: Cómo Construir Vida Saludable*, Edición Panamericana, Bogotá Distrito Capital, Colombia, pp. 120–137.
Organización Panamericana de la Salud/Organización Mundial de la Salud, 1996, *Encuesta de Recursos de Sistemas de Información sobre Servicios de Salud*, OPS/OMS, Washington, DC. Cited by: López-Acuña, D., and Rodríguez, R., 1998, *Sistemas de Información y Tecnología de la Información en Salud: Desafíos y Soluciones para América Latina y el Caribe*, Programa de Sistemas de Información sobre Servicios de Salud, OPS/OMS, Washington, DC, pp. 55–59.
Organización Panamericana de la Salud/Organización Mundial de la Salud, 2000a, El Progreso en la Salud de la Población, Informe Anual del Director 2000 (March 20, 2001); http://www.paho.org/Spanish/D/AnnReport_00.htm.
Organización Panamericana de la Salud/Organización Mundial de la Salud, 2000b, Escuelas Promotoras de Salud en las Américas (March 9, 2001); http//www.paho.org/spanish/HPP/HPM/HEC/hs_about.htm.
Organización Panamericana de la Salud/Organización Mundial de la Salud, 2000c, Vigilancia en Salud Pública en las Américas: Sistemas Nacionales de Vigilancia Epidemiológica y de Información Estadística (March 20, 2001); http://www.paho.org/English/SHA/shavsp.htm.
Pan American Health Organization, 1998, *Health Conditions of Adolescents and Youth in the Americas*, PAHO/WHO, Washington, DC.
Singh, S., and Wulf, D., 1990, *Today's Adolescent, Tomorrow's Parent: A Portrait of the Americas*, Alan Guttmacher Institute, New York. Cited by: Camacho, A. V., 2000, Perfil de Salud Sexual y Reproductiva de los y las Adolescentes y Jóvenes de América Latina y el Caribe: Revisión Bibliográfica, 1988–1998, Organización Panamericana de la Salud, Washington, DC (Serie OPS/FNUAP No. 1).
Tognoni G., ed., 1997, *Manual de Epidemiología Comunitaria*, Edición CECOMET, Quito, Ecuador.

CHAPTER 15

CREATING A SYNTHETIC BEHAVIOURAL RISK FACTOR INDEX TO ASSESS TRENDS IN SURVEILLANCE DATA

An Index of Risk for Cardio-Vascular Disease as an Example

Stefano Campostrini and David V. McQueen[*]

1. INTRODUCTION

The causal web that relates to cardio-vascular disease (CVD) is highly complex, consisting of a mixture of biological, genetic, cultural, and behavioural determinants. It is well appreciated that the behavioural risk factors—such as obesity, lack of physical activity, and smoking—have an important impact on the etiology of CVD. These behaviours are multiple, often clustered (Raitakari et al., 1995), and presumably act in some sort of complex synergistic pattern in enhancing the possibility for CVD in any given individual as well as in the population as a whole. Nonetheless, the dimensions and patterning of these behaviours in relation to CVD are not as well understood as one would like.

Many public health interventions in heart disease have addressed multiple risk factors for CVD at the community and societal levels (see, for example, Multiple Risk Factor Intervention Trial, 1982; Farquhar et al., 1990; Winkleby et al., 1994; Puska et al., 1995; Luepker et al., 1996); the arguement is that addressing single risk factors is insufficient (Castelli, 1983). Yet attempts to satisfactorily evaluate the effectiveness of multiple risk factor interventions often have not been as successful as hoped. The reasons the evaluations are often inconclusive are many. A leading reason may be inappropriate measurement of the pattern of risk factor behaviours. Thus the need for evaluations is still relevant (Noble and Modest, 1996).

Despite the widely recognized need for appropriate measurement of behavioural risk factors, the number of attempts to develop comprehensive measures to

---

[*] Stefano Campostrini, University of Pavia, 27100 Pavia, Italy; David V. McQueen, Centers for Disease Control and Prevention, Atlanta, Georgia 30341-3717, USA.

accompany comprehensive CVD interventions remains limited. Most of the risk indices found in the literature (see, for example, Bao et al., 1994; Gran, 1995; Byers et al. 1998) combine behavioural risk factors such as smoking or lack of exercise with outcome measures such as high blood pressure or high concentration of blood cholesterol.

Measuring multiple CVD risk factors has several inherent difficulties. Two are especially prominent. (1) Outcome measures interact with other factors (mainly with the demographic composition of the population and genetic factors). This interaction can be addressed statistically, but it is not a simple matter. (2) Measurements frequently are based on current data and do not take into account that CVD outcomes are often effects of past behaviours and past behavioural patterns.

2. CREATING A SYNTHETIC BEHAVIOURAL RISK FACTOR INDEX

What is an index? Essentially an index is a conception, based nonetheless on some concrete measures that taken together provide a number. This number is a quantity that shows, through its variation over time, the operation of an abstraction that is not directly or easily measurable. An index is always a proxy. There are many well known indices in common practice, such as indices of business activity (e.g., the Dow Jones Index) or in psychometrics (e.g., intelligence is measured indirectly with the intelligence quotient [I.Q.] and produces a single number). Producing a precise number does not free the researcher from the many problems of interpreting an index, but it does allow for a larger concept to be introduced and considered in its own right. We term this exercise the "creation of a synthetic index" to emphasise the conceptual nature of an index.

Why build an index based on behaviour? In the United States half of all deaths due to the major chronic diseases have been attributed to modifiable risk factors (McGinnis and Foege, 1993); CVD constitutes the main cause of mortality. The modifiable risk factors for the major chronic diseases are well documented and include the primary behavioural risk factors for CVD (i.e., smoking, physical inactivity, and poor diet). The importance of the contribution of each modifiable risk factor and its precise relationship to cardiovascular morbidity and mortality may be debated, but the contributions are inarguably profound. Constructing an index represents an attempt to summarise and numerically represent this contribution in a way that is understandable and useful to decision-makers in public health.

Why tie an index to an ongoing surveillance system? Public health practitioners have little doubt of the role that surveillance has played in public health and chronic disease control. It is the classic means of providing the intelligence on which public health interventions and programmatic efforts towards disease control may be based (Teutsch and Churchill, 2000). In recent years the analysis, interpretation, dissemination, and use of data gathered have been increasingly recognized worldwide as part of a larger role for surveillance in public health. Surveillance is now generally seen as an integrated system of related actions ranging from recognising causal factors and relevant epidemiological parameters in chronic diseases to applying evidence-based public health programmes. It is in the best use and application of surveillance data that the true meaning and usefulness of a synthetic index come into play.

Tracking behavioural risk factors of a population relies principally on the survey as a methodology. When carried out in a continuous series of surveys over time, such as the U.S. Behavioral Risk Factor Surveillance System (BRFSS), one has a surveillance system designed appropriately enough to consider the creation of synthetic indices.

3. THE U.S. BEHAVIORAL RISK FACTOR SURVEILLANCE SYSTEM

The BRFSS, which was developed and is run by the Centers for Disease Control and Prevention (CDC), is an ongoing, random-digit-dialed telephone survey used to determine the prevalence among adults (i.e., persons aged 18 years and older) of behaviours and practices—such as cigarette smoking, seat belt use, blood cholesterol screening, control of high blood pressure, physical activity, weight control, alcohol use, and drinking and driving—related to the leading causes of death in the United States (CDC, 1998). To maximise comparability, methods and questionnaires are standardised across participating states and over time.

3.1. History of the BRFSS

By 1980, telephone surveys had emerged as a reliable and affordable method for determining the prevalence of behavioural risk factors in the U.S. population. Accordingly, the CDC began working with state health departments to develop a system for ongoing surveillance of behavioural risk factors in the population by using random-digit-dialed telephone techniques. The goal of the system was to collect, analyse, and interpret state-specific behavioural risk factor data in order to plan, implement, and monitor public health programmes. From 1981 through 1983, random-digit-dialed, one-time telephone surveys were conducted in 29 states and in Washington, DC, by state health department personnel.

Beginning in 1984, the surveys were conducted in a 7- to 10-day period every month throughout the year and came to be known collectively as the BRFSS. The number of participating states increased from 15 in 1984 to 22 in 1985, 26 in 1986, 34 in 1987, 37 in 1988, 40 in 1989, and 45 in 1990. During the 1990s all states in the United States participated in the BRFSS. In 1998, the median yearly sample for states was 2,648 (Center for Injury Prevention Policy and Practice, 2002).

3.2. BRFSS Methodology

BRFSS methodology is fairly straightforward. Respondents are selected randomly from adult civilian residents with telephones. In most states, the telephone number is selected using a multi-stage cluster design known as the Waksberg method. After a household is contacted, a person is randomly selected from among the adults residing in the household and is interviewed. If the adult selected is not available, the interview is done during a follow-up telephone call. To improve efficiency in contacting eligible respondents, the interviews are conducted primarily weekday evenings, but also during the day and on weekends. Beginning in 1985, most states began using computer-assisted telephone interviewing (CATI) to facilitate the interview, data coding and entry, and quality control procedures.

The BRFSS questionnaire has three components: core questions, standardised modules, and state-added questions. The core questions and the standardised modules are developed jointly by states and the CDC. For comparability, many of these questions have been selected from national surveys such as the National Health Interview Surveys and the National Health and Nutrition Examination Surveys. All states are expected to ask the core questions and may choose to add any or all of the standardised modules. States with interests beyond the core and standardised modules may develop their own questions. These questions are attached at the end of the questionnaire to maintain comparability between states and over time. At the end of the interviewing cycle each month, the data are keyed and sent to CDC for editing. The results are weighted to take into account the effects of telephone non-coverage, non-response, refusals, and sampling design and to adjust the survey data to the age-, race-, or sex-specific population counts from the most recent census or inter-censal estimate in each state.

Because comparable methods are used from state to state and from year to year, states can compare risk factor prevalence with other states and monitor the effects of interventions over time. Also, the use of consistent methods in a large group of states permits the assessment of geographic patterns of risk factor prevalence.

3.3. Using BRFSS Data to Create a Synthetic Index

The availability of BRFSS data is of course a great advantage, but these data have obvious limitations. The BRFSS presents variables to measure the modifiable risk factors for the major chronic diseases, but generally such data sets are not developed with the idea of creating an index. Thus, not all of the BRFSS variables are ideal for an index. Nevertheless, reality requires that one must work with the best available data.

Consider the chief variables of interest in CVD. For smoking behaviour the measure used in the BRFSS is quite accurate and reliable, with extensive documentation in multiple studies on the validity and reliability of the questions used. In contrast, the measure of physical exercise presents many challenges. For example, the BRFSS, like most surveillance systems to date, considers only leisure-time physical activities, which could give an inaccurate estimate of the amount of physical activity in the population, particularly in places where walking to work is possible. Dietary behaviour presents even greater challenges. Even though historically the BRFSS has included diet in the core questionnaire, this topic has been surveyed in only a few states and a few time periods, offering limited information on dietary risk factors. In developing a risk index, using body mass index (BMI; computed as the ratio of weight in kilograms to the square of height in meters) as a proxy measure of diet and eating habits is preferable. BMI is an outcome measure and not a behavioural measure, but it may be used as a proxy because changes in diet behaviours have an almost immediate effect on BMI and because the link between BMI and diet is strong (Stamler and Dolecek, 1997; Stamler et al., 1997).

Because the BRFSS has produced a large, cumulating data set of behaviours in the U.S. population and because the data have been rigorously collected over time, the system serves as an excellent data source with which to develop a synthetic index. Despite the obvious advantage of using such a data source, attempts at index development are uncommon—chiefly because of the time and effort that must go into such development but also because most risk factors are treated separately (historical and funding considerations favor the analysis and presentation of results with one variable at a time).

4. METHODS

4.1. The Cardiovascular Disease Behavioral Risk Index (CaDRI)

The behaviours that put a person at some risk for CVD are smoking, lack of physical exercise, and poor diet and eating habits. Social factors (e.g., stress, psychological factors) due to complex behaviours could influence the development of CVD (McQueen and Siegrist, 1982), but these factors are difficult to define, measure, and address in a public health intervention. After careful review of the measures available in the BRFSS data set, we set out to develop CaDRI by using combinations of the risk variables (i.e., behaviours) listed in Table 1.

The cutoff points used to define categories for each risk variable are important, but their importance must not be over-emphasised particularly when one considers the combinations of several variables. The sensitivity lost by collapsing some

Table 1. Definition of categories for each variable used in constructing CaDRI

Variable	Definition	
Cigarette smoking		
Non-smoker	Have smoked <100 cigarettes in one's entire life	
Light smoker	Smokes ≤3 cigarettes a day	
Smoker	Smokes 4–19 cigarettes a day	
Heavy smoker	Smokes ≥20 cigarettes a day	
Physical activity		
Active	Either ≥5 times per week and ≥30 minutes per occasion of physical activity of any type at any intensity, or ≥3 times per week and ≥20 minutes per occasion of physical activity involving rhythmic contractions of large muscle groups performed at ≥50% of estimated age- and sex-specific maximal cardio-respiratory capacity	
Not regularly active	Reports some activity, but not enough to meet the "Active" definition	
Sedentary	No reported activity during the previous 2 weeks	
Body mass index		
Optimal	<25.0 kg/m^2	
Acceptable	Women: 25.0–27.3 kg/m^2	Men: 25.0–27.8 kg/m^2
Overweight	Women: 27.3–30.0 kg/m^2	Men: 27.8–30.0 kg/m^2
Obese	>30.0 kg/m^2	

variables into a few categories is regained when one considers combining several variables. Furthermore, too many categories would lead to a risk index with fuzzy categories and to problems for the panelists who assign different levels of risk to closely related situations (i.e., for which the differences do not result in a clearly conceptually assessable risk). The cutoff points presented in Table 1 are based on examination of the literature, analysis of the chosen variables and their relationships in the BRFSS data to several outcome variables (e.g., reported high cholesterol concentration and high blood pressure), and discussions with an ad hoc panel of experts at the CDC National Center for Chronic Disease Prevention and Health Promotion. In constructing the index all the variables inter-acting with each behavioural risk were considered, whereas confounders (e.g., age, sex) were set aside and considered only in the data analysis.

The CDC expert panel ranked all possible combinations of behavioural variables from 1 (lowest risk) to 48 (highest risk). For the ranking process we adopted a particular Delphi technique (see Section 4.2). In this ranking the "distances" between ranked situations may be equal (i.e., multiple risks are additive) or unequal (i.e., multiple risks are not additive). We do not address this matter in this chapter: a ranked risk index can potentially meet both assumptions. Actually, a further study observing the relationship between the risk index and output measures could show the effect of multiple risks.

4.2. The Delphi Technique

Since its appearance in the 1970s, the Delphi technique, initially designed for future planning purposes, has become widely used whenever expert judgement is needed or information needs to be collected and analysed for strategic planning. The technique assumes that interaction among experts can produce more knowledge than the simple collection of single experts' opinion can. This method seeks to avoid the typical negative effects of social interaction (e.g., conflicts, steering by a leader) by conducting several rounds in which information is collected through questionnaires and anonymously shared. The technique has been used to construct other indices using continuously collected behavioural surveillance data (see, for example, Campostrini and McQueen, 1993).

In creating CaDRI, the Delphi technique was particularly useful because of the lack of epidemiological data about the effect of multiple risk behaviours on CVD and the need to share the evidence acquired in different fields on the effects of single risk behaviours. In constructing the expert panel, we considered the different disciplines and sectors that have studied CVD risk factors and invited epidemiologists, sociologists, statisticians, and medically trained persons from several public health settings.

A total of 15 panelists answered the questionnaires. Three rounds were required to achieve the final ranking. The first two rounds were necessary to debate the importance of smoking as a CVD risk factor. A discussion meeting (joined by some panelists through teleconferencing) was held before we constructed the third questionnaire. In the final ranking the panelists' median was considered. Agreement on each ranking was assessed by computing the intra-quartile distance (i.e., the difference between the third and first quartiles of the distribution): the greater the intra-quartile distance, the less the agreement.

To have a more synthetic index and a measure that took into consideration the interaction among behavioural risk variables and some personal characteristics linked to CVD (sex, age, geographic area, and race and ethnicity), we asked the panelists to define for each group cut points to create four risk categories (low, medium, high, very high). Using their expertise, the panelists grouped the different situations on the basis of the actual risk for developing CVD in a certain period of time. This task was more difficult because it involved assessing the link between risk behaviours and development of a disease.

4.3. Data Analysis

Other chapters in this book discuss in detail the relevance of appropriate analysis of a data set such as the BRFSS. Therefore our results focus strictly on the analysis of CaDRI. We present only the first results from simple analyses, made principally to exemplify the relevance and the possible uses of CaDRI. Trend analyses using auto-regressive integrated moving-average (ARIMA) models, which are applicable to BRFSS data (Smith, 1978), illustrate how data from states with high-quality, uninterrupted data can use such an index over time.

5. RESULTS

We created CaDRI from the results of the third round of the Delphi surveys. Although the level of agreement among panelists was not high (i.e., the intra-quartile distance was not low) overall, the level of agreement was considerably higher in the final round than in the first two rounds, and the panelists were quite satisfied with the final ranking (Table 2). The major difference was over the combination of conditions in which heavy smoking was the only risk factor.

We proffer a tentative analysis on the basis of actual outcome data, useful only as a broad view of CaDRI and its possible uses. When CaDRI was broken down by sex, age group, geographic area, and race and ethnicity, situations already known by

Table 2. CaDRI: final ranking of the combination of cardio-vascular disease risk behaviours, and level of agreement among expert panelists

Combination				Intra-quartile
Cigarette smoking	Physical activity	Body mass index	Rank	distance
Non-smoker	Active	Optimal	1	0
Light smoker	Active	Optimal	8	3
Smoker	Active	Optimal	23	6
Heavy smoker	Active	Optimal	29	11
Non-smoker	Not regularly active	Optimal	4	2
Light smoker	Not regularly active	Optimal	14	4
Smoker	Not regularly active	Optimal	26	3.5

Table 2. (continued)

Combination				Intra-quartile
Cigarette smoking	Physical activity	Body mass index	Rank	distance
Heavy smoker	Not regularly active	Optimal	34	4
Non-smoker	Sedentary	Optimal	7	3.5
Light smoker	Sedentary	Optimal	17	4.5
Smoker	Sedentary	Optimal	29	2.5
Heavy smoker	Sedentary	Optimal	39	5
Non-smoker	Active	Acceptable	2	0
Light smoker	Active	Acceptable	12	4.5
Smoker	Active	Acceptable	25	3
Heavy smoker	Active	Acceptable	32	6.5
Non-smoker	Not regularly active	Acceptable	5	1.5
Light smoker	Not regularly active	Acceptable	17	1.5
Smoker	Not regularly active	Acceptable	29	3
Heavy smoker	Not regularly active	Acceptable	38	3.5
Non-smoker	Sedentary	Acceptable	9	3.5
Light smoker	Sedentary	Acceptable	20	1
Smoker	Sedentary	Acceptable	32	2.5
Heavy smoker	Sedentary	Acceptable	40	3.5
Non-smoker	Active	Overweight	6	4
Light smoker	Active	Overweight	15	0
Smoker	Active	Overweight	27	1.5
Heavy smoker	Active	Overweight	39	5
Non-smoker	Not regularly active	Overweight	10	4.5
Light smoker	Not regularly active	Overweight	20	5
Smoker	Not regularly active	Overweight	33	4
Heavy smoker	Not regularly active	Overweight	43	2
Non-smoker	Sedentary	Overweight	18	5
Light smoker	Sedentary	Overweight	23	3.5
Smoker	Sedentary	Overweight	36	4.5
Heavy smoker	Sedentary	Overweight	45	1.5
Non-smoker	Active	Obese	10	2.5
Light smoker	Active	Obese	22	0.5
Smoker	Active	Obese	34	1.5
Heavy smoker	Active	Obese	43	4.5
Non-smoker	Not regularly active	Obese	15	5
Light smoker	Not regularly active	Obese	24	6.5
Smoker	Not regularly active	Obese	38	3.5
Heavy smoker	Not regularly active	Obese	46.5	1
Non-smoker	Sedentary	Obese	20	10.5
Light smoker	Sedentary	Obese	26	10.5
Smoker	Sedentary	Obese	43	5.5
Heavy smoker	Sedentary	Obese	48	0

epidemiological data were confirmed by the prevalence of the "very high" risk level (Table 3):

- men indulged in riskier behaviours than women did,
- older age was correlated with worse behaviour, although the oldest age group showed better behaviour than the previous one, perhaps because of retirement,
- persons in the West had healthier behaviours, while the South registered the highest percentage of persons at high risk of CVD, and
- the black population was at highest risk of CVD, while the white population did not differ from the general population.

All the differences reported here were statistically significant. Further analyses revealed that the racial and ethnic differences remained statistically significant even when the effect of possible confounding variables (e.g., age, sex, education) was considered (data not shown). This result exemplifies how such indices applied to similar data files allow for interesting studies on social determinants of health risk behaviours.

One of the more interesting uses of such an index is studying the evolution of clustered risk behaviours over time. The mean CaDRI value of four states for which all the needed observations were collected continuously for 5 years (Arizona, Illinois, South Carolina, Virginia) are presented in Figure 1. The mean value increased over time in all four states, indicating the populations behaved riskily overall. This overall increase appeared to be due to a decrease in the proportion of the population

Table 3. Percentage distribution of risk level for cardio-vascular disease as determined with CaDRI, by sex, age group, geographic area, and race and ethnicity[*]

	Risk level			
	Low	Medium	High	Very high
Sex				
Male	59.50	13.00	8.80	18.70
Female	64.40	8.10	10.60	16.90
Age group				
18–34 years	72.87	9.25	10.80	7.08
35–44 years	62.40	12.15	10.38	15.08
45–54 years	54.72	15.29	12.04	17.95
55–64 years	50.64	4.89	9.10	35.36
≥64 years	56.16	9.94	5.03	28.87
Geographic area				
West	65.26	9.95	9.86	14.93
Central	60.33	11.03	9.67	18.97
Northeast	63.71	10.46	8.45	17.37
South	60.10	10.57	10.27	19.06
Race and ethnicity				
White, non-Hispanic	62.95	10.74	8.78	17.53
Black, non-Hispanic	52.37	11.25	13.99	22.40
Hispanic	59.61	9.52	12.93	17.95
Other	74.07	7.41	7.64	10.88

[*] CaDRI was based on 1998 Behavioral Risk Factor Surveillance System data (N=141,112).

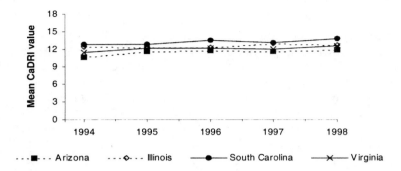

Figure 1. Mean CaDRI value in four states that collected the needed BRFSS data from 1994 through 1998.

at low risk of CVD (i.e., an increase in the proportion that had unhealthy behaviours), as in Arizona (Figure 2). Perhaps people gave up smoking (a high risk) but took on other unhealthy behaviours. The small but steady increase in the percentage of the population at very high risk of CVD is worrying. It could be a sign of the tendency for persons already at risk to indulge in additional risk behaviours.

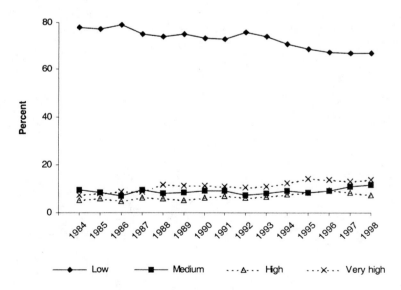

Figure 2. Risk levels for cardio-vascular disease in Arizona, according to CaDRI, 1984–1998.

6. DISCUSSION

Certainly most of the data presented here require more analysis and deeper discussion, but these would go beyond the aims of this brief chapter. We have tried to illustrate the method used and how the literature supports the choices made at every step of the construction of this index. We recognise that a more reliable and valid index could be constructed and that some of the choices the expert panelists and we made could be criticised or debated; however, our point was to illustrate possibilities on how to use an ongoing surveillance system. The major task of data analysis in a surveillance system is that of providing synthetic, quick, and broad views of the ongoing situation of the health behaviour of a population. Also, the simple first analyses of the BRFSS-based CaDRI do show the importance of considering the combination of risk behaviours and how this could offer "good enough" information for disease prevention and health promotion. Data users need simple (i.e., simple to interpret for them, not necessarily methodologically simple) information that could support their health programmes and initiatives. We believe CaDRI is a first tentative answer for their knowledge needs linked to the control of clustered risk behaviours for CVD.

7. REFERENCES

Bao, W., Srinivasan, S. R., Wattigney, W. A., et al., 1994, Persistence of multiple cardiovascular risk clustering related to syndrome X from childhood to young adulthood, *Arch Intern Med.* **154**:1842–1848.

Byers, T., Anda, R., McQueen. D., et al., 1998, The correspondence between coronary artery disease mortality and risk factor prevalence among states in the United States, 1991–1992, *Prev Med.* **27**:311–316.

Campostrini, S., and McQueen, D. V., 1993, Sexual behavior and exposure to HIV infection: estimates from a general-population risk index, *Am J Public Health.* **83**:1139–1143.

Castelli, W. P., 1983, Cardiovascular disease and multifactorial risk: challenge of the 1980s, *Am Heart J.* **106**:1191–1200.

Center for Injury Prevention Policy and Practice, 2002, Behavioral Risk Factor Surveillance System (BRFSS) (January 27, 2003); http://www.safetypolicy.org/hp2010/brfss.htm.

Centers for Disease Control and Prevention, 1998, *Behavioral Risk Factor Surveillance System User's Guide,* U.S. Department of Health and Human Services, Centers for Disease Control and Prevention, Atlanta.

Farquhar, J. W., Fortmann, S. P., Flora, J. A., et al., 1990, Effects of communitywide education on cardiovascular risk factors. The Stanford Five-City Project, *JAMA.* **264**:359–365.

Gran, B., 1995, Major differences in cardiovascular risk indicators by educational status: results from a population based screening program, *Scand J Soc Med.* **23**:9–16.

Luepker, R. V., Rastam, L. Hannan. P. J., et al., 1996, Community education for cardiovascular disease prevention. Morbidity and mortality results from the Minnesota Heart Health Program, *Am J Epidemiol.* **144**:351–362.McGinnis, J. M., and Foege, W. H., 1993, Actual causes of death in the United States, *JAMA.* **270**:2207–2212.

McGinnis, J. M., and Foege, W. H., 1993, Actual causes of death in the United States, *JAMA.* **270**:2207–2212.

McQueen, D. V., and Siegrist, J., 1982, Social factors in the etiology of chronic disease: an overview, *Soc Sci Med.* **16**:353–367.

Multiple Risk Factor Intervention Trial, 1982, Multiple Risk Factor Intervention Trial: risk factor changes and mortality results, *JAMA.* **248**:1465–1477.

Noble, J., and Modest, G. A., 1996, Managing multiple risk factors: a call to action, *Am J Med.* **101**(Suppl 4A):79S–81S.

Puska, P, Tuomilehto, J., Nissenen, A., et al., 1995, *The North Karelia Project: 20 Year Results and Experiences.* National Public Health Institute, Helsinki.

Raitakari, O. T., Leino, M., Rakkonen, K., et al., 1995, Clustering of risk habits in young adults: the Cardiovascular Risk in Young Finns Study, *Am J Epidemiol.* **142**:36–44.

Smith, T. M. F., 1978, Principles and problems in the analysis of repeated surveys, in: *Survey Sampling and Measurement*, N. K. Namboodiri, ed., Academic Press, New York, pp. 201–216.

Stamler, J., Caggiula, A. W., and Grandits, G. A., 1997, Relation of body mass and alcohol, nutrient, fiber, and caffeine intakes to blood pressure in the special intervention and usual care groups in the Multiple Risk Factor Intervention Trial, *Am J Clin Nutr.* **65**(1 Suppl):338S–365S.

Stamler, J., and Dolececk, T. A., 1997, Relation of food and nutrient intakes to body mass in the special intervention and usual care groups in the Multiple Risk Factor Intervention Trial, *Am J Clin Nutr.* **65**(1 Suppl):366S–373S.

Teutsch, S. M., and Churchill, R. E., eds., 2000, *Principles and Practice of Public Health Surveillance, Second Edition,* Oxford University Press, New York.

Winkleby, M. A., Flora, J. A., and Kraemer, H. C., 1994, A community-based heart disease intervention: predictors of changes, *Am J Public Health.* **84**:767–772.

CHAPTER 16

PERSPECTIVES ON BUILDING INFRA-STRUCTURE, COMPARING DATA, AND USING SURVEILLANCE DATA IN DEVELOPING COUNTRIES

David V. McQueen, Mary Hall, and Kelli Byers Hooper[*]

1. INTRODUCTION

Imagine being given the task of documenting the behaviour of elephants in the African savannah. Certainly this is an enormous task. No one would consider merely going into the field and taking a few pictures as sufficient work to accomplish the task. In the same regard, the task of developing an international surveillance system requires more than just selecting a questionnaire and translating it; surveillance activities also require a tremendous amount of planning, analysis, and evaluation to assess the health behaviours of the individuals being studied. Surveillance is a form of evidence-seeking behaviour concerned with broad population factors, not with individuals per se. It is epidemiologically based, which is to say that surveillance is based on the evidence that ties together epidemiological findings and related behavioural issues.

2. BACKGROUND

Several meetings were held in 1999 and 2000 out of a recognised need to bring together representatives from organisations and countries involved in surveillance activities to discuss the current efforts of their organisations and how these efforts could inform the development of a surveillance system that could be used worldwide. The meetings functioned as a forum for sharing information among countries with various levels of surveillance expertise. The ultimate goal was to increase surveillance capacity for less developed countries and to promote dialogue between partners and countries about sharing resources.

The first of these meetings was held in Atlanta, Georgia, in September 1999 on "Global Issues and Perspectives in Monitoring Behaviors in Populations: Surveillance of Risk Factors in Health and Illness." At this inaugural meeting, an international group of

---

[*] Centers for Disease Control and Prevention, Atlanta, Georgia 30341-3717, USA.

public health professionals met and discussed the role of data collection in the development of a surveillance system. The attendees discussed new techniques for data collection
and heard from users of data regarding the types of information that were most helpful.
The next meeting, "Analysis, Interpretation, and Use of Complex Social and Behavioral
Surveillance Data: Looking Back in Order to Go Forward," was held in Savannah,
Georgia, in June 2000. This meeting brought together people who work with or analyse
advanced survey and surveillance systems. Most of the systems represented at the meet-
ing had been operating for several years and had subsequently accumulated a lot of data.
Participants in this meeting grappled with several issues, such as:

- What do we do with the enormous amount of data that have been collected in
  these surveillance systems?
- How much data are enough?
- For how long should data be collected?
- Who really uses the data to set policy (politicians, political staffers, advocates,
  programme planners, the media)?

The September 2000 meeting held in Atlanta, on "Capacity Building, Comparability,
and Data Use in Behavioral Risk Factor Surveillance: Focus on Global Surveillance
Issues," focused discussion on capacity, comparability, and data use in developing countries. The purpose of the meeting was to open a dialogue with representatives from
countries new to risk factor surveillance and thereby to inform the World Health Organization, the World Bank, and the U.S. Centers for Disease Control and Prevention of
potential areas for collaboration. The following sections outline the discussions and key
issues raised during the deliberations of each discussion group of this meeting.

3. ISSUES

3.1. Capacity

Issues related to capacity can be stratified into four distinct dimensions necessary to
the development of a surveillance system. The first dimension involves the activities
required to set up a surveillance system, such as the development of questionnaires and
financial and intellectual resources. Next is methodology and technology, which involve
the actual operation of the system, including data collection. Third is education and
technical assistance, which include activities to develop the surveillance skills of individuals in developing countries where risk factor surveillance systems are planned. The
fourth—and perhaps most important—dimension is politics, which involves providing
information so that politicians and policy-makers understand the value of surveillance
systems and continue to provide resources for the programmes.

In an international approach to surveillance, the role of capacity in building health
information systems must be discussed. Ideally, health information systems all over the
world would be linked, allowing data to be shared. One barrier is the lack of an international inventory of existing surveillance systems that might be collecting parallel
data. This problem is especially relevant within developed countries, such as the United
States, where hundreds of systems may be collecting data on similar topics. Developing

countries can learn from these mistakes and organise their data collection systems so duplication is kept to a minimum.

Investment in risk factor surveillance systems has gained a lot of support in the last few decades because of a number of public health policy documents, such as Canada's *Health for All* and the United States' *Healthy People*. In those documents, objectives are defined by the nation to reflect the population's current state of health and to set goals. Often, surveillance data are used to measure progress towards national objectives. As a result of this practice, policy-makers may develop a one-dimensional view of surveillance. This attitude is problematic in regards to the development of sustainable surveillance activities.

Sustainability encompasses issues of financial resources, technology, and stakeholder support. In developing countries, the nemesis of surveillance systems is the political environment, where support for a programme may disappear as the political system changes. To combat this threat, a mechanism must be in place to clarify for whatever political system is in power that surveillance and monitoring of health behaviours are vital.

Over the last 5 to 10 years public health professionals have discussed quite a bit the development of best practises for surveillance systems. Very similar to the "good clinical practises" or "good medical practises" used in medical settings, best practises for surveillance systems would provide guidelines on optimising the information generated by surveillance in the communities or countries in which they are conducted. While agencies like the World Health Organization and the Centers for Disease Control and Prevention continue developing protocols for work in progress internationally, there is also a real need to work towards a common protocol for risk factor surveillance activities. A best practises document could describe good examples of surveillance from already existing systems. This document could not only support the development of new programmes, but also help increase advocacy among policy-makers in countries where support for surveillance systems is not extant. Additionally, the document could provide examples of how data from risk factor surveillance have been linked with disease and injury prevention programmes.

3.2. Comparability

Issues of comparability are paramount in global surveillance. Geographic regions have specific issues with language, technology, culture, and beliefs that affect the way data are collected and analysed. Countries are also in very different stages of technological and resource development. The purpose of surveillance is not to provide depth of understanding regarding any one topic area but an overview of the problems. Surveillance is interested in quantity, frequency, and variability.

Issues of methodology are increasingly important in the development of a surveillance system for international use. Methodology involves frequency of data collection, minimum precision of estimates, and technological concerns. Of note is the impact of technological advances on methodologies, which in turn may affect the quality and type of data collected. Historically, risk factor surveillance systems have used random-digit-dialed telephone sampling, but this is not the optimal methodology internationally, especially in developing countries. In developing countries data collection is best accomplished via random household surveys or other low-technology methods. Ultimately, the

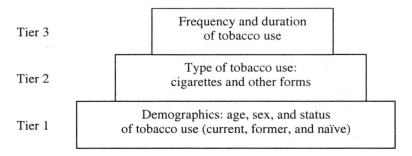

Figure 1. Tiered data collection method, with tobacco use as the variable.

methodology selected should be based on appropriateness, feasibility, and expense and left up to each country. However, there should be a global move towards synchronicity of data collection that would support data sharing among countries and promote information sharing among organisations that support surveillance activities.

To reach the goal of a systematised comparable surveillance system, participating countries must agree on minimum standards that address sampling techniques, types of demographic information collected, and frequency of data collection. This is best conceptualised as a three-tiered process in which there are minimum indicators to be collected, with the complexity of data increasing with each tier (Figure 1). Minimum indicators (tier 1) are those that could be collected even by countries with the least available resources.

Whether data are collected once a month, every 2 months, or every 5 years, behaviour should be understood as a function of time. As behaviours change, surveillance systems must be constructed so that relevant background information is captured. When the proper data are collected, the influence of external events (e.g., natural disasters, new legislation, or emerging social movements) can be documented. For instance, the U.S. Behavioral Risk Factor Surveillance System was able to document an increase in HIV testing and greater use of prevention services in the weeks following the announcement that Earvin "Magic" Johnson, a popular sports star, had disclosed his HIV-positive status.

Monitoring background information can be likened to using a seismograph to monitor earthquake activity. In the study of earthquakes, a seismograph must be running continuously. When an earthquake occurs, the machine registers the event. If the seismograph was not turned on when an earthquake occurs, the data collection is not of much use. While it would indicate that an earthquake had occurred, the machine would not be able to provide much data about the events prior to the earthquake. Likewise, a surveillance system operates at its optimum level when it is always "turned on," collecting data at small enough intervals to provide the necessary information regarding disease incidence and behavioural risk.

3.3. Data Use

Data collected via a surveillance system have two functions. The first function includes providing baseline measurements and monitoring variation between different population groups. The second use of data is for policy development, community action, and research. When a new surveillance system is being built, these two functions of data must be kept in mind, especially when stakeholders are involved.

Stakeholders of surveillance systems are a diverse group comprising experts, academics, community members, policy-makers, and members of special interest groups and social action organisations. Because of the diversity of the individuals involved, the strengths and limitations of surveillance must be communicated to the stakeholders. This information enables all participants to operate with realistic expectations of the data that will be collected and to plan for uses of the information. Stakeholders must be made aware that surveillance is a multi-dimensional task that could provide a wealth of information about the health status of a population. The main strengths of surveillance are that it:

- is inexpensive compared with other forms of public health research,
- is very flexible,
- has established methods for standardised questions and procedures,
- can be used to produce local estimates of health behaviours and risk, and
- can be used to monitor trends.

The limitations of surveillance include:

- data collected through random sampling methods may inadvertently exclude parts of the population at risk if the sample is too small,
- data are often self-reported, and
- surveillance provides an overview of a health problem but does not provide specific information about individual risk.

Once data have been translated into useful information, stakeholders should be guided on how to best use the information. This guidance could be provided in a best practises document, similar to the one described in Section 3.1. Included in this document would be instructions on quality data collection methods and suggestions on how to interpret the data to influence public policy and programme development. Obstacles to data use include insufficient resources, lack of commitment by stakeholders, and failure to demonstrate effectiveness of the system. Conditions that could enhance data use are strong leadership, strong stakeholder involvement, and established links to policy-makers.

Surveillance is a vertical process in which data are collected, analysed, and disseminated in a continuous pattern. It is a constant system, with a vertical hierarchy that keeps moving forward in time. Many health education, health promotion, and community programmes are often limited to 6 months, 1 year, or 2 years. If data are collected only every 5 years, the effects of a programme cannot be seen without an evaluation system that monitors what is happening in that country.

4. THEMES

Six dominant themes from the meeting deliberations regarding the development of an international surveillance tool bear repeating.

4.1. Time as a Variable

The one thing that distinguishes surveillance from other forms of public health research and data collection is that time is a significant variable. Behaviour changes over time—some slowly, others quickly—but time is always a key variable. Surveillance is not just a single survey, just three or four surveys, or something done every 5 years; it is an ongoing, systematic data collection system.

4.2. Sampling Methods

One size does not fit all. Sampling methods vary depending on the country's economic, political, and technological profile. Good data collection is a function of using appropriate sampling methods.

4.3. Data Collection

Various data collection techniques could be used in a surveillance system. An international surveillance system should have a flexible data collection system to accommodate the numerous techniques available.

4.4. Data Analysis

Methods for data analysis should be thorough and enable comparability between data sets.

4.5. How Data Are Used

When used effectively, data can influence public policy and legislation. A best practises document could guide public health officials on using surveillance data to demonstrate links between public health programmes and activities.

4.6. Limitations

In developing a surveillance system, the strengths and weaknesses of the proposed data collection activities must be communicated to stakeholders to ensure they maintain realistic expectations of the system.

5. CONCLUSION

As indicated by discussions at the September 2000 meeting "Capacity Building, Comparability, and Data Use in Behavioral Risk Factor Surveillance: Focus on Global Surveillance Issues," issues of capacity, comparability, and data use are relevant in the development of data collection systems. Further, meeting participants provided practical recommendations about how stakeholders, health organisations, and partners can support international surveillance activities.

CHAPTER 17

NON-COMMUNICABLE DISEASE SURVEILLANCE IN LATIN AMERICA AND THE CARIBBEAN

Advances Supported by the Pan American Health Organization[*]

Stephen J. Corber, Sylvia C. Robles, Pedro Orduñez, and Paz Rodríguez[†]

1. THE PAN AMERICAN HEALTH ORGANIZATION

The Pan American Health Organization (PAHO) is the oldest continuously serving international health institution in the world. It began as the International Sanitary Bureau, formed by the Second International Conference of American States in 1902 when countries of the western hemisphere agreed to work together to prevent the spread of infectious diseases. The World Health Organization (WHO) was established in 1948, and in 1949 the Pan American Sanitary Bureau (the successor to the International Sanitary Bureau) became the WHO Regional Office for the Americas. In 1950, this office became the specialised agency for health for the inter-American system, and in 1958 it was renamed PAHO. PAHO is thus a specialised agency of both the United Nations and inter-American systems.

PAHO headquarters are located in Washington, DC. The Organization has offices in 28 Member States throughout the Americas, as well as eight scientific and technical centres. As an agency of technical co-operation, PAHO works closely with the ministries of health of Member States in designing programmes to improve the health of the most vulnerable populations and to reduce health inequities throughout the region.

---

[*] Address delivered by Dr. Stephen J. Corber, Director, Division of Disease Prevention and Control, Pan American Sanitary Bureau, Regional Office of the World Health Organization, to the "Non-Communicable Disease Surveillance in the Americas—Second International Conference on Monitoring Health Behaviors: Towards Global Surveillance," at Tuusula, Finland, 1–3 October 2001.

[†] Stephen J. Corber and Sylvia C. Robles, Pan American Health Organization, Washington, DC 20037, USA; Pedro Orduñez, Hospital Dr. Gustavo Albereguia Lima, 55100, Cuba; Paz Rodríguez, Hospital Gregorio Marañon, 28010 Madrid, Spain.

2. SURVEILLANCE OF NON-COMMUNICABLE DISEASES

Non-communicable diseases (NCDs) are responsible for the greatest health burden in most regions of the world. For example, NCDs are responsible for almost half of disability-adjusted life years lost in Latin America (Murray and Lopez, 1997). It is therefore important to plan and implement programmes to try to reduce this burden. Several risk factors related to lifestyle behaviours are causally associated with the major NCDs. These include tobacco consumption, poor diet, sedentary lifestyle, obesity, and hypertension. These risk factors usually occur many years before the onset of disease.

An important aspect in developing effective disease prevention and control programmes is understanding the distribution of the disease and its risk factors, as well as their trends over time. The establishment of an effective surveillance system is therefore fundamental. Epidemiological surveillance can be defined as "a systematic gathering, analysis, and interpretation of health data to describe and monitor health events for the purpose of public health action" (Centers for Disease Control and Prevention, 1988, p. 1). To be effective a surveillance system must do more than collect data once. Surveillance should be based on a regular, ongoing collection of the data most helpful in providing information for public health decisions. The method of collecting the data must be valid and reliable (PAHO, 1999). The data should be collected in the same way each time; that is, using the same "standardised" methodology (the same questions should be asked, the same population surveyed, etc.). The data should be analysed, and decision-makers should use this analysis when making policy or planning decisions.

In deciding how best to provide technical co-operation on surveillance to Member States, PAHO reviewed the existing situation. There are three major categories of data for NCDs: mortality, morbidity, and risk factors. (1) Mortality data reflect past behaviours. PAHO's technical information system receives regular mortality reports from Member States. (2) Morbidity data are usually produced from hospital data. This information also reflects past behaviours. As well, it may distort the real incidence, as only people with the most severe cases of a particular disease enter hospital and the same patients may present on numerous occasions. Eleven countries of the western hemisphere have population-based cancer registries, which provide morbidity information. Therefore, information on these NCDs is available to some extent. (3) Risk factor data can predict future disease and deaths. In the Americas, a number of one-time surveys have been carried out in various countries. These surveys have been carried out by different groups, even within the same country, studying different populations and measuring variables in different ways. That is, the methodology has not been standardised.

With this information, PAHO determined that the development of risk factor surveys is a priority for Latin America and the Caribbean. Such development is important because risk factors are and will be the target of many NCD prevention and control activities. Knowing the extent of these risk factors and their changes over time will be important in planning these activities. In addition, one would expect to see changes in risk factors well before changes in morbidity or mortality are evident. Because of the lengthy period between the adoption of a risk factor and the manifestation of morbidity or mortality, it will take years before improvements in risk factors are reflected in a reduction in morbidity or mortality. Moreover, regular monitoring of risk factors will provide information about trends. It is clear that such information is lacking and that risk factor surveys need improved quality and standardisation.

With these needs identified, work began in two areas: development of a standardised questionnaire which could be used and adapted by Member States (Silva et al., 2001), and evaluation of existing activities in countries to determine what technical aspects need improvement (Orduñez et al., 2001).

2.1. Questionnaire Development

In developing a model questionnaire for PAHO, 30 experts from around Latin America and the Caribbean were involved for two rounds of consultation. They considered the risk factors to be studied, the population to be sampled, the sampling methods to be recommended, and logistical issues to be addressed. It was agreed that the general population would be surveyed and that a probabilistic sampling method would be used. Factors to be surveyed included physical activity, nutrition, tobacco consumption, alcohol consumption, body mass index, blood pressure, blood lipid concentrations, blood glucose level, and preventive services for women. In selecting appropriate indicators, PAHO reviewed the nine questionnaires that had been in use in the region: PAHO's Conjunto de Acciones para la Reducción Multifactorial de Enfermedades No Transmisibles (CARMEN), the WHO Standard Risk Factor Questionnaire, the U.S. Behavioral Risk Factor Surveillance System (BRFSS), Cuba's Proyecto Global de Cienfuegos, the binational Mexico–U.S. Border Diabetes Survey, Brazil's Encuesta Domiciliaria sobre Factores de Riesgo y Detección Precoz de Cáncer, the WHO International Physical Activity Questionnaire for Young and Middle-Aged Adults (IPAQ), PAHO's SABE and ACTIVA projects, and the WHO stepwise approach questionnaire.

As a result of this analysis, PAHO was able to produce a model questionnaire consisting of core questions and optional questions. The indicators for each risk factor were selected, and the recommendations for preventive actions are indicated. This information is now available on the PAHO web site (http://www.paho.org).

2.2. Survey Evaluation

To assess the work that has been done so far and the needs for future technical cooperation, PAHO developed a tool to evaluate surveys. The following process was undertaken: develop an evaluation tool, apply the tools in general, and evaluate surveys and assess quality of data for six specific risk factors.

2.2.1. Development of a Survey Evaluation Tool

Six technical aspects of surveys were studied: declared objective, population under study, sampling design, methods of gathering information, processing of information, and communication of results. Using this basis, PAHO developed 19 questions that can be used to evaluate existing surveys. Four questions apply to all surveys: Is it population based? Is the sampling design described? Is it a probabilistic sampling design? and, Are the data de-segregated by age and sex? These four questions constitute the first-stage assessment. If a survey does not comply with all of them, it is not considered for the next step—application of a scoring system. The remaining 15 questions were developed specifically for each risk factor included in the survey. To assess the usefulness of the questionnaire, points are assigned based on how well the survey meets these criteria.

2.2.2. General Application of the Evaluation Tool

A search was made of electronic databases for publications in all four official languages (English, Spanish, Portuguese, French). As well, a search was made in the PAHO document database and through the Member States' offices for reports relating to risk factor surveys. A search was made for "prevalence," "risk factor," and "countries." There were no restrictions placed on the search other than dates (1962–2000). Two hundred and nine reports, covering 63 studies conducted in 19 countries in Latin America and the Caribbean, were found (Figure 1). Most of the studies took place between 1990 and 2000 (Figure 2).

PAHO decided to look at two behavioural risk factors, two physical measures, and two biochemical measures. This classification was used to be able to follow the WHO stepwise approach to surveillance of NCD risk factors (see Chapter 3). Of the 209 reports identified through the search, 11 belonging to national surveys were excluded from further analysis because the results were not officially published. In the remaining 198 surveys, physical measures were studied more frequently than behavioural aspects (Table 1). This may reflect the fact that many of the studies took place in clinics and were conducted by researchers interested particularly in physical measures. It may also reflect important operational aspects related to Latin American and Caribbean countries: in these countries, telephone service may be less extensive than they are in North America or western Europe, and interviewers may be requested to conduct the survey in the presence of the respondent. In such cases, physical measures may be easier to collect and more accurate than questions related to behaviour.

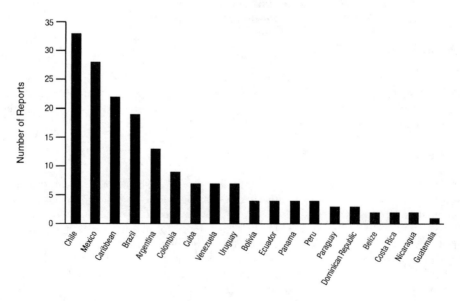

Figure 1. Number of reports in Latin American and Caribbean countries on NCD risk factor surveillance surveys.

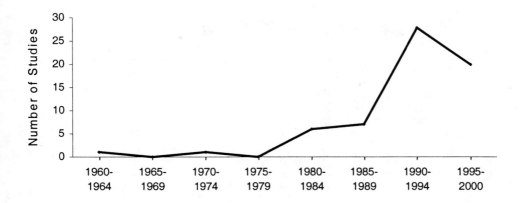

Figure 2. Number of NCD risk factor surveillance studies conducted in Latin American and Caribbean countries, according to year of publication, 1962–2000.

2.2.3. Survey Evaluation for a Specific Risk Factor: Hypertension

The surveys were then evaluated with regard to hypertension, the most frequently studied NCD risk factor. There were 58 papers that estimated the prevalence of hypertension. Two independent evaluators applied the assessment tool described in Section 2.2.1. to these 58 questionnaires. Although the majority were population based, described the sample design which was used, used a probabilistic sample, and reported the prevalence by age and sex (Table 2), only 28 (48.3%) of these surveys met all four criteria of the first-stage assessment. In the evaluation of the data collection, the strongest element among the 58 reports was that known diagnostic criteria, or definitions, were used. However, staff training and quality control of the primary data, in particular, could be improved. In the assessment of data analysis, the majority of surveys studied did not meet the criteria established, particularly with regard to sampling design when estimating prevalence and standard error.

Table 1. Variables assessed in NCD risk factor reports retrieved, 1962–2000

Risk factor	No. of studies	Percentage
Behavioural		
Smoking	48	22.9
Physical activity	2	1.0
Physical		
Blood pressure	58	27.8
Obesity or overweight	30	14.4
Biochemical		
Blood glucose concentration	47	22.4
Cholesterol level	13	6.2

Table 2. Percentage of NCD risk factor surveys (N = 58) assessing blood pressure that met criteria of PAHO survey assessment

Criterion	Percentage
First-stage assessment	
Population based	75.9
Sample design described	74.1
Probabilistic sample	69.0
Prevalence by age and sex	67.2
Data collection	
Problem under study well defined	63.8
Known diagnostic criteria or definitions	84.5
Staff trained in data collection	58.6
Quality control of primary data	41.6
Data analysis	
Estimates made according to sample design	25.9
Error estimated according to sample design	10.3
Stratification by place of residence, occupation, or education	50.0
Extrapolation framework	53.4

3. CONCLUSION

There is a growing interest in NCD risk factors in Latin American and Caribbean countries, as evidenced by the increase in the number of PAHO Member States conducting surveys in recent years and in the number of surveys themselves. Physical measures are studied more frequently than behavioural risk factors. The surveys which have been carried out have not been standardised, nor have they been conducted regularly. In addition, they exhibit important methodological flaws, particularly in data analysis. PAHO's next steps for technical co-operation will therefore be in the area of data analysis and use of data. Behavioural risk factor surveys, of course, are only one component of an NCD surveillance system. The ultimate goal is to establish behavioural risk factor surveillance in countries and to link this with mortality and morbidity databases to provide a more complete NCD surveillance system.

4. REFERENCES

Centers for Disease Control and Prevention, 1988, *CDC Surveillance Update*, CDC, Atlanta.
Murray, C. J., and Lopez, J. A., 1997, Alternative projections of mortality and disability by cause 1990–2020: Global Burden of Disease Study, *Lancet.* **349**:1498–1504.
Orduñez, P., Silva, L. C., Rodriguez, M. P., et al., 2001, Prevalence estimates for hypertension in Latin America and the Caribbean: are they useful for surveillance? *Pan Am J Public Health.* **10**:226–239.
Pan American Health Organization, Program on Non-Communicable Diseases, 1999, *Networking for the Surveillance of Risk Factors for Non-Communicable Diseases in Latin America and the Caribbean*, PAHO, Washington, DC (Publication PAHO/HCP/HCN/99.05).
Silva, L. C., Orduñez, P., Rodriguez, M. P., et al., 2001, A tool for assessing the usefulness of prevalence studies done for surveillance purposes: the example of hypertension, *Pan Am J Public Health.* **10**:152–160.

CHAPTER 18

PERSPECTIVES ON GLOBAL RISK FACTOR SURVEILLANCE
Lessons Learned and Challenges Ahead

David V. McQueen*

1. THE WATERSHED

In the last decade of the 20th century we witnessed a watershed in public health. Three seminal events occurred that changed the landscape for public health surveillance. The first was the rise of chronic disease and health promotion into the mainstream of public health. A great epidemiologic transition occurred throughout the 20th century. At the beginning of the century in the United States the average life expectancy was less than 50 years; by the end of the century it was nearly 80 years. In 1900 most people died from pneumonia, tuberculosis, and other infectious disease; by the end of the century the overwhelming majority died from heart disease, cancer, and stroke—pneumonia and influenza being relegated to causes of death in the elderly and the frail. With this transition we realised that the actual causes of death could be attributed to lifestyle behaviours, notably tobacco use, poor eating practises, substance abuse, and lack of exercise. Furthermore, we realised that these behaviours are often highly associated ways of living linked to social determinants.

The second seminal event was the recognition of the burden of chronic disease globally. Chronic physical and mental afflictions rob individuals of valuable quality time in an ever-lengthening lifetime, ultimately affecting the overall population. Thus this event was the realisation of the incredible impact of morbidity on populations, a morbidity directly related to the combination of increasing susceptibility to chronic illness and the disability resulting from that illness. It was now clear that people across the globe are living longer and need extensive care for and alleviation of the ravages of ageing and disease. Again, we realised there is a strong relationship between this burden and certain risk behaviours.

The third seminal event was the rise of the debate stemming from efforts to develop evidence-based medicine. Public health is not immune to this call for an evidence-based

* Centers for Disease Control and Prevention, Atlanta, Georgia 30341-3717, USA.

practise, and numerous efforts have been undertaken to demonstrate the effectiveness of public health interventions.

These three events alone are powerful reasons to develop a global effort of behavioural risk factor surveillance. It is risk factor surveillance that tracks the change in behaviours related to the epidemiologic transition, assesses the impact of the morbidity of illness, and provides the evidence of changes over time—changes that, we hope, are in response to population-based public health and health promotion interventions.

2. THE POWER OF BEHAVIOURAL MONITORING

Appropriately used, behavioural surveillance data can be a powerful tool for public health. Many examples could be given, but a recent one will suffice. The data described below come from the U.S. Behavioral Risk Factor Surveillance System (BRFSS), which has collected data continuously since the mid-1980s and systematically in all the states since the early 1990s. The system is well described in other chapters of this book.

A growing global concern has been the rapid spread of obesity, which has even been characterised as an epidemic. If we plot the percentage of U.S. adults who have a body mass index equal to or greater than 30 kg/m^2 (a traditional cut point for obesity) by state over a 10-year period, a remarkable and strong increasing trend is revealed. If we superimpose the prevalence of obesity over time onto a map of the United States, the picture is powerful and generally produces a gasp from any audience viewing this moving picture of the growing adiposity of the American people. This map is the direct result of the appropriate analysis and use of the kind of data produced by the BRFSS. Such maps and the results of this tracking were published in prestigious medical journals, but it was the cover of *Newsweek*, multiple articles in community and regional newspapers, and media attention that captured the public imagination. Surveillance is not a topic that easily grips the attention of the public or of policy-makers, but this highly visual and pertinent presentation caught the public's attention and with it an enhanced interest in obesity and diet as a problem to be addressed.

My point is that the impact of the media on powerful findings, presented appropriately, can be enormously influential. Over time data can hit hard, telling us where we have been and where we are going. To address such issues related to chronic diseases at local, national, and global levels we must establish a sound socio-behavioural monitoring system for public health (SMSH).

3. TERMINOLOGY

Throughout this book many terms are used to characterise behavioural risk factor surveillance. During the many meetings of the past few years a number of people have expressed discomfort with the word "surveillance," arguing that it carries some negative political baggage, particularly in countries that have experienced repressive political regimes. The term "monitoring" has come to be used as a more acceptable term. It is not my aim to enter this debate over terminology. The term "surveillance" has a long and distinguished history of use in public health and epidemiology, and those educated in these fields probably have little difficulty with the term. It is, of course, an English word and one has to be aware of the possible unfortunate direct translation of this term into many other languages. In any case, many of us dedicated to surveillance have come to be sensitised to the term in a given context.

The perils of language also come into play with regard to risk factors for disease. In the early stages of behavioural surveillance these were largely seen as individual behavioural risk factors, tightly bound to the individual and free of the social context in which they were set. The evolution of approaches to surveillance has since been heavily influenced by social epidemiology and the social sciences, with the result that the social context of the behaviour is also a prime determinant of or risk factor for disease. For example, we now well understand that the social status of an individual is highly related to health-related behaviour.

Finally, there has been a considered effort in public health over the past few decades to recognise that public health is concerned with the triad of detection, prevention, and promotion—that is, the detection of diseases and their causes in the population, the prevention of disease, and the promotion of a healthy lifestyle that leads to a compression of morbidity in the population into a short period.

For all these reasons, this closing chapter puts behavioural risk factor surveillance under the general rubric of SMSHs. This placement is a compromise to address global concerns and in no way suggests that well-established systems such as the BRFSS are not appropriately named. Each country will have to solve the nomenclature problem in its own fashion. The important thing is that there is a common understanding of the essentials of these pursuits.

4. FOUR ESSENTIALS OF A SOCIO-BEHAVIOURAL MONITORING SYSTEM FOR PUBLIC HEALTH

In the myriad discussions about surveillance with regard to behaviour and health, four essential elements are fundaments: a theoretical base, time as a variable, a systems approach, and enduring partnerships in the execution of the effort. Although surveillance is in practise a very complex undertaking, it is essential to understand the basics that underpin all of this work. Public health practitioners and researchers, faced with the demand to get on with the pressing public health tasks at hand, often do not reflect on why activities are carried out the way they are. Surveillance is no exception to this pressure, but over the past few years and as a result of the meetings that generated so much of the content of this book, we have reflected more on the primary reason to carry out socio-behavioural monitoring of the population.

"Theory" is a big word. What exactly is meant when we talk about a theoretical base for socio-behavioural monitoring? Historically the theoretical base for behavioural risk factor surveillance was straightforward: certain behavioural practises were viewed, from an epidemiological standpoint, to be causally linked to key chronic diseases. Therefore, the logical, theoretical approach would be to ask questions about these specific behaviours and show how that "causal" connection varies over time. The deeper theoretical foundation for this connection lay within the well-established etiological literature of chronic disease epidemiology.

As such risk factor surveillance developed in the Western world, increasingly persons trained in the social and behavioural sciences became involved, leading to a modified theoretical approach that argued for the concept of "lifestyles" as the critical causal factor. This approach continued the focus on individual or personal behaviour, but it ultimately included the theoretical notion of "social determinants" as an exogenous factor to be considered. This debate was very pronounced, for example, at the October 2001 conference in Tuusula, Finland. In many ways, however, many epidemiologists and social scientists in their analysis of data from systems already operating had anticipated this theoretical view. Such analyses almost always took into account the sociodemographic variables measured in the questionnaires, thus introducing social context and social determinants into the discussion of data. Nevertheless, much of this theoretical debate lies at the level of what might be termed "little" theories because they arise primarily out of the theoretical literature of personal behaviour and interactions, in contrast to the theoretical literature of sociology, economics, or anthropology.

Today many larger scale theories are being considered worthy of consideration in risk factor monitoring—theories arising from concepts such as social capital, urbanisation, globalisation, and deprivation. These concepts could be critical to understanding the socio-behavioural causal mix related to chronic diseases. For example, urbanisation leads to urban sprawl, which leads to long commuting times, which leads to less physical activity, thereby leading to weight gain. Such causal relationships may be complex; nonetheless, they are plausible and represent a distinct challenge for an SMSH to accommodate.

The essence of surveillance is that it tracks change over time. Therefore time must be a variable within the surveillance effort. Which means data should be collected as often and regularly as possible, minimising the time period between discrete data collections and approximating a continuous stream of data. In the real world of data collection, this is a tremendous theoretical, logistical, and technical challenge. At the heart of the behavioural surveillance effort is the survey-based data collection approach, which stems almost totally from the social science-based survey that collects point-in-time data. Surveillance requires that this point-in-time basis be transformed into a series of point-in-time surveys in which the time intervals between surveys approach zero. Given the statistical and practical constraints on such data collection, the unit of time that is obtainable reaches a limit of 1 day and practically is more feasible at 1 week or 1 month. In global efforts, many agencies carrying out surveillance simply may not have the resources to collect data on such a routine, short-time basis.

In analysis of surveillance data, time becomes an essential variable in trend analysis. Every single variable in a surveillance system that is analysed over time has its peculiarities. Behavioural variables vary over time at both the individual and population levels. For example, cigarette smoking by an adult individual will oscillate dichotomously over 20 years; that is, either that person is or is not smoking at any point in time. At the population level the percentage of adult smokers in the population is increasing, decreasing, or remaining stable. The shorter the time interval of data collection, the more accurately individual and population variations will be tracked. Other variables may be much more complex at both the individual and population levels in terms of quantity, variability, and frequency of the behaviour—physical activity, for example. However, I must point out that all of the many variables in a surveillance system have their own dimensions of variance with respect to time and their own particular relationships to each other that vary over time. Unfortunately the variable of time is often reduced, or removed entirely, by analysing data on a broad time measure such as 1 or 2 years. When over time surveillance data are "collapsed" to yearly analysis, it appears that all the data were collected at one point in the year, thus obliterating the temporal dynamics in the data.

The third essential of an SMSH is a systemic approach. Surveillance should be seen as a seamless system where data collection, analysis, interpretation, and use all inter-relate. Unlike typical survey research approaches in which each of these activities is often separate in time, surveillance calls for all of these activities to be going on at the same time. Thus a surveillance team would consist of some people concerned with data collection and some with information release and data use; at the same time, management would be making certain that all these phases of surveillance are integrated. This is certainly a classic approach to surveillance of any type in public health: while pursuing an event detected by surveillance, we continue to carry out the basic detection process. Time enters directly into the systemic approach in that if we collect data continuously, we also analyse it on a timely basis.

The fourth essential of an SMSH is the development, fostering, and maintenance of partnerships. The idea of partnerships seems to be the sine qua non of modern public health, and the practise of surveillance illustrates very well the necessity of partnerships. Furthermore, the role of partnerships is critical to the systemic functioning of surveillance. Data collection and analysis require partners to agree on which approaches to take, which questions to ask, and which analyses to undertake. The use of data involves health departments at every level, health intervention programmes, academic researchers, the media, and many other entities. It is hard to imagine a successful surveillance programme that does not have interests generated across a broad spectrum of public health entities.

I emphasise these four aspects of risk factor surveillance because some public health practitioners believe that surveillance is only about the technical aspects of data attainment. Many, if not the majority, of those interested in surveillance and believing surveillance to be an essential function of modern public health practise were trained in universities and schools of public health to be scientists, with a strong emphasis on epidemiology, biostatistics, and the technical aspects of data collection. It is only through years of practical experience in surveillance that skills in management, policy development, and communications are seen as equally relevant and important. The many meetings of the past few years have also revealed this truth.

5. TWO MAJOR AREAS OF CONCERN FOR SOCIO-BEHAVIOURAL MONITORING

The chapters in this book illustrate different areas of concern in designing and carrying out socio-behavioural monitoring in a population. Most of these concerns can be grouped under two broad dimensions, one dealing with the technical aspects of surveillance, and the other with what may be termed the "structural" aspects. Both of these dimensions are complex and are discussed in myriad writings ranging from standardised textbooks, current journal articles, and research protocols to research reports. The literature on the technical aspects far outweighs the literature on the structural aspects. Historically attention has focused on questionnaire construction, sampling, data collection method and mode, data analysis, data dissemination, and the interpretation of data. Less prominent is the body of literature dealing with how one obtains "buy in," how surveillance is linked to the public health infra-structure, how data are used for health promotion, and how surveillance systems can obtain and sustain resources to maintain the system. Unfortunately there is wide anecdotal evidence that the global success of socio-behavioural monitoring depends on the degree of public health infra-structure in countries and the leadership of agencies charged with monitoring health.

In this section I consider a few of these technical and structural concerns, namely those that have been discussed predominantly in the global meetings held in Atlanta, Savannah, and Tuusula. These issues have raised considerable discussion over time, and this chapter may not adequately represent all the viewpoints raised. Rather, I intend to distill the essence of the issues raised. The views expressed are mine and are not a formal consensus of the meetings or the institutions involved with the meetings.

Many discussions of the technical issues arising in behavioural risk factor surveillance focus on sampling. Long-operating systems base sampling on a classic statistical approach. The BRFSS, for example, makes use of modern sampling techniques and the final sample is weighted by telephone selection probabilities and demographic characteristics. Such approaches are standard in countries with highly developed lists of households, telephones in most homes, and a high level of understanding of the population parameters. At the global level, however, all the classic assumptions about sampling need to be re-evaluated for practicality. For example, in the BRFSS one randomly chosen adult is interviewed in each household, whereas in many countries the meaning of a household is very different. The household may be more extensive, consisting of far more than the nuclear family that characterises the typical American household. Or the household may have a head (or spokesperson) who speaks for everyone and it is difficult to interview a randomly chosen member who is not the head. Quite often, the arguement—and practise—is to interview every adult in the household. Of course this practise introduces a kind of sampling that is less familiar to many Western observers. In point of fact, decisions on sampling issues are powerfully influenced by cultural considerations, in all cultures. Thus, sampling is one of the first issues to enter into the larger discussion of standardisation and, ultimately, comparability. The hopeful resolution of the questions related to sampling is that it remains a technical, but solvable, problem as long as those in surveillance take a broad perspective on what is practical and feasible to obtain the most representative data from a population.

Data collection itself remains a huge area of concern because it involves both technical and structural issues, and the area is not without considerable controversy. The first issue is self-report. To a great extent risk factor surveillance grew out of traditional survey research, an area fostered and developed more extensively by social and behavioural scientists. A basic assumption of this approach is that individuals are the carriers of the data we want and that the best way to know what an individual does is simply to ask that person. Indeed, in the case of attitudes, opinions, and beliefs, alternatives to asking an individual directly are limited. With behaviours, however, observation is possible as well. For example, if we want to know whether someone smokes, we can ask and presume that the responses are valid, observe traits that indicate one is a smoker (e.g., stained teeth and yellow fingers), or perform various laboratory tests on samples from the individual. Each procedure requires a different approach to data collection that has its strengths and weaknesses. In behaviour surveillance we are generally not interested in great depth of understanding of the behaviour, but only its dynamics. In the case of smoking, we may just want to know whether a person smokes and if so, how much and how frequently. We are really interested not in any individual's smoking pattern, but in patterns in the population and how they change over time. For this purpose, self-reported behaviour is more than adequate. In fact, with some behaviours—for example, sexual behaviour—self-reported data might be the only way to get the information. Physical measurements such as weight, height, blood pressure, and so on may be obtained only in a direct invasive interview. Obviously taking any physical measure requires a face-to-face interview, which implies a mode of data collection that is more problematic, time-consuming, and costly than telephone interviewing.

Any decision on the approach to data collection will define the time parameters of a surveillance system. Telephone interviewing, particularly the use of computer-assisted telephone interviewing (CATI), allows for a much more efficient and rapid data collection system and seriously affects the time variable. Theoretically, with CATI the time unit of data collection can be reduced to even a single day, thus allowing for a dynamic data collection system that approximates continuous data collection. Nevertheless, this approach presents a number of challenges with regard to sampling, sample size, and data analysis. Many of these challenges were discussed in depth during the June 2000 meeting in Savannah, Georgia, and there is little doubt that exploring innovative approaches in data collection, tied to innovative analytic approaches, could be possible in the future. At present, however, no country has the dedicated resources to mount such an elaborate data collection approach.

Sampling and data collection present considerable challenges for any global surveillance effort, but probably the most discussed and contentious area of data collection is the instrument (or questionnaire) for data collection. In most meetings on surveillance the questionnaire not only dominates the discussion, but seems to provide the most animated discussions as well.

6. HISTORY AND DEVELOPMENT OF QUESTIONNAIRES USED IN RISK FACTOR SURVEILLANCE

In general the history and development of questionnaires in risk factor surveillance reflect the paradigm shift from disease prevention to health promotion and a changing theory underlying surveillance. Surveillance may be understood as a type of "evidence-seeking" behaviour in public health. It has been a well-established practise, particularly in tracking infectious diseases, and was firmly based in the epidemiological approach to public health. In a sense, behavioural risk factor surveillance is the child of this epidemiologically based surveillance. Over time, particularly with the need to incorporate social and behavioural variables, the relevance of the social survey (rooted in the social science disciplines) became incorporated into the approach of risk factor surveillance. The confluence of these two approaches—one stemming from the world of biomedicine, the other from the social sciences—yielded a new and powerful tool in approaching population health. In a sense the two merged most fruitfully in the concept of "lifestyle" as a risk factor for chronic diseases. During much of the 1980s and well into the last years of the 20th century, lifestyles were seen as highly related to non-communicable diseases. At the same time, social epidemiologists and social scientists became concerned that the social context in which the behavioural or lifestyle risks were operating be recognised. By the time of the Tuusula conference in October 2001, social determinants of risk factors was a leading topic of debate.

The other issue increasingly recognised in the history and development of the questionnaire was data use, which would inevitably have to address the types of questions placed on surveillance systems. This concern was shared globally by countries with highly developed surveillance infra-structures as well as those in the early stages of infra-structure development. Indeed, the use of data became a prominent theme in all the meetings, summits, workshops, and discussions held during and since the September 1999 conference in Atlanta, Georgia. For the developed systems, the concern was making use of an enormous amount of already collected and rapidly accumulating data. For this mountain of available data, the question of use translated into issues of what types of questions to analyse, how to analyse the data, how to interpret these data, and how to translate this information to persons who need it. For the developing systems, the question loomed largely because of economic considerations. Faced with limited resources, developing economies must choose their data-gathering approaches wisely. The usefulness of data in improving population health becomes the paramount economic consideration and, ultimately, the primary public health consideration.

Structurally, the form of the instrument used in behavioural risk factor surveillance has evolved and generally stabilised around four basic components: the fixed core, recurring questions, optional modules, and local questions. More recently the need has arisen to add rapid deployment questions. Most discussion globally is about the core questions. The hallmark of surveillance is a stable set of questions that vary little over time, so that any changes and trends detected over time can be attributed to true changes in the population rather than to questionnaire effects. There is fairly widespread agreement that all behavioural risk factor surveillance systems should include basic questions on risk behaviours and demographics. With regard to behavioural risk factors, there is general agreement that tobacco use, diet, physical activity, and substance abuse should all be included. Following the rise of the AIDS epidemic, many systems include sexual behaviours as a part of the essential core. Although we agree on what should constitute an acceptable "fixed core" for surveillance, agreement on the actual questions to be used remains problematic.

Recurring questions are those that enjoy fairly widespread agreement as to their usefulness in risk factor surveillance. In general these questions revolve around specific chronic disease topics, ranging from cancer screening to activity limitations and quality of life. They are usually more sensitive than core questions to country policies and to public health practises. Standardising such questions across countries remains problematic.

Optional modules arrive in conceptual bundles. In practise these modules generally arise in fairly developed surveillance efforts where a particular constellation of risk factors related to a chronic disease needs to be tracked. Examples are a battery of questions attempting to assess dietary fat intake, self-assessed quality of life, or social capital in a population. Optional modules need to be adapted as a totality, as they are generally the product of a conceptual measurement research effort and produce some type of indicator. Such bundles may take up a large amount of space on a questionnaire, and to some extent they detract from the stability and reliability of the core questions over time.

Over the years we have been subjected to the mantra "think globally, act locally." This wisdom is reflected in the development of behavioural risk factor surveillance. Whereas comparability with neighbouring states, cities, and countries may be interesting and important, the information that motivates decision-makers and individuals appears to be local data. This assumption manifests in the BRFSS state-added questions. The arguement is that some issues really are geo-politically critical. For example, questions on fish consumption from the Great Lakes are important only for the states bordering the Great Lakes. It is difficult to make a case against adding local questions in any surveillance system. Indeed, this component and the use of these local questions often sell the surveillance system to policy people at all levels of government.

Finally, critical events may arise that need to be tracked. Some of these events may be planned, such as the initiation of a major, population-wide public health intervention; some may be anticipated, such as expectation of certain legislation; some may be somewhat anticipated, such as the potential for a flood, earthquake, or other natural disaster; and some may be unanticipated, such as terrorist attacks. In all these cases the need arises to plan exactly what type of questions should be asked and how they should be introduced into an ongoing surveillance system without affecting the system's stability. This is a truly challenging area for risk factor surveillance, and discussions are still in early stages.

7. CHALLENGES IN QUESTIONNAIRES

This topic area is so large that I can only point to some of the more critical challenges and opportunities for questionnaire development. Behavioural questions related to lifestyle will undoubtedly remain the critical core of behavioural risk factor surveillance related to chronic disease and health promotion. The amount of effort that has gone into developing questions on alcohol consumption, tobacco use, food habits, physical activity, and sexual behaviours is enormous. Despite this effort, agreement on the exact questions to be used to monitor these behaviours has never been reached globally. Given all the political, technical, and linguistic considerations that need to be taken into account, complete agreement may never be obtained. However, interest is widespread on pursuing questions that are as comparable as possible when analysed in joined sets of data. This is a laudable and important goal. For example, when smoking behaviour is compared from country to country we want to be fairly certain we are comparing like data. Determining exactly how comparable the data are will probably remain an analytic research problem. Smoking appears relatively straightforward, in contrast to diet and eating patterns, which probably more than any of the behaviours we are interested in are highly contextual and culturally bound. Still others areas such as physical activity remain a challenge to measure in a small number of questions. The challenge of any behaviour is that it varies temporally in any individual in terms of quantity, frequency, and variability. For behavioural surveillance the task is to identify the parameters of the behaviour in a population. Unfortunately we cannot interview the population—we can only interview individuals as proxies for the population. Nonetheless, we must always remind ourselves that our primary interest is in the population parameters.

Over the years of risk factor surveillance development certain demographic variables have become standard. Age, sex, race, income, education, marital status, and employment are routinely collected in most operating surveillance systems and are often accepted as variables that do not need to be scrutinised like the behavioural variables. In the recent meetings on surveillance this routine acceptance has been questioned, however. The social science literature has made it much more apparent that these demographic variables have their own complexity. For example, we now appreciate that a variable such as "age" is not a simple linear function, but that different periods in a person's life span form their own contextual patterns that relate to health and illness. In point of fact, very few of these variables are now viewed as simple linear functions. We have come to understand that years of education are not equal for all groups of people, not all secondary school graduates are equal, and a college education may be highly contextual. Similarly, we now discuss the meaning and measurement of income and wealth. Although apparent in some of the heated discussions at the surveillance meetings, notably in Tuusula in October 2001, much of this type of discussion has not yet permeated the public health surveillance literature. Finally, I would be remiss to not point out that some of the demographic variables may be based on non-scientific classifications. The oft-used variable of "race" is such an example. When we take a global perspective, the issues get even more complicated and muddled. Our realisation that many of the demographic variables that were once seen as rather basic and immutable are actually very conceptual and context related has been sobering, with considerable implications for the possibility of global standardisation. Future meetings will consider this issue in more depth.

8. OPPORTUNITIES IN QUESTIONNAIRES

Questionnaires in survey research have always provided an opportunity to introduce new concepts through building social constructs defined by a cluster of questions based on definitive variables that can be validly measured. This research effort usually requires considerable time to design the questions. In the best of worlds the questions are developed with the help of a cognitive laboratory that rigorously tests the questions on panels of appropriately chosen respondents. Then the questions are pre-tested in a series of pre-surveys, followed by their use on established valid surveys. This is the ideal background scenario for deciding on the eligibility of questions to be used in surveillance systems.

Surveillance systems are generally not designed for questionnaire development. That is a task relegated for research. Ideally, questions ready for use on established surveillance systems should already possess proven characteristics of reliability and validity. In the world of public health, issues and opportunities may arise before the labour-intensive, time-consuming research has been completed. We must then judge the extent to which such new question areas should be incorporated into ongoing or new surveillance systems.

Many of the opportunities for questionnaire development lie in the realm of tracking knowledge and attitudes. For example, even though risk factor surveillance is based on assessing the risk behaviours of the population, we know little about how people assess their behaviour in relation to attributed risk, their perception of the risk associated with urbanisation, or how they link various social phenomena to risk behaviours. Certain emerging behaviours have health consequences but remain to be developed as question areas, such as road rage, commuting, internet and video use, and use of over-the-counter and alternative medicine. Finally, perhaps the most under-developed area of behaviour relates to mental health. All of these areas are being raised in global public health discussions. Eventually surveillance systems will need to track these emerging areas.

9. ANALYSIS OF SURVEILLANCE DATA

In the many discussions and presentations that took place in the various meetings in Atlanta, Savannah, and Tuusula, data analysis—especially the more complicated analytic approaches, beyond the use of basic statistics and statistical packages—was not uniformly seen as a critical issue in risk factor surveillance. In part this hubris may be because these issues are a luxury for well-advanced systems with mountains of data to analyse. Furthermore, many surveillance systems struggle to merely produce the routine reports demanded by funders and expected by those working in public health. Yet in my opinion, analysis is the most critical problem in behavioural risk factor surveillance for both well-developed and newly emerging behavioural surveillance systems. Many of the reasons are discussed in the chapter summarising the June 2000 Savannah meeting and will be touched upon only briefly here.

The first analytic problem is that behavioural surveillance data often are not analysed with regard to the dynamic time aspect of the data. Even when such surveillance is conducted on a timely basis (for example, with a monthly data collection interval), the data are often analysed on a yearly basis. The effect of analysing such data this way is to remove the variable of time from the analysis, in which case all of the data logically may have been collected on a single mid-year date. All of the dynamics of every variable measured in the system are lost: if the data vary considerably by time of year, that variation cannot be seen. Thus the true behaviour of the variable in the population is not expressed in the analysis.

The second analytic problem is that quite often only single behavioural variables are analysed over time. We have many reports that cross-tabulate smoking with every demographic variable, physical activity with every demographic variable, and so on. But we generally lack analyses that look at the inter-relationships of the various behaviours and at the risk constellations in some type of index. This is a real weakness because of the purported additive importance of risk factors for chronic disease. The analytic possibilities have simply not been explored to their fullest. If we added time as a variable to these constellations, the potential insights of surveillance would be enhanced.

Both of these problems fall under the larger issue of analysing highly complex data. To date the analytic approaches taken to behavioural surveillance data have been fairly standard descriptive statistical approaches that are more appropriate for simple cross-sectional surveys. The reasons for this limited approach are manifold and have been discussed throughout the surveillance meetings. One reason is the amount of time that can be devoted to analysis—so much time and effort go into managing large data collection systems and preparing required routine summary reports that little staff time is left to pursue more enhanced analyses. Second, many persons who analyse surveillance systems are under-trained in the use of advanced statistical packages that could provide more appropriate analyses. Third, many of the analytic techniques and new innovative approaches that might be more appropriate come from fields outside the traditional training of people working in public health; they may more likely be found in the physical and social sciences. Finally, the advanced analytic procedure that yields more in-depth and appropriate analyses is not necessarily amenable to being simplified in a way that would be meaningful to policy-makers and other end users of the data. After all, most of us are accustomed to seeing simple bar charts, graphs, and cross-tabulations with appropriate p values and statistical tests.

All of these reasons for the lack of better analysis of surveillance data are debatable, but they also apply to both highly developed systems and newly emerging ones. The first two reasons have implications for the infra-structure and design of surveillance systems; that is, how many staff should be relegated to collecting data, how many to analysing them, how many to interpreting them, and how many to preparing them for end users. These are resource issues. The third reason presents the general challenge of how the field of public health should broaden to include sectors not usually involved in public health. This is a generic problem for public health as it enters a new century and new challenges. The final reason relates to the use of data, much discussed in our surveillance meetings and covered in this book in depth. With the realisation that the use of data involves many potential end users, health departments, public health programmes, communities, academic researchers, policy-makers, legislators, the media, and many others, it is clear that we have only begun to explore what type of analysis best relates to each and every one of these users.

10. CONCLUSIONS

It is a daunting task to sum up in a few concluding remarks all the discussions at the surveillance meetings, the many papers presented, and the formal chapters in this book. Nevertheless, certain key ideas re-occur and form a general centre for the debates and discussions on the conduct of behavioural risk factor surveillance. I have tried to address some of these in this concluding chapter.

The debates and discussions initiated in Atlanta in September 1999 have been lively and important. As a result the global concern with and interest in behavioural risk factor surveillance for disease, illness, and health promotion has benefited. This is seen in the prominence now given to behavioural risk factor surveillance in the agendas of global organisations such as the World Health Organization as well as at the national levels of ministries of health.

It is a sobering reminder of the work that needs to be done that we as yet have no uniform commitment to such surveillance around the globe. This is despite the widespread recognition of the global burden of chronic illness, the epidemiologic transition to diseases of lifestyle, the role of social determinants in poor health, and the continued growth of behaviour patterns leading to the burden of disease. One cannot identify many ongoing surveillance systems in the economically highly developed world and even fewer in the poorer countries. Thus it is critical to focus on what it is that we are doing, collectively, to build systems of behavioural risk factor surveillance throughout the world.

First and foremost we need systems that are true surveillance systems. In the classic sense of surveillance in public health, these are not elaborate efforts to carry out research but systems of data collection and analysis that track dynamic changes in the reputed causes of diseases and illnesses at the population level. Like any good monitoring system, surveillance systems are there to detect, in as timely a fashion as possible, significant changes from the norm and to provide decision-makers and action-oriented public health practitioners with data that allow them to act expediently on a public health problem. In practise this means surveillance systems in which collection, analysis, interpretation, and use of data are an integrated package ready to respond to public health needs and emergencies. Systems that are slow, time independent, and generating mounds of data without rapid and useful analysis are anathema to the idea of surveillance. Rather, monitoring constitutes the ideal learning and information system for informed decision making. Fortunately, the current and continuing efforts offer the hope that we will soon see such surveillance systems established across the globe.

INDEX